D1281757

Functional Restoration
for Spinal Disorders:
The Sports Medicine Approach

Functional Restoration
for Spinal Disorders:
The Sports Medicine Approach

Tom G. Mayer, M.D.

Associate Clinical Professor of Orthopaedic Surgery
The University of Texas Southwestern Medical Center at Dallas, Texas

Robert J. Gatchel, Ph.D.

Professor of Psychology, Psychiatry, and Rehabilitation Science
The University of Texas Southwestern Medical Center at Dallas, Texas

Lea & Febiger   *Philadelphia*   *1988*

Lea & Febiger
600 Washington Square
Philadelphia, PA 19106-4198
U.S.A.
(215) 922-1330

LIBRARY OF CONGRESS
Library of Congress Cataloging-in-Publication Data
Mayer, Tom G.
    Functional restoration for spinal disorders: the sports medicine
approach / Tom G. Mayer, Robert J. Gatchel.
      p.   cm.
    Includes bibliographies and index.
    ISBN 0-8121-1137-0
    1. Backache–Exercise therapy. 2. Spine–Abnormalities–Exercise
therapy. 3. Backache–Patients–Rehabilitation. 4. Sports
medicine. I. Gatchel, Robert J., 1947-   . II. Title.
    [DNLM: 1. Backache–rehabilitation. 2. Spinal Diseases–
rehabilitation. 3. Sports Medicine.   WE 725 M468f]
RD771.B217M39 1988
617'.5606–dc19
DNLM/DLC
for Library of Congress   87-29859
                                              CIP

Copyright © 1988 by Lea & Febiger. Copyright under the International Copyright Union. All rights reserved. This book is protected by copyright. No part of it may be reproduced in any manner or by any means without written permission from the publisher.

PRINTED IN THE UNITED STATES OF AMERICA

Print Number 4 3 2 1

With love to our wives,
Holly Mayer and Anita Gatchel,
who contribute so much to our
lives and work

FOREWORD

There is no more devastating medical ailment than chronic low back pain when measured by socioeconomic impact. It costs more in lost productivity and payments for inability to work than any other single entity. Yet it is a "disease" specific to the mechanized and scientifically based societies. Chronic low back pain, unrelated to tumors or infections, is a rare entity in the primitive societies of the world. Why? Surprisingly, that question remains unanswered by current scientific evidence. Common sense dictates that the answer must have something to do with physical activity. This book presents an extensive documentation of the role of physical activity in chronic low back pain. Specific details of a new "functional restoration" treatment approach are presented which deal with problems such as physical deconditioning in chronic back problems. Ultimately, this philosophy may remove chronic back pain from the list of significant medical ailments, and be able to return the complaint of chronic back pain to the minimal significance it had for our forefathers and the less developed societies.

The comments above, of course, are meant to be bold and provocative. What innovations could there be which can reverse a problem which has been increasing in impact over the past several decades? What technical innovation could have appeared to change the "natural history" of a disease process? What "penicillin" for backache has been discovered? The innovation, the technical advance, the new concept for backache is, of all things, based on the ability to accurately measure dynamic function. This provides the foundation for the functional restoration approach. This is the scientific basis for sports medicine as well.

The musculoskeletal system is measured in the real world by physical performance. Although there are some objective investigative tools, such as x rays, blood tests, and even physical examination, these are all "snapshots" at an instant of time. Really, the question of all health or "sickness" of the musculoskeletal system revolves around function as portrayed by dynamic activity. How does one's individual function compare to the expected norm? When we evaluate extremities, there is generally some clue to identify deviation from normal. How does the left arm compare to the right? This comparison test, however, is unavailable in evaluation of the spine, especially the low back, which we cannot even see in ourselves. Thus, to achieve the goal of measurement of spine dynamic function, we must compare performance at different points in time and to expected norms.

The focus on human physical performance is sharp in the area of athletic activity. The specialty of sports medicine has grown up evaluating the numerous links in the mechanical chain of human physical function. The summary of this smooth-running human machine is clearly identified by athletic performance. When there is a defect in the mechanical links, the deviation from normal or supernormal performance can be measured. The efficacy of treatment can be defined by progress from the baseline measurements identified on the occasion of injury. Safe return to competitive activity may be anticipated once the measured performance returns to normal. The sports medicine community has developed numerous assessment devices to assemble a large number of data points relative to musculoskeletal performance. The computer now allows efficient assemblage, storage, and correlation of many of these data points. Essentially, this technical development has made it possible to measure dynamic human performance. The measurements can now be accomplished with such accuracy that, in the sports medicine world, precise predictors as to expected performance can be assembled.

The obvious success of this philosophy of measurement of human performance noted with improving athletic performance is easily demonstrated. Athletes return to their sports sooner and more safely than in earlier eras. Thus, it was a natural conceptual step to transfer the philosophy of the human machine performing at above normal levels of activity (competitive sports) to the other end of the spectrum—chronic physical disability—in which suboptimal physical performance is the rule.

The authors of this text justify this transfer of philosophy by first pointing out what we know about the physiology and pathology of back injuries. They also point out the characteristics of benign chronic pain. The potentials for disability and inactivity habituation within our psyches can well be demonstrated, as can potentials for emotional and motivational deconditioning. Once the mechanisms for both physical and emotional underperformance have been put into place, the stage is set for a functional restoration treatment approach.

The use of measurement of function as an assessment tool for the lumbar spine is demonstrated by several techniques. Certainly, the lumbar disc does not sit alone, but functions in cooperation with multiple other anatomic parts, and it is coordinated towards movement by an even more complex nervous system. The engine of this nervous system—the mind—also has multiple impacting factors interfering with its potential for effective action. The measurement of these factors is also identified. Since such wisdom, skill, and methods for evaluation seldom reside in one individual, it is probably inefficient to ask that a single specialty do all of this assessment. All participants must recognize that effective measurement is the key to efficient treatment, leading to the concept of the therapeutic team. It is the chemistry of this team working together with the injured individual that creates the success of physical restoration using sports medicine principles. In treatment, the measurement of function is used as a guide for the patient's progress. The injured individual can now work with something objective and concrete such as a number contrasted to the often unreliable self-report of pain. Attitudes and emotions can so greatly alter pain perception that it is difficult to measure by self-report. Function is far more germane. A level of activity done today can be compared to that of a week ago, and how far from normal the individual remains can also be shown to him or her for motivational purposes.

And where does this take us? First, it allows many performance dimensions to be clarified when we look at the injured individual. Certainly, pain is worthy of consideration, but is highly variable. Some individuals are physically so impaired that they cannot be expected to return to previous levels of function.

Society may wish to make a judgment on future work capacity. A just contribution for financial support can be identified once true functional impairment can be factored into the other components of disability such as structural damage, age, education, and opportunity. Until now, there were no good ways of objectively measuring physical capacity. Now this piece can be filled into the disability puzzle.

Thus, I am very pleased to introduce this new look at the problem of chronic back pain. There is every reason to hope that the philosophy presented here will have an important impact on health care delivery and the cost of this significant medical problem. We have not been honest with ourselves in the past when we have supported months of passive modality "care" that can offer no long-term benefit. We have not been fair to our patients when we have focused on pain rather than function. We, as medical clinicians, have relied only on the science available to us for the care of structural disorders and not for functional deficits. Perhaps, because nobody dies of back pain, its presence in the arena of medical concern has been left relatively unnoticed. The time has come to develop rational principles of care. Now we can do it because we can measure the essence of the problem: variation in human performance. This book provides an excellent presentation of the rational principles and performance measurement techniques that are involved in the functional restoration treatment approach. It is of crucial importance to all physicans, surgeons, psychologists, and physical and occupational therapists interested in a team approach to deal with up-to-date methods for testing long-standing, disabling back pain.

Vert Mooney, M.D.
Professor of Orthopedic Surgery
The University of Texas Southwestern
Medical Center at Dallas, Texas

PREFACE

Chronic low back pain is a far greater socioeconomic problem than is commonly suspected. During their lifetimes, 80% of people in industrialized countries develop low back pain. Of this group, 10% go on to chronic unremitting or episodic back pain, incurring 80% of the cost of treatment, and undergoing a variety of difficulties from minor loss of recreational capabilities to total occupational disability. Surgical procedure is appropriate in only 1 to 2% of back pain patients, while the vast majority must be treated conservatively for lack of a correctable lesion. Rehabilitation for this group has consisted, over the past 25 years, of "pain clinic" treatment involving primarily psychologic intervention and is currently represented by more than 2000 such facilities across the United States. Yet, despite voluminous literature, research, and understanding of the psychosocioeconomic factors impinging on disability, these facilities have not succeeded in developing a treatment that effectively negates the disabling consequences of low back pain.

In recent years, a revolutionary approach termed functional restoration, which utilizes sports medicine principles, has been developed and has been demonstrated to have unique efficacy in spinal rehabilitation. Not only is pain assuaged, but major improvements in return to work, settlement of litigation, and reduction of unnecessary use of the medical care system for desperate or prolonged treatment have been accomplished. This approach emphasizes the recognition, through objective quantitative assessment of physical function, of the loss of physical capacity that accompanies disuse following injury (termed the deconditioning syndrome). The treatment algorithm is an amalgam of a number of well-understood technologies: a sports medicine approach to musculoskeletal disability for restoring physical function; pain management and other psychologic approaches for understanding the psychosocioeconomic processes underlying chronic back pain; work capacity evaluations using new technology to quantify physical capacity.

In this text, we have carefully delineated how functional restoration works, and what techniques are used. Integrated with this amalgam of well-documented therapeutic strategies is the careful objective quantification of spine function utilizing newly developed technologies, such as computerized range-of-motion, trunk strength, and lifting devices, which are just now beginning to be marketed. This new technology is revolutionizing the field of objective noninvasive assessment of back functioning. No longer will the physician have to rely solely on structural measures, originally designed only to identify the small percentage of back sufferers requiring surgical treatment. Nor will subjective and unverifiable patient self-report be the anchor of spine diagnosis. Although this is a relatively new technology, it is being embraced throughout this country and the world.

The purpose of this text is to provide physicians and other health professionals with a comprehensive introduction to this functional restoration approach to chronic low back pain. This will provide them with a better understanding of how to diagnose and treat these patients more effectively, with important implications for treatment of less severe disorders throughout the spine and musculoskeletal system. It will also offer them an understanding of the theory behind this approach, its recent scientific documentation, and practical *step-by-step* descriptions of the assessment and treatment components involved in it. Both of us have been actively involved in developing and running the prototypical functional restoration program, the Productive Rehabilitation Institute of Dallas for Ergonomics (PRIDE). This experience has provided us with the ability to communicate the important everyday clinical concerns and issues that arise in dealing with chronic low back pain patients, and which can be effectively dealt with by this method. We have also been active in conducting research aimed at evaluating the clinical utility and reliability of this approach. The reader will therefore be exposed to a balanced mixture of material on basic theory, assessment, treatment, and specific practical issues.

We have written this text with the primary-care and general practitioner in mind, though it should be of interest to physical and occupational therapists, psychologists, spine surgeons, and pain treatment specialists. Nonetheless, we are cognizant of the fact that the readers will have differing levels of expertise in orthopedics. We have attempted to present the material in clear, understandable language without introducing overly technical or complicated jargon or, conversely, oversimplifying basic concepts and issues. Our aim has been to provide the reader with a working knowledge of this new functional restoration treatment philosophy.

Dallas, Texas

Tom G. Mayer
Robert J. Gatchel

CONTENTS

Part I

The Problem of Low Back Pain

Chapter 1

Introduction and Overview of the Problem

The term "functional restoration" refers not merely to a treatment methodology for chronic low back pain, but to a wider conceptualization of the entire problem, its diagnosis, and management. Rather than accepting current limits in history-taking based solely on patients' self-report of pain and diagnosis through skeletal imaging technology, the methodology involves reliance on more objective information. Structured interviews, quantified self-report measures, and batteries of psychosocial tests provide problem-oriented information for patient management. Moreover, objective assessment of physical capacity and effort, with comparison to a normative data base, adds a new dimension to diagnosis. This permits the development of treatment programs of varied intensity and duration aimed primarily at restoring physical functional capacity and social performance. The previous goals of merely attempting to alter pain complaints, decreasing medications, and "improving the quality of life" are greatly enlarged by a focus on the vast societal problems associated with low back pain. This attention to realistic goals has already helped to alter the focus of treatment programs, as well as the evaluation process for its effectiveness.

This book is clearly not intended as a comprehensive review of thought on all the problems of chronic low back pain. It will, however, present a summary of multiple historical perspectives, and a synthesis of current thinking on both active and passive treatment approaches. Most of all, though, it will integrate the recent research contributions of the authors and others for viewing the problem, providing subjective and objective assessment, and developing treatment and evaluation approaches never previously systematized for low back pain. We hope that the reader will obtain a clear and unbiased overview of the problem of degenerative lumbar spine disease. Furthermore, we hope to provide a definitive way of handling not only the expensive chronic problems, but insight into approaches for the extremely commonplace acute problems.

SCOPE AND COST OF THE PROBLEM

Low back pain is the most expensive benign condition in industrialized countries. It is also the number one cause of disability in persons under age 45. Over this age, it is the third leading cause of disability, becoming progressively less of a factor during the later years when function and productivity become of less concern than survival. It has been estimated that in any one year, about 3 to 4% of the population has a temporarily disabling low back pain episode in all industrialized countries, and that more than 1% of the working age population is "totally and permanently disabled" by this problem.

3

With these compelling statistics in mind, we are at the core of the social and medical enigma addressed by this book. While the financial and human costs to all industrialized societies are staggering, the clinician's view of the problem has been limited. The medical profession, which should be expected to devote a great deal of attention to a problem of such major public health magnitude, has ignored its significance almost completely until recently. The research community neither requests nor receives significant funding for work in this area relative to the magnitude of the low back problem. The National Institutes of Health (NIH) virtually ignore degenerative low back pain, while only a few other agencies pay slightly more attention to it.

The vast majority of internal medicine, occupational medicine, and family physicians recognize only the acute self-limited conditions, and treat them with relative indifference. Furthermore, they are often discouraged and baffled by the behavior of a small minority of patients who go on to become chronically disabled and whose physical basis for symptoms can neither be accounted for by their diagnostic skill nor dealt with through commonly available treatment approaches. The attendant frustration frequently leads them to conclude that these individuals are "malingerers," "fakers," or have "low motivation," often in spite of countervailing evidence from the patient's occupational history. The presence of compensation and legal factors in such cases lends credence to this impression, and fosters similar beliefs on the parts of plaintiffs and defense attorneys and claims representatives of insurance organizations.

Meanwhile, the orthopedic surgeon and neurosurgeon tend to be involved in the process as experts for referral. They perform the structural imaging tests designed to discover what is "seriously wrong"; i.e., a surgically correctable lesion. Yet, the patient's legal involvement may prevent the surgeon, who is viewed by patient and referring physician alike as the "court of last resort," from seeing other alternatives to his or her standard approach. The traditional methods of diagnosis have been based on skeletal imaging, operating on those with a "real problem" (i.e., a positive CT scan or myelogram) and rejecting those with negative imaging tests as "only having a strain." Moreover, patients assessed as having depression or "difficult personalities" are additionally labeled as having a "psychologic problem." At its best, orthopedic diagnosis leads to surgical treatment which allows for more rapid pain relief and more complete return to function when indicated. At its worst, it can lead to crippling, multiple surgeries, and inaccurate judgments, and patient labeling based on inadequate information.

From a financial point of view, the most recent data reveal the bill for medical care for low back pain to be $16 billion annually, slightly more than one-half of which is expended for surgical treatment (Holbrook, Grazier, Kelsey, Stauffer, 1984). This should be contrasted to the total of only $27 billion yearly for diagnosis and care of *all* musculoskeletal trauma. Though there are no firm statistics available, it has been estimated that the total cost of all aspects of low back pain care, including medical, compensation, legal, vocational retraining, occupational modifications, and lost industrial productivity, may be in the range of $40 to $50 billion annually.

TRADITIONAL VIEW OF LOW BACK PAIN AS AN INJURY

Much of this high cost centers around the acceptance of low back pain as an injury, rather than as an inevitable part of the aging process. This general acceptance of a loose definition of "injury" has permitted the authorization of most low back pain developing on or near the job site as compensable under workmen's compensation statutes. Similarly, the appearance of such symptoms around the time of an accident involving one party's negligence (classically an auto accident or product liability situation) has also become viewed as compensable. Of course, the frequent counterpoint view of low back pain taken by many insurance companies and attorneys is that "secondary gain," or even fraud, motivates the patient. The physician's inability to quantify the "hidden impairment," and to develop a consensus with colleagues on disability rating, only succeeds in adding weight to this perception. Employers and unions also take sides in what becomes a contest of beliefs rather than science. When all is said and done, the claimant/patient's interests are usually unlikely to be served.

On the one hand, a higher incidence of low back pain report appears to occur with certain jobs and movements (twisting, bending), recreational activities or physical somatotypes. On the other hand, it appears that individuals who are most fit tend to have fewer injuries (Cady, 1979), and workers performing regular medium lifts have fewer injuries than sedentary workers with intermittent light lifting. Furthermore, recent evidence from a large-scale study conducted by the Boeing Corp. suggests that the only statistically significant predictor of a reported industrial back injury may be a preceding poor job performance report by a supervisor, irrespective of any other occupational factors (Bigos, Spengler, Martin, Zeh, Fisher, Nachemson, 1986). Scandinavian workers, for whom compensation is unaffected by occurrence on or off the job, report much lower incidences of "injury" prior to low back pain episodes, though low back pain occurs with equal frequency in the United States.

The assumption that imagable degenerative changes in the spine, including discs, are the cause of most back pain may lead to spurious conclusions. The peak incidence of back disability is in the middle years, but the degenerative process continues to increase in severity well into the 7th and 8th decades, generally accompanied by a decrease in spine-related disability. Is it reasonable to believe that the asymptomatic older patient with severe degenerative joint disease has "something wrong," while the 20-year-old back-crippled worker with a negative CT scan "has nothing wrong" or may be "malingering?" Clearly, skeletal imaging tests fail to evaluate the soft tissues and are inappropriate for identifying the cause of pain in the vast majority of cases. Yet, they are misused for this purpose daily.

Even more noteworthy is another time factor in chronic low back pain. The term "chronic" refers to a persistent problem, not generally self-limited, which may continue on an episodic or progressively unremitting course. Table 1–1 presents the conventions to be used in this book concerning duration of injury. It is the time course of low back pain that leads to a great deal of the perceptual distortion among medical observers. More than 90% of the time, back pain is a brief time-limited condition for which the treatment chosen often appears to be irrelevant to the outcome. From the onset of symptoms, about half of the patients with acute low back pain are no longer disabled within 2 weeks, 70% have recovered in 1 month, and about 90% within 3 to 4 months. Yet, of those whose symptoms persist for more than 3 to 4 months, about 50 to 60% will continue to be disabled at the end of the year, and the majority of this group

Table 1–1.   Conventions Used for Duration of Injury

Description	Duration of Symptoms
Acute	Onset to 2 months
Subacute	2 to 4 months after onset of present episode
Chronic	More than 4 months after onset of present episode
Chronic episodic	More than 2 disabling episodes occurring one or more times annually, regardless of symptom duration

will continue to be disabled even afer 2 years. These individuals often go on to extensive medical treatment, compensation costs, and settlement awards that make their contribution to the problem disproportionate to that of the entire group suffering acute low back pain. In fact, 10% of the cases cost about 80% of the money in a variety of industries (Fig. 1–1) (Bigos, Spengler, Martin, Zeh, Fisher, Nachemson, Wang, 1986; Bigos et al., 1986; Spengler, Bigos, Martin, Zeh, Fisher, Nachemson, 1986).

If we scale the cost of all compensable low back pain cases from the lowest to the highest, the cost of the case in the middle (or *median* cost) is only about $600. By contrast, the average or *mean* cost of a case has risen in 10 years from $6200 to more than $7500. Clearly, this represents a tremendous discrepancy between the most costly and least expensive cases (Snook, Jensen, 1984). Thus, the chronic back case, as is true in most other chronic medical conditions, produces the greatest financial costs. Yet, unlike the sympathy shown for the chronically disabled in which the medical issues are well understood, chronic back patients, with their "hidden impairment," arouse a great deal of suspicion in their fellow citizens.

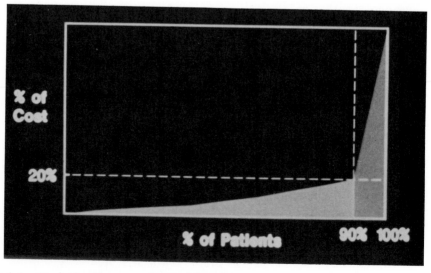

Fig. 1–1.   Graph of cost increase as length of disability increases.

PRESENT THERAPEUTIC ALTERNATIVES

Since the practicing physical therapist and primary care physician tend to view the surgeon as the locus of referral for chronic or "problem cases," we must ask ourselves if surgical treatment has solved many of the problems. While this subject will be discussed in greater depth in a subsequent chapter, it must be recognized that surgical treatment really is appropriate for only a small percentage of low back pain patients. The discectomy is by far the most common surgical procedure, and may be performed on 2 to 4% of the low back pain population in the United States. Yet, there appears to be a great disparity across cultures; specifically, those with alternate medical provider systems, such as England and Sweden, present an incidence rate of only 0.5% per year. In third-world countries, discectomy is virtually unknown. While it is clear that differing priorities and attitudes to medical care affect surgical treatment rates in many areas, it is unusual to find a disparity of an eight or more times greater rate of surgical care for such a common ailment.

Quite naturally, as the chronicity of the process increases, the prevalence of surgical treatment, particularly secondary procedures such as fusions, also increases. Yet the reporting of results of delayed or multiple spine surgery is inconsistent with outcome reports on other types of musculoskeletal surgery (Waddell, 1979; Spangfort, 1972). These often discouraging summaries tend to dissuade many surgeons from devoting much time to the practice of spine surgery.

Through brilliant analysis of the effects of psychosocial, economic, and stress factors on the central nervous system, a series of behavioral treatments, based on the perspective that chronic low back pain has cognitive, in addition to physical, components, have been developed (Fordyce, 1985; Turk, 1983; Sternbach, 1983). The behavioral conceptual framework has led, over the past 25 years, to a proliferation of "pain clinics" devoted to management, among other things, of chronic low back pain utilizing a form of multidisciplinary assessment and treatment. They have succeeded in focusing attention on many important psychosocial issues, especially those related to pain medication abuse and, more recently, to treatment of depression. However, as these clinics began to proliferate over the years, there was a tendency to lump all "hidden disabilities" such as low back, neck, headache and phantom limb pain into a vast dissimilar array, all supposedly yielding to the same behavioral or psychologic approach. It is not surprising, then, that many failed to alter the critical societal outcomes dealing with the financial and human cost. In fact, the vast pain clinic literature that subsequently developed rarely demonstrated an interest in exploring its accountability regarding disability, litigation and cost, preferring instead to focus on "quality of life" issues generally based on subjective patient self-report. Since such patient report is generally viewed as notoriously unreliable, and subject to change from one moment to the next, reports of outcome have been viewed with a great deal of skepticism among the legal, insurance, and medical communities not directly involved in pain management.

THE ISSUE OF ASSESSMENT

The issue of assessment is another "weak link" in this field, made more so by lack of recognition of deficits of present techniques. The absence of quantifiable assessment techniques for the low back is only infrequently recognized by the medical community, and almost never by nonmedical groups. The need for an objective arbiter of "What is wrong?" "Who has really been injured?" and "Is there something that needs to be fixed?" has been noted, but no scientifically validated test has emerged to resolve the need. Standard radiographic imaging techniques have been used to make judgments about all of these factors since many specialists often find it difficult to utter the words "I don't know." However, these techniques have been mostly inappropriate and unreliable. Misuse of CT scan, x ray, and new MRI technology continues specifically because no valid test is available to answer these questions, and because the answers have such great socioeconomic importance. The discriminatory aspects of x-ray screening for pre-employment evaluation have now been widely documented, yet this is still the most common technique utilized in industry for keeping certain workers out of certain jobs (Rockey, Fantel, Omenn, 1979). The practice has repeatedly been attacked in Equal Employment Opportunity Commission proceedings and yet, so desperate is the need for "objective assessment," it continues to be used for worker selection even though it is inaccurate and invalid.

Invasive radiographic techniques such as myelograms and discograms have been used to make judgments about whether or not an injury has occurred, or whether or not there is "anything wrong." Yet, at best, these tests provide a static view of the degenerative process which may be totally irrelevant to the injury that has occurred. The injury that cannot be seen (the sprain, strain, or "soft tissue injury") and that is probably responsible for the inception of back pain in the vast majority of cases, is viewed as a minor aberration of such insignificance that its compensation is frequently questioned. However, if there is a "bulge," "facet arthritis," "spur" or a "disc disruption," then it is assumed that the radiographic change confirms a link between an injury that has occurred at the time of symptom onset and an explanation for symptom persistence. This change is viewed as in some way responsible for the symptoms, and its persistence is inconsistent with resolution of symptoms. At this time, however, there is no evidence to support any of these contentions. Yet these contentions are taught daily to therapists, medical students, and residents and form the basis for a belief system about spine pathology which often leads to incorrect conclusions and ineffective management.

Documenting the "Deconditioning Syndrome"

The absence of visual feedback to the low back area has been the major factor forcing us to accept the evidence of radiographic screening in spite of its inconsistencies. Patient pain complaints in the spine are unverifiable and fail to lead to a pain source that can be noted on a physical examination such as is done in other musculoskeletal conditions. In a knee, for instance, the location of pain and tenderness may correlate with findings such as instability or a meniscal click. In the spine, however, we are confounded by peculiar deep-seated anatomy with its small, complex hidden joints and muscles, and an absence of a contralateral side for comparison. In fact, our only standardized physiologic test available for the back is range-of-motion, which has become the standard for determining disability under both American Medical Association and American Academy of Orthopedic Surgeons guidelines. While this test features great simplicity with the use of a two-piece plastic goniometer, measurements are subject to considerable imprecision. Among other problems, the technique fails to identify the endpoints adequately, fails to distinguish between segmental spine motion and hip motion (which may be a huge component of sagittal movement), fails to identify an "effort factor" that identifies patients demonstrating less than their true physiologic limits, and finally fails to be supported by a large normative data base from which inferences regarding variance from accepted values can be drawn (Mayer, Tencer, Kristoferson, Mooney, 1984).

Other important factors that have been found to have substantive impact on function of extremity joints, such as periarticular strength, stability, endurance, cardiovascular fitness, and coordination have also been virtually ignored. It is one of the central contentions of this book that new technology may provide an insight into the physiology of the lumbar musculoskeletal system. Furthermore, it appears clear that deficits of physical functional capacity may play a substantial role in explaining a major part of the dysfunction and persistent pain in chronic back pain cases, and that correction of such deficits may lead to major alterations in outcome.

Physiologic measurements of true lumbar motion, trunk strength, cardiovascular fitness, and lifting capacity have all demonstrated a significant difference in performance between chronic low back pain patients and age-, gender-, and body weight-matched normals. This finding remains true even when variations in effort have been accounted for. The phenomenon is termed the *"deconditioning syndrome,"* and is of great importance in functional restoration. It has now been shown empirically that its correction leads to major improvements in physical capacity and functional outcomes, as well as to a reduction in pain self-report. Even more importantly, however, such physiologic deficits are amenable to treatment which is active, participatory, and noninvasive. This should be contrasted to modality, injection, or surgical procedures, which lack most or all of these features. Furthermore, the understanding of the role of disuse in producing the deconditioning syndrome leads to a new awareness that medical advice has frequently added to the problems of the chronic low back pain patient, rather than improving it. Even the "back school," which was devised to educate back patients, has frequently been responsible for spreading misinformation and further confusing the patient through a misguided and poorly standardized curriculum. Education appears to be of great value in a condition requiring such extensive measurement technology, but it must be guided by coherent concepts that are internally consistent.

With disuse of the musculoskeletal system, joint immobility becomes progressively more complete. Muscle atrophy, with attendant loss of fatigue resistance, is noted. A process placing a patient at bedrest for prolonged periods of time will affect cardiovascular fitness, just as a brace or a body cast limits mobility. It has been shown, utilizing biplanar radiographic techniques, that back injury leads to hypomobility even in segments previously considered "unstable." (Rockey, Fantel, Omenn, 1979; Pearcy, Sheperd, 1985). Muscle atrophy is noted after only short periods of cast immobilization in the extremities, yet cannot be seen by the clinician in the low back and therefore is rarely recognized as a factor in chronic disability. Other factors, even more opaque to modern measurement (balance, neuromuscular inhibition and coordination), are also clearly vital to restore extremity function and may also be of importance in lumbar dysfunction. This deconditioning syndrome is directly addressed by the functional restoration approach, and will be discussed at great length throughout this text.

FUNCTIONAL RESTORATION USING A SPORTS MEDICINE APPROACH

Programs that assist individuals to progressively regain functional aptitudes have been promulgated in the extremities for 30 years, and have followed a variety of sports medicine principles. A general program of physical training usually restores range-of-motion by stretching joint contractures and periarticular scar while stimulating production of synovial fluid, thus assisting lubrication and cartilage nutrition. Muscle atrophy is combatted through progressive resistance exercise, and subsequently through endurance training. Aerobic training assists extremity endurance and improves cardiovascular fitness. Neural inflow and coordination is developed by performing specific tasks to simulate work/sport activities in repetitive training geared to the patient's capabilities and future demands. It is also always associated with slight "overuse" to stimulate through increasing resistance. Clearly, certain structural abnormalities cannot be corrected (however, when one considers the severity of the degenerative process in the later years, which can be consistent with mild symptoms, one must wonder whether such structural anomalies are significant or relevant to the back disability process). These same sports medicine principles provide the core ingredients of the functional restoration approach to low back pain.

This functional restoration training program must be guided by something other than subjective patient self-report. Because of the lack of visual feedback from the spine, the patient is aware only of the pain and its qualities, i.e., location, intensity and whether burning, dull, stabbing, or tingling. This perception leads inexorably to overprotectiveness in a significant minority of the vast pool of back pain patients who may resist strenuous therapist efforts to re-educate. Therefore, specific goals of improvement on quantitative physical function tests must be the principal objective guiding the patient in the treatment program. As long as the patient, therapist, and clinician are relying on self-report to progress treatment, the management must inevitably be nonstandardized and related primarily to the pain sensitivity of the patient. The patient population involved in chronic pain processes may also be dealing with substantial psychosocial problems in addition to the physical ones, making objective measurement an even more important part of functional restoration to provide patient reassurance. These objective measurement techniques will be fully discussed in Part II of this text.

In passing, it should also be noted that until now, we have said relatively little about psychosocial and economic factors involved in low back pain. When dealing with a chronic back pain patient, it is tempting to delve into the manifold developmental and personality factors leading to their disabling dysfunction. The therapy involved may be costly and also unnecessary, since most such disabled individuals will previously have displayed a capacity for performing as productive citizens. If the goal of treatment is to restore such individuals to a level of productivity similar to that attained prior to their disabling back problem, it should not be necessary to delve into premorbid psychopathologic conditions which may be extraneous to the specific treatment process, even though it may be of great interest to the psychotherapist. What does appear to be extremely important, however, is a knowledge of the patient's current psychologic profile in anticipating responses to disease and treatment. A variety of test measures to detect neuropsychologic deficits, psychotic behavior, characterologic disorders, depression, anxiety neurosis, self-perception of pain and disability, and other personality factors are available and are utilized in a functional restoration program. Some of these tests may be performed on multiple occasions through the treatment process to mark changes in perception and coping mechanisms available to the patient. These psychologic measures are used to help tailor the treatment program to each individual (rather than applying the same inflexible program across all patients). The way in which this assessment is integrated with treatment will be discussed in Chapter 13.

A COMPREHENSIVE FUNCTIONAL RESTORATION TEAM APPROACH

The functional restoration treatment process involves a team approach modeled after that usually utilized in dealing with more catastrophic musculoskeletal rehabilitation. However, because of the lack of physical visual feedback and the desperate psychologic, social and economic factors peculiar to the low back "hidden disability," even closer staff inter-communication is essential.

As we will be discussing in greater detail later in the book, the critical elements of such a program are physical therapy, occupational therapy, psychology, nursing and physician direction. In the program developed at the Productive Rehabilitation Institute of Dallas for Ergonomics (PRIDE), certain specific roles have evolved for staff over the past several years. The unique effectiveness of this program attests to the appropriateness of such roles, though clearly there is room for development of other models. The much-abused term "interdisciplinary" may also be applicable, although it often implies a hodge-podge of inputs to a program with no coherent guiding principles (i.e., multiple physician specialties providing consultation in areas such as psychiatry, neurology, etc., are often termed interdisciplinary). Staffing of patients, guided by a physician-arbiter, is essential. The leadership ability of the physician in cutting to the heart of the critical "barriers to functional recovery" present in some patients, and focusing the team's attention on objective assessment rather than pain complaints, can make the treatment process an exciting and rewarding one for all the participants. The higher the quality of individual staff members, and the more incisive they are in "getting to the issues," the more successful the facility is likely to be.

THE ASSESSMENT OF IMPORTANT OUTCOME MEASURES

Ultimately, the functional restoration program will be judged on its performance. Just as patient self-report is unreliable as a measure of the severity of injury and adequacy of progress, so too is it insufficient to help judge outcome. Attention *solely* to such issues as medication usage, pain level, like or dislike for staff members and the treatment program, and objective views of families and employers, should be avoided. Instead, since we are dealing with a problem of major social and economic significance, more realistic outcome measures should be sought.

Return to Work

One of these measures which has gained a great deal of attention since publication of several articles over the past few years (Mayer, Kishino, Keeley, Capra, Mayer, Barnett, Mooney, 1985) is the subject of *return to work*. In this one issue, we summarize several of the critical problems of financial costs, human waste, and loss of productive skills to society. Yet, paradoxically, many of the participants in the low back "disability system" may find this medical goal of less than primary interest. Juries may be convinced that inability to work represents "real" disability, sometimes motivating the legal system to encourage clients to remain disabled longer in hopes of greater settlement awards. This may be particularly true if weekly benefits make up a substantial part of their lost income.

Surprisingly, insurance companies and employers may inadvertently "feed" the system. They have been educated to the fact that those who have had a previous back injury or surgical procedure are far more likely to have a subsequent injury at additional cost. Coupling this recognition with the previously noted prejudice within these organizations against back patients as "malingerers," and with evidence that certain multiply injured workers really *do* "play the system," the employer and insurance carrier may not wish to allow the injured worker back into their industry. This attitude is commonly termed "Use a back, lose a back," and serves as further justification by the plaintiff's attorney in work-injury cases that the system discriminates against the client with regard to re-employment. Finally, in heavily unionized industries, the union may also resist a return-to-work outcome, since the injured worker is being compensated while off duty, and his or her place has been taken by a previously unemployed union member. At no cost to itself, the union has placed two men on the equivalent of 1½ to 2 wages, whereas previously only one worker was employed at a single wage. A rush to "get the worker back before he is ready" may not be in the self-interest of this organization either, at least in the short run.

Of course, from a "big picture" point of view, all of these attitudes are short-sighted in that they ultimately hurt industry. Our economy and society as a whole fail to benefit when we pay individuals for being nonproductive and set incentives or negative examples that encourage disability in our potentially most productive society members. However, while the return to work would seem to be one of the simplest, most laudable and easily attainable goals if it could be accomplished by the patient, there are often substantial societal barriers to this outcome. Furthermore, many injured workers are participating in blue collar trades requiring heavy materials handling and assuming unusual positions that place considerable biomechanical loads on the back. International economic competition places severe financial constraints on companies attempting to use expensive equipment to replace manual materials handling, with government regulations stymied by the same factors. The general decrease of physical capacity with age in the face of unchanging job demands can make the worksite a progressively more dangerous place over time if promotions to less arduous tasks are not forthcoming.

Further complicating the issue may be limited cognitive skills and intercurrent disease. Even those individuals of high intelligence and multiple areas of interest are often "phased out" by industry-wide business problems. The injured worker may be facing much more common and serious problems based on such factors as limited education, limited skills in less arduous fields, limited intelligence for retraining, and other age-related deficits. Furthermore, intercurrent disease such as cardiovascular limitations and organic brain dysfunction from a variety of causes may further complicate the return to work issue. Yet, in spite of all of these negative factors, attention to this critical societal outcome is one of the most important standards of success for functional restoration.

Litigation

Another major high cost factor in low back pain is the litigation attendant upon the settlement award. Though the rules are different for each particular legal venue, litigation is frequently involved in state and federal workmen's compensation, Social Security Disability, personal injury and product liability cases. Back disability represents a substantial percentage of cases in each of these areas. It is arguable whether economic factors initiate back injuries, though most of the literature would tend to refute this idea. However, there can be no doubt that compensation is a critical factor in the persistence of disability (Beals, 1984). Thus, the prompt and fair resolution of disability compensation issues would appear to be important to help resolve disability.

In an effective treatment program, rehabilitation cannot be viewed as taking something away from the patient. The restoration of function and decrease in pain must be seen as a benefit, not an economic hardship. It must be understood by both the medical and the legal professions that the "hidden disability" cannot be quantified solely on the basis of radiographic imaging techniques, as this will incompletely describe the underlying structural damage. Clearly, the more aggressive the surgical intervention, the more likely other structures will be damaged and scar tissue formation will be more extensive. The key point is that compensation is currently based primarily on the structural injury and the impairment that is so created. However, the amount of disability is potentially related to many physical *and* psychosocial factors, but can be overcome to a great extent by patient effort in functional restoration. The impairment is "permanent" and may be the factor upon which compensation is based, but it should not be used to penalize efforts designed to decrease disability.

Medical Care

Additional medical care following rehabilitation is another outcome that can be measured in many ways. The chronic pain patient is a heavy over-utilizer of the medical care system. In their search for "the magic cure," medication use, multiple therapies, chiropractor care, and multiple surgical treatments are frequently sought and obtained. After restoring high levels of physical functional capacity, patients generally seek only necessary and reasonable medical care, and strains on the medical system can be diminished.

Injury Recurrence

Finally, the improvement in physical functional capacity should also have an effect on recurrence rates. If, as has been suggested, high levels of physical functional capacity correlate with lower risk of reinjury, then many of industries' problems with the returning worker will be resolved, and the prejudices currently noted will slowly disappear. Even if the multi-factorial etiology of compensable back injury includes psychosocial characteristics that are more preponderant in one group than another, a treatment approach that educates the individual patient to the negative consequences of back disability as a coping mechanism may help the patient deal with more than the physical causes of disability. We know that under most circumstances, acute back pain resolves within weeks; it is likely that a patient previously functionally restored who sustains a new injury may have enough appropriate education to arrest the process in the acute stage. By converting a new injury from a potentially high-cost one to a minor acute problem, tremendous prevention benefits are realized.

Throughout this text, we will be discussing these important outcome assessment issues. As will be seen, the functional restoration program has been developed to actively address and deal with these issues. It does not rely solely upon patient self-report. Indeed, in a recently completed 2-year follow-up study of patients undergoing the functional restoration program at PRIDE, the assessment of these important realistic outcome measures was carefully documented (Mayer, Gatchel, Mayer, Kishino, Keeley, Mooney, 1987). Table 1–2 summarizes these data, and contrasts the program patients to a comparison group of patients who did not receive treatment. As can be seen, at the 2-year follow-up, 87% of the treatment group was actively working, as compared to only 41% of the non-treatment comparison group. Moreover, about twice as many of the comparison group patients had both additional spine surgery and unsettled workmen's compensation litigation relative to the treatment group. The comparison group continued with approximately a 5 times higher rate of patient visits to health professionals, and had high rates of recurrence or reinjury. Thus, the results demonstrate the striking impact that a functional restoration program can have on these important outcome measures.

Table 1–2. Summary of Important Outcome Measures (from Mayer, Gatchel, Mayer, Kishino, Keeley and Mooney, 1987)

	Functional Restoration Treatment Group (n = 116)	Non-Treatment Comparison Group (n = 72)
% Return to work	87%	41%
% Additional surgeries	9%	20%
% Visiting additional health care professionals	34%	60%
Average number of visits to health care professionals	3.6	16.0
Average % of recurrent back-related injuries	3.5%	12%
% Unresolved workmen's compensation litigation cases	19%	32%

CHAPTER REFERENCES

Beals R: Compensation and recovery from injury. West J Med *140*:233–237, 1984.

Bigos S, Spengler D, Martin N, Zeh J, Fisher L, Nachemson A, Wang M: Back injuries in industry: a retrospective study II. Injury factors. Spine *11*:246–251, 1986.

Bigos S, Spengler D, Martin N, Zeh J, Fisher L, Nachemson A, Wang M: Back injuries in industry: a retrospective study III. Employee-related factors. Spine *11*:252–256, 1986.

Cady L, Bischoff D, O'Connel E, Thomas P, Allen J: Strength and fitness and subsequent back injuries in firefighters. J Occup Med *21*:269–272, 1979.

Fordyce W, Roberts A, Sternbach R: The behavioral management of chronic pain: a response to critics. Pain *22*:112–125, 1985.

Holbrook T, Grazier K, Kelsey J, Stauffer R: The Frequency of Occurrence Impact and Cost of Selected Musculoskeletal Conditions In the United States, American Academy of Orthopedic Surgeons, 1984.

Mayer T, Gatchel R, Kishino N, Keeley J, Capra P, Mayer H, Barnett J, Mooney V: Objective assessment of spine function following industrial injury: a prospective study with comparison group and one-year follow-up; Volvo Award in Clinical Sciences. Spine *10*:482–493, 1985.

Mayer T, Gatchel R, Mayer H, Kishino N, Keeley J, Mooney V: A prospective randomized two year study of functional restoration in industrial low back injury utilizing objective assessment. JAMA *258*:1763–1769, 1987.

Mayer T, Tencer A, Kristoferson S, Mooney V: Use of noninvasive techniques for quantification of spinal range-of-motion in normal subjects and chronic low-back dysfunction patients. Spine *9*:588–595, 1984.

Pearcy M, Portek I, Sheperd J: The effect of low back pain on lumbar spinal movements measured by three-dimensional x-ray analysis. Spine *10*:150–153, 1985.

Pearcy M, Sheperd J: Is there instability in spondylolisthesis? Spine *10*:175–177, 1985.

Rockey P, Fantel J, Omenn G: Discriminatory aspects of pre-employment screening: low-back x-ray examinations in the railroad industry. Amer J Law and Med *5*:197–214, 1979.

Snook S, Jensen R: Cost in Occupational Low Back Pain (Ed. J Frymoyer). New York, Praegen Press, 1984.

Spangfort E: The lumbar disc herniation: a computer-aided analysis of 2,504 operations. Acta Orthop Scand Suppl *142*:1–95, 1972.

Spengler D, Bigos S, Martin N, Zeh J, Fisher L, Nachemson A: Back injuries in industry: a retrospective study 1. Overview and cost analysis. Spine *11*:241–245, 1986.

Sternbach R: Pain Patients: Traits and Treatments. New York, Academic Press, 1983.

Turk D, Meichenbaum D, Genest M: Pain and Behavioral Medicine: A Cognitive-Behavioral Perspective. New York, Gilford Press, 1983.

Waddell G, Kummel E, Lotto W, Graham J, Hall H, McCulloch J: Failed lumbar disc surgery and repeat surgery following industrial injuries. J Bone Joint Surg *61*A:201–207, 1979.

ADDITIONAL REFERENCES

Florence D: The chronic pain syndrome. Postgrad Med *70*:217–228, 1981.

Hult L: Cervical, dorsal, and lumbar spinal syndrome. Acta Orthop Scand (Suppl) *17,* 1954.

Leavitt S, Johnson T, Byers R: The process of recovery: patterns in industrial back injury. Indust Med Surg *40*:7–14, 1971.

Nachemson A: Prevention of chronic back pain: The orthopedic challenge for the 80's. Bull Hosp Joint Dis Orthop Inst *44*:1–15, 1984.

Nachemson A: Work for all. Clin Orthop *179*:77–82, 1983.

Nordby E: Epidemiology and diagnosis in low back injury. Occup Health Safety *50*:38–42, 1981.

Chapter 2

A Review of the Basic Anatomy, Physiology and Biomechanics of the Lumbar Spine

Before discussing the specific assessment and treatment components of the functional restoration approach in Part II of this text, a review of some basic information concerning the lumbar spine and the pain-disability process will be provided. Such a review is vitally important in any text of this type in order to provide the reader with a full appreciation of the psychophysiologic complexities involved in the assessment and treatment process. In this chapter, we will review the basic anatomy, physiology, and biomechanics of the lumbar spine.

THE LUMBAR SPINE

The lumbar spine is but one portion of an axial supporting structure for the head, upper extremities and internal organs placed over a bipedal stance. It represents a series of five segments, each connected by a "three-joint complex," and seated, at its lower end, over the five fused segments of the sacrum and vestigial coccyx. The sacrum is connected through the sacroiliac joints to the pelvis which, in turn, transmits loads through hips to the lower extremities.

Sitting above the first lumbar segment are the 12 thoracic spine segments, each of which is connected to a rib that provides circumferential stability to this portion of the spine, and a primarily soft tissue connection to the upper extremities. Superiorly, the seven segments of the cervical spine support the head.

The cervical and lumbar portions of the spine each carry heavy loads in relation to their cross-sectional area. Since they are posterior structures, they each resist an anterior gravitational moment and display a lordosis, or anterior convexity, in neutral posture. Because they are unsupported laterally by other skeletal members, these segments display considerable mobility in both sagittal (flexion/extension) and coronal (lateral bend) planes. While rotation is more restricted in the lumbar area, the differences are not so great when one considers that most rotational cervical motion occurs in the upper two motion segments, whose articulations are considerably different from that of the rest of the spine.

The basic unit of the spine is the vertebra (Fig. 2–1). This basic building block of the spine provides the inflexible bony support for transmitting loads. The three-joint complex linking one vertebra to another consists of the unique, avascular intervertebral disc, whose motion is guided by the bilaterally sym-

16

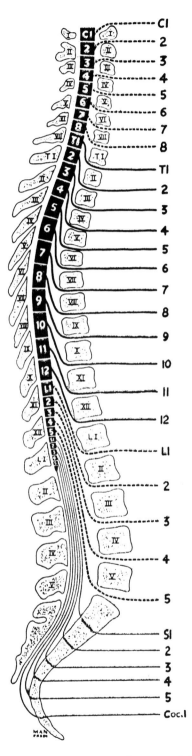

Fig. 2–1. Sagittal hemisection of the spine. (From Haymaker, W., and Woodhall, B.: Peripheral Nerve Injuries. 2nd Ed., Philadelphia, W.B. Saunders, 1953.)

metrical facet joints. Ligaments provide passive support to these vertebrae, while muscles, often with multiple tendinous connections, provide active control over single or multiple segments. Finally, a neural canal posterior to the vertebral body transmits the nerves from brain to body, with neural foramena permitting exit of a pair of nerve roots between each segment just anterior to the facet joints.

COMPONENTS OF SPINAL ANATOMY

All support system structures in the spinal canal are of mesothelial origin, and thus have several things in common. While we will be most interested in the aspects of the support system under voluntary control, namely the neuromuscular system, we should be aware that all of the support structures share a common collagenous underpinning. The properties of the different structures are greatly affected by the alignment and method of collagen cross-linking. Tissue narration also depends on the appended components such as calcium hydroxyapatite (bone), and proteoglycans (cartilage), as well as water, lipid, cellular elements, elastic fibers, and traversing blood vessels or nerves.

There are at least three types of collagen: *Type I,* found in most tissues such as skin, bone, ligaments and tendons; *Type II,* found in cartilage; and *Type III,* found in the walls of the large blood vessels. Despite these differences, it is important to keep the basic similarities of all mesothelial tissues in mind. Since there is an underlying collagenous structure, the essential property of high tensile strength, resistance to deformation with low elasticity, and the potential for fibrous repair after tissue disruption must be borne in mind. Let us consider these properties of the various components of the spine.

The Vertebrae

The vertebrae consist of specialized stable structures for transmitting load through the spine, becoming progressively larger in cross-sectional area as gravitational loads increase from cervical to lumbar spine. The vertebrae provide a protective cover for the spinal nerves, as well as an attachment point for ligament and tendons. The major load-bearing structure is the *vertebral body,* a block-like structure separated from its adjacent segment by the intervertebral disc. This structure, like other parts of the axial skeleton, is made up of cancellous rather than cortical bone. Cancellous bone consists of parallel lamellae of highly vascularized bone formed into trabeculae which are oriented along lines of stress. These lines may be multiplanar, and become thicker where stress is the greatest. A peripheral cortical shell provides significant stability, while the central portion of the vertebra transmits the greatest compressive forces through the disc nucleus and central vertebral endplate. In addition to resisting vertical compression, trabeculae are also oriented to support the posterior elements and resist tensile forces in this area. Trabecular patterns in the vertebrae provide an excellent demonstration of Wolff's Law.

The *pedicles* provide the lateral walls of the spinal canal, containing cancellous bone within a thin cortical shell. They lead, at the posterior margin, to the *pars interarticularis,* a narrowed transition zone or isthmus between the pedicle and the *lamina* or roof of the spinal canal. The contribution of a single vertebra to the superior and inferior facet joints originates from this narrowed area, which is susceptible to a peculiar type of fatigue fracture known as *spon-*

dylolysis. If bilateral, this condition may predispose to segmental instability, allowing a forward slip of the upper vertebrae on the lower known as *spondylolisthesis* (see Chapter 3).

Three projections are common to the lumbar vertebrae. The posteriorly oriented spinous process is generally palpable just beneath the skin and is bordered bilaterally by the large extensor musculature. The laterally projecting transverse processes maintain ligamentous and muscular connections to segments above and below them. They are susceptible to fracture in cases of sudden asymmetric load bearing, or vertebral translation as in falls from a height or high speed collisions. The connection between adjacent laminae consists of a unique ligament of great elasticity and low tensile strength. Its yellow appearance, related to its high content of elastic fibers relative to collagen fibers, yields its name—*ligamentum flavum.* It provides a barrier between the posterolateral muscular structures and the neural contents of the spinal canal, and also constitutes the posterior peripheral margin of the epidural space (Fig. 2–2).

The Intervertebral Disc and Facet Joints

The three-joint complex consists of the intervertebral disc which spans the adjacent vertebral bodies and the bilaterally symmetrical facet joints whose orientation varies from one portion of the spine to another, permitting varying amounts of rotation. The intervertebral disc, a thoroughly unique joint, consists of two components, one completely, and the other nearly completely, avascular. The outer portion, or *anulus fibrosis,* consists of concentric lamellae of collagen fibers oriented in a progressively more oblique fashion as the central anulus is approached. Interestingly, adjacent lamellae are generally oriented at opposing obliquity with microscopic cross-linking of collagen fibers. This feature appears to give unique resistance to torsion, while the tight lining of the anulus to the vertebral endplate strongly resists translation (Fig. 2–3). Vascularity and neural ingrowth (only small, unmyelinated fibers) appear to be present, at most, in the peripheral one-third of the anulus.

The completely avascular *nucleus pulposus* consists of an amorphous gel made up of 90% water in the young adult, with a substrate of proteoglycans containing loose strands of collagen. With aging, the water content of the nucleus declines. Under compressive load, the nucleus is progressively pressurized, acting hydrostatically as an incompressible fluid, to maintain disc height. In this way, the properties of torsion and translation resistance of the anulus fibrosis are preserved even under load. Though Gracovetsky and Farfan (1986) believe that torsional injury is most significant in leading to disc degeneration, such injury would have to occur selectively at the periphery of the disc. Most cadaveric discographic studies, however, reveal that annular tears appear to be generated from the central disc outward in a radial direction with aging, ultimately leading to occasional extrusion of nuclear contents from the disc periphery with complete disc rupture.

Another potential mechanism of degenerative disc injury occurs from the disc's greater relative strength compared to the vertebral endplate under pure compressive loads. Gross or microscopic fractures of the vertebral endplate may lead to neurovascular ingrowth, potentially converting the central disc into a "rotten core" of pain-sensitive granulation tissue.

Asymmetric loading of the spine produces compression (with bulging) of

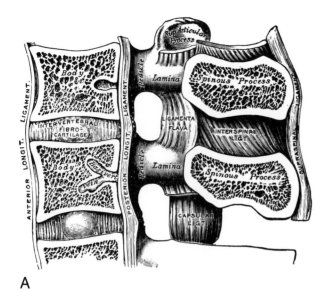

Fig. 2–2. A, Adjacent lumbar vertebrae with supporting structures. B, Lateral view of typical lumbar vertebrae. C, Superior surface of a lumbar spine vertebra. (A from Gray's Anatomy, Lea & Febiger; B and C from Ruge, D., and Wiltse, L.: Spinal Disorders: Diagnosis and Treatment. Philadelphia, Lea & Febiger, 1977.)

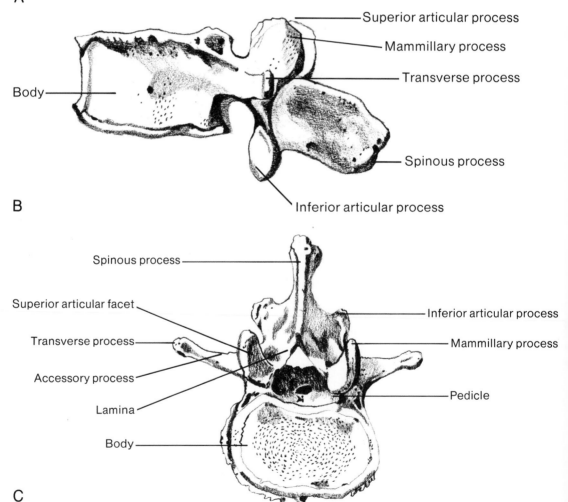

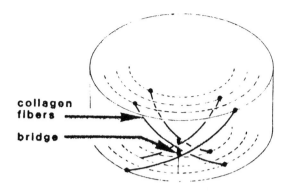

collagen
fibers

bridge

Fig. 2–3.   Anulus fibrosis section showing pattern of alternating orientation of concentric lamellae producing torsional resistance. (From Gracovetsky, S., and Farfan, H.: The optimum spine. Spine, *11*:543, 1986.)

one side of the anulus, but tension on the unloaded side. In this way, the unique structure of the disc can maintain torsion and translation resistance with any combination of multiplanar loading.

Repair of the injured disc is slow at best, as the avascular central disc is almost completely dependent on diffusion through adjacent vertebral endplates for nutrition. The young individual may lose an inch of height in the first 2 to 4 hours of upright posture in the morning as compression "squeezes" fluid into the vertebral circulation. Conversely, height is regained with spine unloading when reclining. This process of fluid transfer occurs with motion throughout the day, but at complete bedrest, the exchange of nutrients and gases is far more sluggish than when motion is present. At the periphery of the anulus, a fine nervous and vascular network may be present, covering up to the peripheral one-third of the radius of the normal disc. Thus, repair may be more rapid, and sensation more complete in this area.

The facet joints, in contrast to the disc, are typical synovial joints similar to those in other parts of the body (Fig. 2–4). The opposing cartilage surfaces are smooth, permitting gliding under the lubricating effect of synovial fluid. Such fluid is generated by the joint synovial lining, which is reinforced by a tough fibrous joint capsule permitting only limited motion. In the lumbar spine, the orientation of the facets is generally in an oblique direction between sagittal and coronal planes. There is extreme resistance to torsion, but relative flexibility in sagittal and coronal motions is permitted. In addition, there is a wedging phenomenon in extension. In this "closed pack" position, there is excellent load-sharing between the intervertebral disc and the facet joints with virtually negligible rotation permitted. By contrast, when the spine is flexed, the "open pack" disengaged position shifts all of the load to the anterior column, with the spine literally "hanging on its ligaments" and the posterior elements and posterior anulus in tension. Like all synovial joints, the facets are subject to degenerative changes in the cartilage, particularly in circumstances of poor nutrition or extremes of compression and shear. Immobility or excessive passive manipulation may produce particularly deleterious effects on the nutrition and wear characteristics of the facet joint cartilage and capsules.

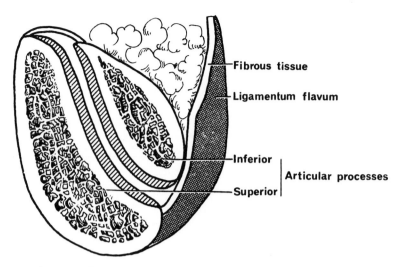

Fig. 2–4. Architecture of a facet joint illustrating similarity to other human synovial joints. (Courtesy of W.H. Kirkaldy-Willis, M.D.)

The Lumbar Nerves

The anatomy of the lumbar nerves reveals that the spine functions both as a conduit and as a source of local innervation. The spinal cord acts as a system of "hard-wired telecommunications" between brain and periphery. In the adult, the end of the spinal cord, or *conus medullaris,* terminates at approximately the level of T12-L1. In the spinal canal distal to this point, the *cauda equina* consists of a dural sac containing the lumbosacral spinal nerve roots which pass from the sac as a bilateral pair at each level. The sac effectively ends at about the S1 level, with individual nerve roots traversing the remaining sacral spinal canal and exiting the sacral foramina at each level as the *filum terminalae.* These lumbosacral nerve roots innervate not only the local musculature, but also the entire pelvis and lower extremities, and are thus of great importance.

Moving distally, the nerve root quickly divides into two components, an *anterior and posterior primary ramus,* whose division is of great significance. The anterior ramus is most important for its innervation of the lower extremity musculature and the production of sciatica. Through a process of direct nerve root compression and/or alteration of the local chemical environment, nerve roots are particularly irritated (in the lumbar region) in the overwhelming number of cases only at the level of the lowest three intervertebral disc spaces. More than 90% of the time, the two lowest intervertebral discs (below L4 and L5) are involved, usually producing unilateral sciatica involving either the L5 or S1 nerve roots. The focus of most books and articles concerning the low back are on the patterns of sensory, motor, and reflex disruption occurring as a result of anterior primary ramus compression, and to its surgical solution through excision of the offending disc fragment or bulge. The reader is here referred to Chapter 3 for information on the dermatome and myotome patterns leading to such surgical intervention.

The *posterior primary ramus* innervates the local structures. Its particular importance is that noxious stimuli from local structures are likely to be modulated through this ramus. In addition, local voluntary muscular control is transmitted by the posterior primary ramus, so that damage to it may also interfere with segmental muscular activity. This ramus also provides sensation to the skin above the segment, the ligaments and facet joints, often with overlapping nerve supply to adjacent segments. Of particular interest is the recurrent *sinu-vertebral nerve of Luschka,* which innervates the posterior vertebral periosteum, posterior longitudinal ligament, and probably the posterior periphery of the disc anulus (Pedersen, 1956; Wyke 1982). This nerve has been implicated in the critical question of the origins of low back pain (as opposed to sciatica), and a panoply of theories is supported by voluminous pain research. The nociceptor is the pain-sensitive end-organ, with transmission usually through small unmyelinated "C" fibers. The issues of peripheral versus central (cognitive) contributions to pain, and the relationship to function, will be discussed in Chapter 4. However, the involvement of the *dorsal* or *posterior primary ramus* in innervating the posterior stabilizing structures of the spine is of great importance in comprehending and formulating theories of spinal structural disorders and physiologic factors in relation to low back pain (Fig. 2–5).

THE VOLUNTARY SUPPORT STRUCTURES: THE MUSCULOLIGAMENTOUS COMPLEX

Since functional restoration is an active process, the anatomy and physiology of greatest interest are those under voluntary control. The musculoligamentous complex provides a control system for other spinal structures, and its capacity to control function can be demonstrably altered through training. For this reason, it is of great interest and will now be discussed at some length.

The Spine Musculature

The spine consists of a series of bilaterally symmetrical joints, phylogenetically adapted for protection of the neural communciations network linking brain to periphery (Hollinshead, 1982). The critical role of the spine musculature in dynamically protecting and vitalizing these articulations, with their passive ligamentous supports and accompanying neural transmission lines, is currently only partially understood. Our appreciation of the evolutionary changes in the role of spine musculature have been greatly enhanced by the theoretical work of Gracovetsky and Farfan (1986). Greatly simplified, their theory begins with the large paravertebral spine muscles providing lateral flexion for propelling a body through water, best exemplified by the lateral tail motion of the fish. This form of locomotion ultimately evolved to the predominantly flexion/extension mode of propulsion occurring in the better-adapted four-footed land animals or mammals who have returned to the sea (whales, porpoises). Conversely, primitive or semi-aquatic land animals may retain the lateral propulsion characteristic of their ocean-limited ancestors (alligator, lizard). Much more recently, it appears that the special adaptation of man to a bipedal stance necessitates a lordotic lumbar spine for balance and ambulation. The unique property of the curved lumbar spine is to convert coronal forces to axial ones. In other words, lateral bending is coupled to axial torque driving the hips forward and producing the unique, smooth gait of man. Changing the lordosis may dramatically alter the stride length but is limited by the spine's maximal tolerance of compressive and rotary loading. It must be carefully borne

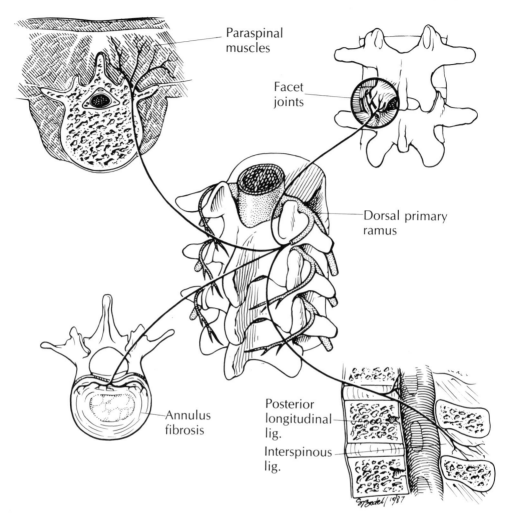

Paraspinal muscles

Facet joints

Dorsal primary ramus

Annulus fibrosis

Posterior longitudinal lig.

Interspinous lig.

Fig. 2–5. Structures innervated by posterior primary ramus.

in mind that this theoretical construct is based on a mathematical model as yet unvalidated by experimental evidence. Countering this particular aspect of the theory, Stokes, Krag, and Wilder (1987) point out the relatively minimal loss of pelvic torque noted clinically in patients with long spinal fusions for scoliosis, eliminating this particular mechanism. Experimental verification in this area of biomechanics is obviously necessary.

Another unique evolutionary factor involves bipedal balance, and the need to bend efficiently to allow hands to touch the ground. A stable "biomechanical chain" transferring forces from hands through arms, shoulder girdle, spine, pelvis, legs and feet to make renewed ground contact is necessary. Controlling static forward bending with muscles alone is inefficient, and space required for abdominal/thoracic contents imposes size restrictions on spine muscles. The evolutionary solution is three-fold: (1) strong, elastic posterior spinal ligamentous structures (midline ligaments, joint capsules and lateral ligaments), producing passive restraint to spine flexion. This allows static "hanging on the ligaments" without muscular effort, subject only to slow "creep"; (2) an "external power pack" of pelvic motors and stabilizers in extension and abduction; and (3) relatively small (compared to gluteal muscles) intrinsic musculature covered by lumbodorsal fascia providing (a) a strong ligamentous component to the tips of the spinous processes (because of its long lever arm), and (b) a weak active force (through attachment to the transversus abdominis and portion of the internal oblique) (Bogduk, Macintosh, 1984; Macintosh, 1987). This combination of a posterior ligamentous complex, powerful motors of the buttocks and posterior thigh, and psoas muscles controlling the degree of lordosis permits the spine to function in a way not generally recognized; that is, as a crane, whose boom is the ligament-stabilized flexed spine, whose fulcrum is the hips, and whose engine is the pelvic extensor musculature.

While this work is mainly theoretical, it is supported by work on lumbar spine mobility demonstrating the pattern of spine and hip mobility through a full forward bend, in which the spine flexes first to "hang on its ligaments" with only gradual engagement of the hip flexion mechanism allowing efficient, limited use of the lumbar paravertebral spine musculature (Mayer, Tencer, Kristoferson, Mooney, 1984). This underlying mechanism is further confirmed by the appearance of an electromyographically "silent period" when the spine is fully flexed in forward bend, a seeming paradox without invoking this theory since the sagittal moment is quite large in this position.

While it is beyond the scope of this chapter to discuss these concepts in greater depth, the reader should come away with an understanding of the spinal musculature as part of the "functional unit" encompassing paravertebral, abdominal, buttock and hamstring muscles critical for bipedal stance, locomotion and balance. Moreover, this spine/pelvis module is inextricably linked to the cervicothoracic/shoulder girdle/upper extremity modules, and to the lower extremity module, providing a complete biomechanical chain allowing manual handling tasks by the upper extremities to be performed while maintaining a stable foot/ground contact (Fig. 2–6).

The small interconnecting vertebrae, with their multiplanar motions and "coupling" through the three-joint complex, make it difficult to assign specific uniaxial functions to individual groups of muscles. For instance, the erector spinae group of muscles are generally thought of as extensors of the spine. However, functioning unilaterally, they may also be powerful abductors or lateral stabilizers (providing power for locomotion), and have also been shown to function to some extent in spine derotation (Mayer, Smith, Kondraske, Gatchel, Carmichael, Mooney, 1985). Similarly, lateral abdominal muscles (external oblique, internal oblique and transversus abdominis) may act as rotators, flexors or extensors of the spine under a variety of circumstances through their actions at various times on the thoracic cage, rectus sheath and lateral raphe of the thoracolumbar fascia (Gracovetsky, Farfan, 1986; Bogduk, 1984). The external oblique, without an attachment to thoracolumbar fascia, lacks potential to effect extension. These muscles may also assist in abduction and lateral stabilization.

Anatomy of Spinal Musculature

In examining the gross anatomy of the spinal muscular functional unit, we must emphasize the role of the long-ignored posterior passive stabilizers, whose functional integrity is of extreme importance. We must also emphasize that the

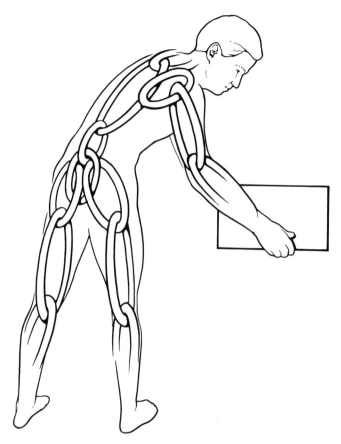

Fig. 2–6.   The "biomechanical chain" of functional units working together to provide efficient manual handling, sensory orientation, and stable ground contact.

intrinsic lumbar musculature is only a part of the functional unit. Just as the surgeon should avoid overly enthusiastic muscle stripping to prevent denervation, so should care be taken when handling lumbodorsal fascia, interspinous ligaments, and facet joint capsules. The cavalier mishandling of these collagenous and elastic structures may be as damaging as muscle denervation for the high rate of recurrence of lumbar dysfunction in the postoperative patient. With the advent of sophisticated techniques of quantifying physical functional capacity, we are, for the first time, gaining an understanding of the marked biomechanical derangements in the postoperative spine, and the need to address these in both preventive and treatment modes (Mayer, 1987).

Through evolution, the spine musculature has developed certain characteristics. The most superficial layers are truly extensions of the shoulder girdle "functional unit," and include muscles such as serratus posterior and latissimus dorsi. Their proximal function is confirmed by their innervation from the proximal spinal cord. The true spinal muscles, by contrast, have a segmental innervation that arises from the posterior rami of the contiguous spinal nerves (Fig. 2–5). While the true spinal motors function together, their most salient differentiating factor is length. The deepest muscles, such as the interspinalis, span only a single segment, while the most superficial muscles may bridge a large portion of the entire spinal column.

Local muscle action to provide motion and stability between adjacent vertebrae is a critically important part of spine function. The loss of such musculoligamentous control probably predisposes the variety of pathologic syndromes such as segmental instability and degenerative disc/facet syndromes. However, we are as yet too unsophisticated to detect discrete intersegmental aberrations, and must rely on measurements of function across several contiguous segments. On the one hand, this is as crude as measuring the function of a leg, rather than of the hip, knee, or ankle separately; on the other, it is a step forward from having no functional capacity assessment capability whatsoever.

Muscle Physiology

Muscle, the dynamic control mechanism of the skeletal system, consists of long cells specifically adapted for shortening. Voluntary, or skeletal, muscle is by far the muscle type of greatest volume. Musculature involved in spinal movement and control is, in turn, the largest complex of skeletal muscles in the body. The muscle fibers may be only a few millimeters in diameter, but may extend 5 cm or more in length. The muscle fiber is surrounded by an external layer known as the *sarcolemma,* which connects the fiber to adjacent fibers or tendon, and is sharply indented by a nerve fibril at the *myoneural junction.* The fiber is filled with many nuclei and smaller myofibrils aligned longitudinally in such a way that alternating light and dark striations are formed, leading to the designation "striated muscle." The myofibrils are made up of even smaller myofilaments of two varieties: one, formed of the protein *myosin,* and the other consisting of *actin* (McComas, 1977).

Under normal circumstances, contraction of striated muscle does not occur without neural stimulus. This is a necessary condition for skeletal muscle, whereas contraction of cardiac and most smooth muscle fibers can trigger firing of adjacent fibers without neural stimulation. The cellular mechanics of contraction are relatively simple: actin filaments (light band) slide over the myosin filaments until, with complete contraction, they are completely overlapped and the light bands of the resting muscles are completely eliminated. However, the biomechanical reactions are far more complex. Contraction is initiated by release of *acetylcholine* (ACL) at the myoneural junction, probably changing the permeability of the sarcolemma to $Na+/K+$ ions through depolarization. The contraction which follows receives energy from the conversion of *adenosine triphosphate* (ATP) to *adenosine diphosphate* (ADP), which in turn is powered by the hydrolysis of glucose into water and carbon dioxide. This process is aerobic and requires oxygen, but in the case where adequate oxygen cannot be supplied (such as vigorous exercise), glucose is converted to lactic acid. The price paid for *anaerobic metabolism* is less energy per unit substrate and an "oxygen debt." The higher the concentration of lactic acid produced, the more time is required for the metabolic poison to be removed, lengthening recovery time.

Over the past 20 years, we came to recognize that distinctly different motor units were present within a muscle. One type was noted to have a slow twitch, with good fatigue resistance and low tension development. Its muscle fibers had rich capillary beds and high concentrations of mitochondrial enzymes, with relatively low concentrations of glycogen and myosin ATPase. They appeared ideally suited for aerobic activity due to their fatigue resistance. A second type showed a fast twitch with good strength, but poor endurance. These fibers had contrasting biochemical characteristics, and appeared organized for high-intensity, short-duration bursts. Finally, an intermediate variety of fiber, melding characteristics of both fast- and slow-twitch fibers, was found. Muscles dominated by the capillary-rich *slow-twitch* or *Group I fibers* (as well as the intermediate fibers) tend to be dark in color, whereas the *fast-twitch* dominated muscles tend to be pale by comparison.

The interrelationship between biomechanical and histo-chemical properties of muscle fibers is a fascinating area for study. It is now clear that the use to which a muscle is put can adapt the muscle by selectively stressing one or another of the types of motor units. However, the concept of actual conversion of one motor unit type to another remains highly controversial. Furthermore, fiber type composition in the spinal musculature is only now beginning to be studied (Gonyea, Moore-Woodard, Moseley, Holmann, Venger, 1985).

With the long human gestation period, an infant is probably born with its full complement of muscle fibers. It appears that the growth in muscle size is due to increase in size of the fibers, rather than increase in numbers. The strength of contraction, however, appears to be related not only to muscular factors such as muscle size, fiber type and fiber number, but also (and perhaps to a greater extent) to neural factors. These include the specific characteristics of neural stimulation of motor unit firing including *frequency, extent, order* and *synchrony* which determines *fiber recruitment,* as well as the activity in the *pyramidal tract.* Training may affect several of these factors, as will the effect of certain anabolic hormones (both endogenous and exogenous). The characteristic rapid increase in strength and muscle diameter under the hormonal influence of puberty is a specific example. Muscle hypertrophy appears to occur through two processes which may proceed simultaneously: *myofibrillar hypertrophy* or *splitting.* The degree and sequence in which these changes occur is under study, but it certainly appears clear that *isometric contraction* (in which the contracting muscle is not permitted to shorten) is far more effective in increasing muscle bulk than *concentric (isotonic or isokinetic) contractions.* By contrast, various pathologic factors such as denervation, starvation, or immobilization may produce muscle atrophy. Thus, we may surmise that multiple factors, including a functional nerve supply, good nutrition, and periodic muscle activity are all necessary to maintain and increase muscle bulk.

Electromyography has been used for some time to analyze normal function and pathologic conditions in the spine musculature. Two distinct patterns of EMG activity have clearly been identified in trunk movements: (1) trunk stabilization, and (2) initiation of motion (Basmajian, 1978; Morris, Brenner, Lucas, 1962). Different movements recruit muscles in different patterns of activity, but most spinal intrinsic musculature is involved in the initiation of most movements and maintenance of posture.

Longissimus and other paravertebral muscles are frequently quiet in the "flexion-relaxation" position, in which the flexed spine is "hanging on its posterior ligaments." It is also relatively quiet in gentle extension of the spine, but with full extension, lateral bend or torsion, the role of the intrinsic musculature as a "balancer" of the spine is demonstrated by its prominent activity (Floyd, Silver, 1955). More recently, it has been found that loading of the flexed spine in the posture normally producing EMG silence leads to increasing myoelectric activity in the intrinsic spine musculature in proportion to the loads applied. This is similar to the changes seen in loading the spine in the upright position (Schultz, Haderspeck-Grib, Sinkora, Warwick, 1985). Presumably, these increasing loads sufficiently stress and stretch the posterior ligamentous structures so that compensatory muscle firing is required. The multifidus and rotatores muscles have similar activity in sagittal plane movements. However, they are active in rotation to the contralateral side, in conjunction with bilateral abdominal muscular contraction (Mayer, Smith, et al., 1985). These muscles, however, also achieve flexion-relaxation silence when the spine is in the ligamentous support phase.

The function of the lateral abdominal musculature in affecting sagittal motion remains controversial. Gracovetsky and Farfan (1986) have suggested that the oblique and transverse abdominal muscles attaching to the lumbodorsal fascia may contract to laterally stretch the fascia. The fascia thus tightens in the sagittal plane, thereby exerting an extension moment on the tips of the spinous processes. Their theoretic calculations indicated this might be a potent extensor force in certain postures. Other authors (Bogduk, Macintosh, 1984; Macintosh, 1987) have suggested that only the transversus abdominis has significant attachments to the lateral raphe of the lumbodorsal fascia (with a partial internal oblique attachment). Calculations based on the force-generating capability of the transverse musculature indicate that the extension component is a minimal factor in producing extension through this mechanism (Macintosh, 1987). However, this does not rule out the possibility that a secondary mechanism of "encapsulation" of the erector spinae by the thoracolumbar fascia through contraction of the transversus abdominis might boost efficiency of the spinal extensors.

Equally controversial is the action of the abdominal musculature on intra-abdominal pressure. For a generation, the abdominal muscles have been thought to be primary "pressurizers" of the abdominal contents by acting to increase hydrostatic pressure and thus "float" the upper torso on the pressurized abdominal contents to transfer load from the spine. While abdominal contraction may produce momentarily high peak pressures, sustained levels above that of central venous pressure would almost surely collapse the vena cava and place an unacceptable strain on the cardiovascular system by blocking venous return from the lower extremities and viscera. While the effect of abdominal musculature on sagittal stabilization and mobility remains highly controversial, its importance in rotation is undisputed. The obliques act as the primary rotators of the lower trunk (Mayer, Smith, et al., 1985).

Ligament Anatomy

The posterior ligamentous complex serves as a passive tensile load bearing element in spine flexion. All ligaments act as a "check rein" to limit motion separating the connected surfaces in the spine. Although there are anterior and lateral restraining ligaments, the majority are posterior, presumably to resist flexion moments.

Failure of ligaments is inevitable, when excessive distraction literally "tears the ligament apart." Healing may occur in an overlengthened position, leading to dysfunction if stability is comprised, as may occur in the knee. Failure may also occur at the bony attachment of the ligament in an *avulsion fracture.* Alternatively, when the ligament has a mechanical advantage over the bony structure to which it is attached, this structure itself may fracture, as might occur with spinous or transverse processes. Finally, plastic deformation, or "creep," may lead to elongation of ligaments, but it is unknown whether this truly represents a failure mode in the spinal ligaments.

Two structures already mentioned also possess properties of spinal ligaments. They are the intervertebral disc anulus and facet joint capsules. Their function has already been discussed.

The anterior and posterior longitudinal ligaments are attached to the vertebrae adjacent to the cartilaginous endplate. They provide strong check reins to excessive flexion or extension at each disc level. They have poor mechanical advantage, but their great strength and wide vertebral attachments help them to strongly resist translation and excessive motion in the sagittal plane. By contrast, the interspinous and supraspinous ligaments posteriorly, as well as the intratransverse ligaments laterally, are insubstantial with relatively long moment arms. This provides good mechanical advantage, but has the potential for sudden high stresses leading to pathologic sprain, rupture or fracture. The ligamentum flavum, already mentioned, is strong and extremely elastic, probably functioning more as a barrier between the mesothelial and neural elements than as a true check rein.

Finally, the thoracolumbar fascia may provide a powerful secondary spine control mechanism with both passive and active elements. By its attachment to the spinous processes, ilium, and ribs, it maintains a strong stabilizing effect in limiting flexion. The two ligamentous mechanisms providing passive strength include a long lever arm and interdigitating superficial and deep laminae of the posterior layer attaching to periosteum at either end, primarily to the ilium (either directly or through the lateral raphe) (Bogduk, Macintosh, 1984). The active thoracolumbar fascia component providing extension is probably weak since only the transversus abdominis appears to produce significant forces on the lateral raphe of the fascia (Bogduk, Macintosh, 1984; Macintosh, 1987). Internal oblique exerts its effect only on the lateral raphe opposite the fibers to L3, while latissimus dorsi primarily attaches directly to the spinous processes deep to the lumbodorsal fascia. However, some fibers exert a force on the lateral raphe of the fascia, though with the force partially deflected by iliac attachments (Bogduk, Macintosh, 1984). At this time, it appears that, while the lumbodorsal fascia acts only weakly through its complex muscular-ligamentous attachments, it may provide significant passive sagittal stabilizing effects.

Muscular Anatomy

We will now consider the structure and function of the various spine muscles:
1. *Intrinsic Muscles*
   a. *Erector spinae:* This large and superficial muscle, lying just deep to the lumbodorsal fascia, arises from an aponeurosis on the sacrum, iliac crest and thoracolumbar spinous processes (Hollinshead, 1982). The muscle mass is caudally poorly differentiated, but divides into three

sections in the upper lumbar area: (1) the *iliocostalis* is most lateral and inserts into the angles of the rib; (2) in the intermediate column, the *longissimus* inserts into the tips of the transverse processes of thoracic and cervical vertebrae; (3) the *spinalis* is most medial and inserts into spinous processes of the cervical and thoracic vertebrae (Fig. 2–7).

b. *Multifidus:* This series of small muscles, best developed in the lumbar region, originates on the mammillary process of the superior facet and runs upward and medially for 2 to 4 segments, inserting on the spinous process (Fig. 2–8). This orientation produces greater capacity for rotation and abduction, in addition to extension.

c. *Quadratus Lumborum:* This most lateral of the lumbar musculature originates on the iliac crest and iliolumbar ligament, and runs obliquely to insert into the last rib and transverse processes of the upper four lumbar vertebrae.

d. *Deep Muscles:* The *interspinalis* muscles are pairs of deep muscles spanning one segment on either side of the strong and elastic interspinous ligaments. The *intertransversarii* consist, in the lumbar spine, of a pair of muscles on each side, bridging the transverse processes of adjacent vertebrae. Each side has dorsal and ventral slips.

e. *Psoas Muscles:* The psoas major, though usually thought of primarily as a hip flexor, has a direct action on the vertebral column since it originates bilaterally from the vertebral bodies and transverse processes, and is the only muscle acting anterior to the sagittal axis. Yet,

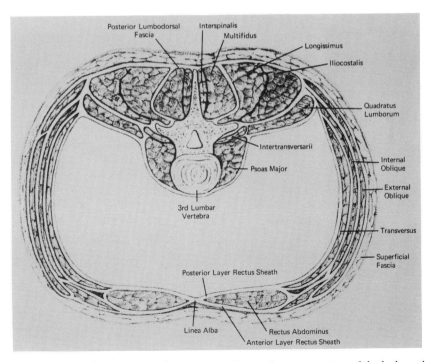

Fig. 2–7. Intrinsic and extrinsic spinal musculature illustrated on cross-section of the body at the L3 level. (From Finneson, B.E.: Low Back Pain. 2nd Ed. Philadelphia, J.B. Lippincott, 1980.)

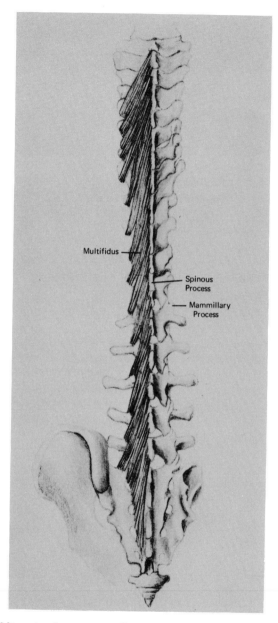

Fig. 2–8. The multifidi consist of numerous small muscular slips that arise from small bony prominences on the articular facet. (From Finneson, B.E.: Low Back Pain. 2nd Ed. Philadelphia, J.B. Lippincott, 1980.)

paradoxically, the psoas is usually an intersegmental extensor in the midlumbar spine, even as it flexes at the lumbosacral junction. In the process, it increases the lumbar lordosis which may be its primary effect. It is an important spine stabilizer in sitting and standing (Nachemson, 1968). Acting asymmetrically, the psoas may produce abduction or adduction resistance to maintain coronal balance.

2. *Extrinsic Muscles*

    a. *Abdominal Musculature:* There are four important abdominal muscles in spine function. The *rectus abdominis* is primarily a flexor, spanning the anterior abdomen from its origin on the pubic crest to its insertion on the anterior rib cage between the fifth and seventh ribs. The obliquely oriented abdominal muscles are, from superficial to deep, the *external oblique, internal oblique* and *transversus abdominis.* They all may act to produce rotation and abduction with the transverse abdominis acting to provide weak extension forces through the thoracolumbar fascial mechanism (Gracovetsky, Farfan, 1986; Macintosh, 1987). The fibers of the external oblique run in an anteroinferior direction from attachments on the lower eight ribs to insert along the anterior rectus sheath and anterior wall of the iliac crest (Fig. 2–9). The internal oblique, on the other hand, has fibers running transversely

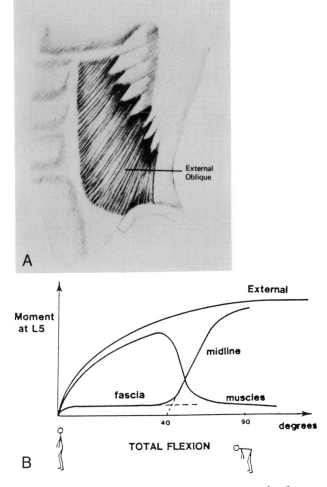

Fig. 2–9. A, External oblique muscle. B, Relative contribution compared to flexion angle of ligaments, intrinsic and extrinsic musculature in spine sagittal mobility (A from Finneson, B.E.: Low Back Pain. 2nd Ed. Philadelphia, J.B. Lippincott, 1980; B from Gracovetsky, S., and Farfan, H.: The optimum spine. Spine, *11*:543, 1986.)

only in its lowermost portion, with most of the muscle running anteriorly and proximally, nearly perpendicular to the external oblique fibers. It originates from lumbodorsal fascia and the anterior two-thirds of the iliac crest, and inserts in the lower three ribs and rectus sheath anteriorly. The transversalis, the deepest muscle of the group, runs transversely like a horizontal girdle from the lumbodorsal fascia, anterior iliac crest, and inner surface of the lower six ribs. The main mass of the muscle inserts into the linea alba in the midline. It is probable that in spine flexion, abdominal muscles not only act to create a ventral sagittal moment with lateral stabilization, but may also produce weak stabilization of the spine posteriorly through action of the transversus abdominis (and perhaps internal oblique) on the thoracolumbar fascia.

b. *Gluteal Muscles:* The large muscles of the buttocks, chiefly the *gluteus maximus, gluteus medius,* and *gluteus minimus* act variously as hip extensors and abductors. As such, they act to motor the spinal "boom" in forward bending and twisting movements around the hip axis (Hollinshead, 1982) (Fig. 2–10).

c. *Posterior Thigh Musculature:* Muscles attached to the ischial tuberosity, such as the hamstrings, are also strong pelvic extensors acting about the hip fulcrum. As such, they provide powerful assistance to the gluteal musculature in raising and lowering the pelvis. Similarly, the hamstrings provide a passive restraint that limits pelvic flexion when the knees are locked and the hamstrings are fully extended.

d. *Latissimus Dorsi:* Latissimus dorsi is a powerful accessory superficial spine muscle originating in the shoulder girdle and running caudally and medially to insert deep to the thoracolumbar fascia on the lumbar

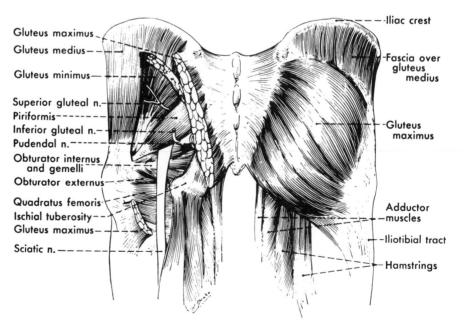

Fig. 2–10. Musculature of buttocks and proximal thigh. (From Hollinshead, W.: Anatomy for Surgeons. Vol. 3. Philadelphia, J.B. Lippincott, 1982.)

spinous processes and the iliac crest. Some fibers of the aponeurosis may deflect from the iliac crest to attach to the lateral raphe of the thoracolumbar fascia. The direct and indirect attachments may provide accessory action in extension and adduction/abduction. The latissimus dorsi may also be active in the proposed "spinal engine" mechanism of ambulation fueled by lateral bend of the spine and hip/shoulder counterrotation (Gracovetsky, Farfan, 1986).

CHAPTER REFERENCES

Basmajian J: Muscles Alive: Their Functions Revealed by Electromyography. 4th ed. Baltimore, Williams & Wilkins, 1978.

Bogduk N, Macintosh J: The Applied Anatomy of the Thoracolumbar Fascia. Spine *9*:164–169, 1984.

Floyd W, Silver P: The function of the erector spinae muscles in certain movements and posture in man. J Physiol (Lond) *129*:184–203, 1955.

Gonyea W, Moore-Woodard C, Moseley B, Holmann M, Wenger D: An evaluation of muscle pathology in idiopathic scoliosis. J Ped Orthop *5*:323–329, 1985.

Gracovetsky S, Farfan H: The optimum spine. Spine *11*:543–573, 1986.

Hollinshead W: Anatomy for Surgeons. Volume 3, 3rd ed. Hagerstown, Md., Harper & Row Publishers, 1982, p. 19–23.

Macintosh J, Bogduk N, Gracovetsky S: The biomechanics of the thoracolumbar fascia. Clin Biomech *2*:78–83, 1987.

Mayer T: Assessment of Lumbar Function. Clin Orthop *221*:99–109, 1987.

Mayer T, Smith S, Kondraske G, Gatchel R, Carmichael T, Mooney V: Quantification of lumbar function Part 3: Preliminary data on isokinetic torso rotation testing with myoelectric spectral analysis in normal and low back pain subjects. Spine *10*:912–920, 1985.

Mayer T, Tencer A, Kristoferson S, Mooney V: Use of noninvasive techniques for quantification of spinal range-of-motion in normal subjects and chronic low-back dysfunction patients. Spine *9*:588–595, 1984.

McComas A: Neuromuscular Function and Disorders, Boston, Butterworth Publishers, 1977.

Morris J, Benner G, Lucas D: An electromyographic study of the intrinsic muscles of the back in man. J Anat *196*:509–520, 1962.

Nachemson A: The possible importance of the psoas muscle for stabilization of the lumbar spine. Acta Orthop Scand *39*:47–57, 1968.

Pedersen H, Blunck C, Gardner E: The anatomy of the lumbosacral posterior rami and meningeal branch of the spinal nerves (sinuvertebral nerves) with an experimental study of their functions. J Bone Joint Surg *38*A:377–391, 1956.

Schultz A, Haderspeck-Grib K, Sinkora G, Warwick D: Quantitative studies of the flexion-relaxation phenomenon in the back muscles. J Orthop Res *3*:189–197, 1985.

Stokes I, Krag M, Wilder D: A critique of "the optimum spine." Spine *12*:S11-S12, 1987.

Wyke B: Receptor Systems in Lumbosacral Tissues in Relation To The Production of Low Back Pain. American Academy of Orthopedic Surgeons Symposium On Idiopathic Low Back Pain (Ed. White A, and Gordon, S) St. Louis, CV Mosby Co., 1982, pp. 97–107.

ADDITIONAL REFERENCES

Anderson C, Fine L, Herrin G, Sugano D: Excess days lost as an index for identifying jobs with ergonomic stress. J Occup Med *27*:740–744, 1985.

Anderson G: Epidemiologic aspects on low-back pain in industry. Spine *6*:53–60, 1981.

Bartelink D: The role of abdominal pressure in relieving the pressure on the lumbar intervertebral discs. J Bone Joint Surg *39*B:718–725, 1957.

Bigos S, Spengler D, Martin N, Zeh J, Fisher L, Nachemson A, Wang M: Back injuries in industry: a retrospective study. II. Injury factors. Spine *11*:246–251, 1986.

Bigos S, Spengler D, Martin N, Zeh J, Fisher L, Nachemson A, Wang M: Back injuries in industry: a retrospective study. III. Employee-related factors. Spine *11*:252–256, 1986.

Gracovetsky S, Farfan H, Helleur C: The abdominal mechanism. Spine *10*:317–324, 1985.

Mayer T, Terry A, Smith S, Gatchel R, Mooney V: Quantitative postoperative deficits of physical capacity following spine surgery. Presented at annual meeting of American Academy of Orthopedic Surgeons, San Francisco, CA, January 24–28, 1987.

Nachemson A, Andersson G, Schultz A: Valsalva maneuver biomechanics. Effect on lumbar trunk loads of elevated intra-abdominal pressure. Spine *11*:476–479, 1986.

Rockey P, Fantel J, Omenn G: Discriminatory aspects of pre-employment screening: low-back x-ray examinations in the railroad industry. Amer J Law and Med *5*:197–214, 1979.

Sander R, Meyer J: The relationship of disability to compensation status in railroad workers. Spine *11*:141–143, 1986.

Chapter 3

Structural Sources of Low Back Pain

In most disease processes, the persistence of a particular symptom (most commonly pain) alerts the patient to its potential seriousness, and commonly initiates physician visits. After taking a history and performing a physical examination, the physician may decide that an obvious, treatable syndrome is present, and may immediately prescribe effective treatment. However, if treatment is ineffective, or if a treatable diagnosis is not easily reached, more complex diagnostic testing is usually called for. Ultimately, though with lower frequency, a specific organic diagnosis, which may or may not be treatable, is obtained. Alternatively, by exclusion, a finding of a "psychosomatic" disorder (usually a wastebasket category providing little information to guide the treatment process), may be appended by the physician.

In the field of musculoskeletal medicine, the diagnostic puzzle is usually not particularly difficult. An "injury" is usually identified, and its physical manifestations can be easily visualized in the extremities: swelling, discoloration, deformity, local tenderness or instability. Treatment is generally symptomatic, but in more severe instances, surgical stabilization may be required. This relatively straightforward diagnosis-treatment process is not the case, however, for low back pain.

THE PROBLEM OF DIAGNOSING LOW BACK PAIN

In the diagnosis of back difficulties, problems are more complex than in the extremities, and are even more complicated by perceptual difficulties. Medical experts have a wide disparity of views, with the opinion that a specific pathologic entity causing low back pain can be identified varying among experts from 10 to 90% of cases. When we analyze the diagnoses that make up the vast majority of "definite entities," we soon realize that these are often ill-defined and physically unverifiable. These include such common entities as muscular strain, ligament sprain, anular tear, or a variety of visualized degenerative changes (disc narrowing, narrow canal, etc.). Naturally, with increasing age, or in the postoperative spine, visualizable disorder becomes considerably more evident. However, there has never been a clear demonstration that this pathologic condition is *the cause* or source of the patient's perceived pain. In fact, there are compelling reasons to believe that the relationship is not one-to-one. For example, the degenerative process becomes gradually worse with increasing age, even as the peak incidence for low back problems is between 35 to 50 years of age. Low back pain is the primary cause of disability for individuals under age 45; this is no longer true above this age.

As another example, most disc procedures are ablative procedures done to relieve sciatica and actually *increase* the damage to the disc. Even the cause of sciatica remains obscure, as most operated discs are nerve root-only localized bulges that do not produce mechanical nerve root compression (though, perhaps, biochemical irritation may be present). Severe biomechanical disruption must be produced by removing 25 to 40% of disc anulus and nucleus, as well as asymmetrical ablation of bone, ligaments and muscles inherent to the exposure. Moreover, scarring is produced by incomplete perineural hemostasis, leaving the spine much more severely degenerated than it was preoperatively. Yet, in the large majority of cases, back pain and leg pain are *both* relieved by the surgery. Even more remarkable is that the nerve root, now exposed to a raw bed of disc anulus, leaking nuclear material, and muscle dorsally (in place of ligamentum flavum), appears to lose its irritability promptly. Clearly, there are many conceptual inconsistencies even in this best understood of spinal therapeutic procedures.

Acute Low Back Pain

Acute low back pain is one of the commonest afflictions of man, with an estimate that 65 to 80% of populations of industrialized countries will at one time succumb to at least one episode. As was discussed in Chapter 1, the natural history of these events is well understood and is depicted in Figure 3–1. Within 2 weeks afer an acute episode, nearly 50% of the group will have recovered. This number of responding patients increases nearly to 70% at 1 month, and to 90% by 3 months following the episode. The timing of termination of disability may be affected by the socioeconomic environment, but this 3-month end-point will occur between 2 to 4 months under most circumstances in most

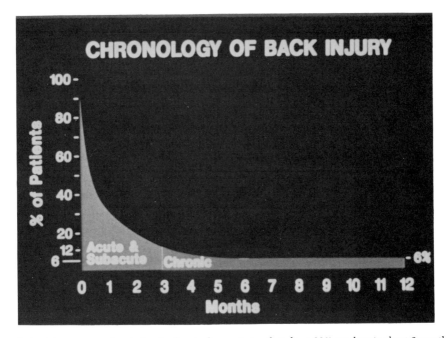

Fig. 3–1. Time course of acute low back pain demonstrates that about 90% resolves in about 3 months.

industrialized countries. Of this group of responders, however, nearly 50% will go on to have recurrent episodes of acute back pain (Mayer, Kishino, Keeley, Mayer, Mooney, 1985; Bergquist-Ullman, Larsson, 1977; Troup, 1978).

Chronic Low Back Pain

Figure 3–2 illustrates the fate of the 10% of individuals who have an atypical response to an acute low back pain episode. This group of individuals is the "high cost" group which will produce the greatest societal expense, producing 80 to 85% of the ultimate cost of low back pain (Bigos, Spengler, Martin, Zeh, Fisher, Nachemson, Wang, 1986; Mayer, Gatchel, Kishino, Keeley, Capra, Mayer, Barnett, Mooney, 1985). Of the group who are still disabled at this point, about 50% will *continue* to be disabled 1 year after symptom onset. From this point on, the rate of spontaneous resolution of disability is small. Many of these patients then go on to become the "totally and permanently disabled," leading to long-term disability payment by third party carriers and Social Security, loss of productivity and other societal sequelae.

While this text focuses on this "hard core" group, and the causes, diagnostic tests and treatment approaches involved, we must initially have an understanding of the commonest and best understood structural etiologies. Such understanding will be the goal of the remainder of this chapter.

POTENTIAL STRUCTURAL SOURCES OF LOW BACK PAIN

Acute Trauma

One type of acute trauma involves *spine fractures.* We tend to deal best with those things that we can see. Since spinal structures are not readily accessible

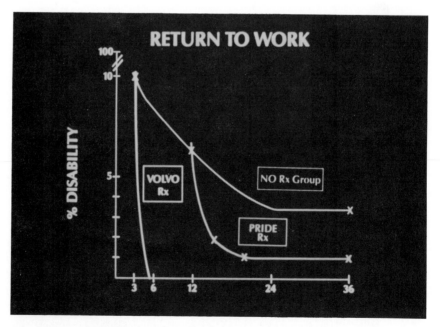

Fig. 3–2. The fate of the 10% of patients still disabled after 3 months demonstrates that more than half will continue to be disabled at the end of 1 year. Also shown are anticipated results of interventions in the acute phase (Volvo study) and chronic phase (PRIDE study).

to palpation or manipulation, as is the appendicular skeleton, we must rely on alternate techniques, usually radiographic. Because bony structures can be easily demonstrated, fractures are injuries we are invariably made aware of when they are present. In the lumbar spine, these are most commonly due to excessive axial loading, producing a typical compression fracture. These are typically wedged anteriorly due to the axial forces transmitted anterior to the sagittal axis and relative strength of the posterior elements, but in severe trauma may result in a "burst" fracture (Figs. 3–3 and 3–4).

These fractures are more common with increasing age, and in the older age groups there is a female preponderance due to the higher incidence of osteoporosis in the postmenopausal female. Common wedge compression fractures, customarily occurring through cancellous bone, generally heal in a relatively short time with minimal treatment. They are usually unaccompanied by neurologic complications or late instability. On the other hand, the severe burst fracture may explode into the spinal canal, leading to a variety of neurologic sequelae. Severe compression fractures with disrupted posterior elements may lead to progressive kyphotic deformities.

Pure compression fractures are usually produced by loads in a single plane, typically by a fall from a height on buttocks or heels. Multiplanar loading may also occur, however, and result in fracture-dislocations. These more severe

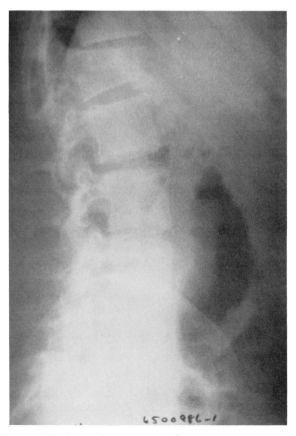

Fig. 3–3. X-ray of a typical lumbar wedge compression fracture.

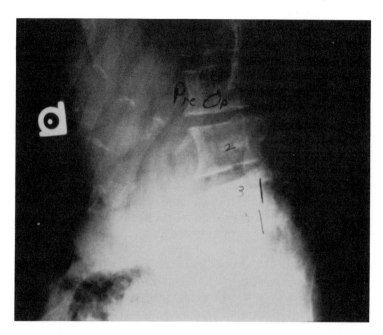

Fig. 3-4.   X-ray of a severe "burst" fracture sustained under extreme loading.

injuries are often associated with neurologic sequelae, and may involve disruption of the "three-joint complex," necessitating surgical stabilization. Trauma produced by significant momentum, usually involving motor vehicle collisions, is usually responsible and may disrupt other important structures involved in spine biomechanics such as hips or sacroiliac joints (Malgaigne fractures).

Spondylolysis or Spondylolisthesis may represent another type of acute trauma. While there may be many causes of these common entities, prolonged, repetitive microtrauma or a single traumatic event seem to be a common thread through the different types. In the commonest isthmic spondylolysis, the thin area of the pars interarticularis may have a congenital deficiency. This appears to be subjected to trauma, generally in the second decade, leading to the persistent defects probably representing fibrous union and predisposing to an anterior slip of the involved vertebra on the one below (most generally at the L5-S1 level). Spondylolisthesis may also be viewed as acutely traumatic in origin, often leading to a major slip and severe symptoms. However, other forms of spondylolisthesis due to an elongated pars, degenerative instability, or to pathologic fracture through a metabolic or neoplastic process, may also be traumatically produced (Wiltse, Newman, MacNab, 1976, Wiltse, Widell, Jackson, 1979).

While the incidence of spondylolisthesis is relatively variable among populations, with an incidence as high as 10% among Eskimos, populations of most industrialized countries have a spondylolysis incidence of 4 to 5% and spondylolisthesis of 2 to 3% (Allen, Lindm, 1950; Kettelkamp, Wright, 1971; Splithoff, 1953). No controlled study has ever demonstrated an increased risk of injury in patients with pre-employment evidence of spondylolysis or spondylolisthesis. This has not kept radiographic screening from being used by employers, desperate to reduce their incidence of work-related injury, to screen potential workers. Such practices are increasingly being recognized as discriminatory and contrary to U.S. Equal Employment Opportunities Commission guidelines (Rockey, Fantel, Omenn, 1979).

Soft Tissue Trauma

The vast majority of acute "traumatic" incidents associated with the onset of low back symptoms are generally ascribed, rightly or wrongly, to "soft tissue" origin (ligaments, muscles, tendons, joint capsules, disc anulus). The relationship of trauma to these "injuries" is a highly controversial point. There is a marked discrepancy in the reporting of a precipitating traumatic event between varying socioeconomic situations. In American industry, where compensation is dependent on reporting a specific injury on the job, low back pain onset is accompanied more than 90% of the time by a traumatic complaint. In practice, such statements can rarely be disputed. However, in parts of Scandinavia where compensation is unaltered by the circumstances of symptom onset, traumatic events are reported only about 25% of the time. Furthermore, there is considerable latitude in understanding what constitutes a "traumatic" event: from a single bending, lifting or twisting incident, to pain developing after repetitive lifting over the course of a day, or even back pain developing several days or weeks following an event which produced injury to another body part. Since these "soft tissue injuries" cannot be visualized, their existence can almost never be verified on physical examination or radiographic studies, and are almost always imputed merely on the statement of the patient. As the reader might imagine, this persistent lack of injury verification is one of the primary "root causes" of the conundrum of industrial low back pain.

In the past, the terms "sprain" and "strain" were used presumptively to categorize the vast majority of low back "injuries." In the absence of pathologic verification, however, a variety of "syndromes" has been proposed and often substituted for these more structurally specific diagnoses. A "sprain" (ligament injury), "strain" (muscle/tendon injury), or anular tear may well be the inciting cause for many low back incidents. Even granting the relatively poor blood supply to many low back structures slowing healing, and the difficulty in relieving the tremendous loads that must be borne through the spine, it still strains the credulity of most physicians that such a high proportion of these relatively insignificant injuries take so long to heal, or frequently "persist without cure" indefinitely. The seemingly logical conclusion accepted by most physicians (and subsequently by employers, attorneys, and claims adjusters) is that persistent disability following sprain/strain implies a "head case," conscious malingerer, or both. However, if surgical procedure is performed, regardless of medications or number of previous negative surgical consultations, it validates the injury as "real" and increases the value of the case. No wonder that results of surgical treatment are so much worse in the litigation group (Dzioba, Doxey, 1985; Waddell, Kummel, Lotto, Graham, Hall, McCulloch, 1979). This conceptual gap is expressed in physician skepticism concerning the motivation of back-injured workers, and the adversarial/litiginous relationships that evolves subsequently.

Yet, it is an inescapable conclusion that, if trauma is truly important in producing low back pain, soft tissue injuries must account for the vast majority of such events. Until soft tissue imaging techniques are dramatically enhanced, the role of trauma in producing low back pain will remain extremely controversial. Unfortunately, the best answer to "What is the source of low back pain?" at this time is "We don't know!"

Degenerative Disease

Degenerative disease generally implies the effects of age, microtrauma, or "wear and tear" on spinal structures (primarily the joints of the three-joint complex). In this series of entities covering osteoarthritis, herniated nucleus pulposus, disc disruption syndrome, anular tears, spinal stenosis (central or lateral recess), facet arthropathy, and a number of other entities, we have the most commonly used diagnoses thought related to low back pain. Unfortunately, however, the demonstration that these pathologic findings, usually demonstrated radiographically, are the *source* of low back pain, is frequently lacking. While it has become traditional, particularly in medicolegal situations, to draw a presumptive link between pathologic conditions and symptoms, there are compelling reasons to doubt this relationship in the majority of symptomatic cases. In fact, this presumption may be extremely misleading and the source of a great deal of confusion. It may also induce unavoidable inequities and increasing cost in the disability evaluation system.

For example, the degenerative process progresses inescapably with age, while the peak incidence of low back pain is prior to age 50. Back pain, as a symptom, is declining in the seventh decade, at a time when degenerative change is almost universally seen. In addition, the prevalence of degenerative changes such as osteophytes is no higher in a low back pain population than in a routine pre-employment screening population. Moreover, surgical disc excision removes 25 to 40% of the disc instantaneously. Despite this sudden, iatrogenic degeneration, disc space narrowing is uncommonly seen on plain x rays for 3 to 6 months, while osteophytes may only occur over years. Yet, once seen in the presence of back symptoms, such changes are usually considered to be the source of pain by most physicians. Patients generally accept the "bad disc" noted on their x rays as a legitimate portrayal of the cause of their pain.

Finally, while disc space narrowing (particularly at L4-5) has been used to predict future injury in workers, the correlation between radiographic narrowing and disc rupture level in proven disc herniations is less than 50% (Pope, Frymoyer, Andersson, 1984; Kellgren, Lawrence, 1958; Hakelius, Hindmarsh, 1972). Thus, while x rays may show changes in calcified spinal structures, there is little evidence that these changes establish a source of pain. Advanced degeneration may be painless, while a radiographically normal spine may be symptomatic. However, the majority of physicians continue to assume a direct relationship in most cases, leading to the greatest single error in low back diagnosis.

Herniated Nucleus Pulposus (HNP)

This is a much discussed and the best understood of lumbar spine clinical entities. It also gives rise to other major misconceptions in low back disease. While the layman understands this entity as the only "real" back disorder, it appears to be the cause of the specific syndrome described by Mixter and Barr (1934) in only about 1 to 2% of low back pain cases. This entity has achieved greatest prominence because it is the only combination of consistent clinical and radiographic findings that results in symptomatic "cure" in a high proportion of cases when adequately dealt with through surgical intervention. The clinical presentation of sciatica, neurologic involvement, root tension signs, with or without backache, combined with confirmatory electrodiagnostic and radiographic testing, consistently leads to a finding of a disc protrusion, extrusion, or sequestration when the appropriate disc level is surgically explored.

It is interesting to note that there is wide disparity between the incidence of such surgery for reported low back pain cases in different countries. It varies from about 0.5% in such countries as England and Sweden to about 4 to 5% in certain parts of the United States. It is obvious that this discrepancy does not occur primarily as a result of varying somatotypes, degree of industrialization, or stoicism of these different populations. Rather, variations in social support and medical care provider systems probably account for much of the difference.

Certain other important observations concerning disc surgery may be summarized as follows:

1. Disc surgery is effective, with prolonged good results ranging from 70 to 95%, if appropriate clinical and radiographic selection criteria are followed.

2. Disc surgery performed without appropriate root tension signs or neurologic involvement (i.e., for backache or symptomatic leg pain only) is associated with a marked decay in results.

3. Operations performed for "midline HNP" or "asymmetrical disc bulges," without appropriate clinical correlation, likewise have unpredictable results.

4. Surgical procedure itself produces damaging effects, including perineural fibrosis, potential instability, lumbar hypomobility and localized damage to muscles, ligaments, joints and bone in an asymmetrical fashion that may lead to impaired lumbar biomechanics. Spine surgery is *not* a harmless procedure, and should be undertaken only if the gains outweigh the risks.

It has also been shown that documented disc rupture (Fig. 3–5), if left untreated, will produce the same long-term results as successful surgically treated disc rupture. Furthermore, surgery performed more than 3 months after sciatic onset has no better short- or long-term results when compared to nonoperative treatment (Weber, 1983). Only in rare cases is disc surgery clearly an emergency, as in the "cauda equina syndrome" involving multiple nerve roots with neurologic findings in extremities, bladder, and bowel. If this syndrome goes unrecognized and is not decompressed within hours, neurologic sequelae of significant degree may persist permanently. The same risks may be attendant upon delay in responding to neurologic complications of chemonucleolysis, though it is unclear at this time whether decompression and lavage can consistently reverse the effects of this unusual toxic syndrome. More commonly, progressive neurologic deficits, particularly muscle weakness in motors of the foot, ankle and hip, is a usual indication for moving ahead with surgical treatment. For lesser degrees of neurologic involvement, however, surgical treatment is primarily advocated to hasten the recovery process; eventual healing with com-

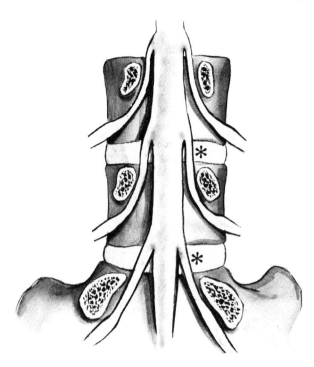

Fig. 3–5. Asterisks mark where disc protrusion compresses nerve roots. Hence, L5-S1 herniated nucleus pulposus would compress S1, not L5, nerve root. (From Ruge, D., and Wiltse, L: Spinal Disorders: Diagnosis and Treatment. Philadelphia, Lea & Febiger, 1977.)

parable outcomes is anticipated with or without surgery. It is beyond the scope of this book to discuss the details of surgical decision-making for this entity, and the reader is referred to a wide variety of other texts (LaRocca, in press).

Spinal Stenosis

Stenosis implies narrowing of a tube or canal. In the spine, it occurs in two forms: central or lateral recess stenosis (Fig. 3–6). In the more typically described central stenosis, there is a narrowing of the spinal canal producing compression of the cauda equina (Verbiest, 1954). The clinical syndrome of spinal stenosis is usually associated with back pain and fleeting multi-level neurologic symptoms that have a postural component not typically fitting a nerve root pattern. Electrodiagnostic tests are usually equivocal, probably related to the fact that the neurologic claudication is postural, not persistent.

While congenital narrowing of the central canal may predispose to symptomatic stenosis with a minor disc herniations, central stenosis is most commonly an entity of the 6th decade and beyond. Degenerative narrowing may arise through a combination of osteophytes resulting from disc degeneration, facet overgrowth, ligamentum flavum hypertrophy or postoperative bony/scar overgrowth and settling. Degenerative spondylolisthesis commonly accompanies this entity. While surgical decompression with or without stabilization may prove beneficial, results of surgical treatment, though apparently appropriately addressed to the specific disorder, are of lower quality than those generally achieved by disc surgery.

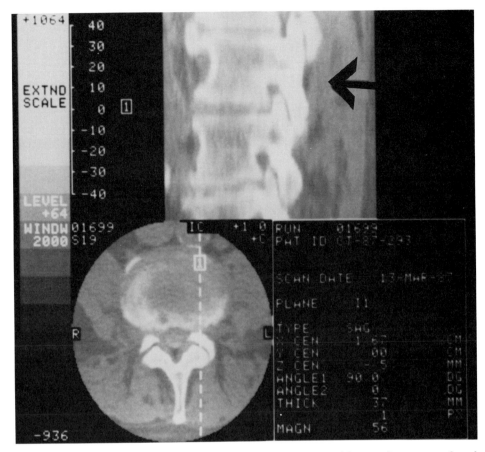

Fig. 3–6. CT scan axial cut and sagittal reconstruction through the neural foramen demonstrating lateral recess stenosis.

Facet Arthropathy and Osteoarthritis

This dynamic clinical entity (Mooney, Robertson, 1976), produced by acute injury, capsular tears, and/or prolonged hypomobility, involves a syndrome of pain with referral presumably through the posterior primary ramus of the involved spinal nerve root. Pain, generally with hip or thigh referral, which is increased by extension and often associated with hypomobility and local tenderness, characterizes this clinical syndrome. Treatment is nonspecific, with the exception of local injection, but since the specific joint cannot usually be identified by radiographic means, relief is usually undependable (Jackson, Jacobs, 1986). With aging, degenerative osteoarthritis can be radiographically demonstrated in these typical diarthrodial joints, but they appear to be surprisingly infrequently the cause of disabling symptoms in the older age group in whom osteoarthritis becomes progressively more common.

Disc Disruption Syndrome

The syndrome of the "painful disc" has gained greater currency, and has provoked considerable controversy in recent years. In the syndrome of Crock (1974), a variety of clinical and psychologic symptoms associated with stereotypical responses to activity and exercise were described. Negative tests on any of the usual structural diagnostics may be seen. However, a positive discogram is necessary for diagnosis, characterized by radiographic abnormalities such as anular tears or epidural flow, in combination with the patient's verification of "concordant pain." There is pain reproduction with injection of the dye material that exactly mimics the patient's customary pain pattern.

Unfortunately, radiographically positive discograms become exceedingly commonplace at multiple levels with aging. Furthermore, "concordant pain" is subjective and may occasionally be reproduced at disc levels that are perfectly normal radiographically. The pathophysiology of why the exceedingly common anular tear continues to produce prolonged symptoms responsive to surgical intervention is far from well understood. At this point in time, the cost/benefit relationship of surgical treatment for this controversial entity is too poorly understood to warrant the performance of large numbers of such procedures.

Segmental Instability

While this entity has been identified as a clinical syndrome for many years, and has been the specific diagnosis leading to multiple posterior and posterolateral fusions over the decades, there is no general agreement on the clinical syndrome, method of diagnosis or proper treatment. As generally understood, a degenerative process leads to an "unstable" level due to advanced single-level degenerative changes, possibly exacerbated by surgical procedure or fracture. The inappropriate translation or excessive mobility may lead to localized deformity including rotoscoliosis. Recurrent episodes of spasm and pain are thought to ensue. If chronicity increases, surgical stabilization, with or without internal fixation, is advocated. In practice, however, it is difficult to demonstrate excessive mobility at a single level when evaluating for surgical treatment. In fact, hypomobility is the common sequela of prolonged lumbar dysfunction. If a generalized hypomobility is inducing excessive load and motion on a neighboring segment, then an obvious initial solution is to restore mobility in the adjacent, uninjured segments. Like "soft tissue injury," segmental instability is a clinical diagnosis without pathologic confirmation, whose very existence remains controversial.

On the other hand, spondylolysis, or defect in the pars interarticularis, may lead to a slip of one vertebra on another, termed spondylolisthesis. Several degenerative or congenital anomalies may lead to this form of instability (Fig. 3–7). Such slips frequently lead to disruption of the intervertebral disc, as demonstrated by discography, when it is felt that symptoms are emanating from the unstable segment. Surgical stabilization may provide pain relief even after a prolonged period in which the degree of "symptomatic" spondylolisthesis has not progressed. Such slips are easily noted on plane radiographs (Fig. 3–8).

OTHER SOURCES OF LOW BACK PAIN

Neoplastic Disorders

Compared to other causes of back pain, neoplasms are quite uncommon. Primary bone tumors, benign or malignant (osteoid osteoma, chondroblastoma, multiple myeloma), are rare compared to metastatic bone disease from another site (commonly breast, lung, prostate, kidney and thyroid). The pain may be

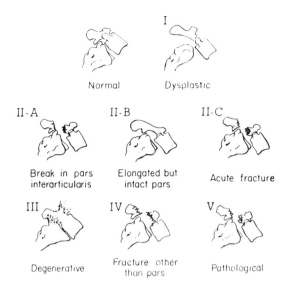

Fig. 3–7. Classification of spondylolisthesis. (From Bradford, D.S.: Spondylolysis and spondylolisthesis. *In* Chou, S.: Spinal Deformity and Neurologic Dysfunction. New York, Raven Press, 1977.)

particularly unrelenting and resistant to postural change, and is often accompanied by other signs such as weakness, weight loss, and findings related to the primary site. Spine involvement is frequently heralded by pathologic fracture, after which a lytic lesion is usually easily identified on standard radiographs. Blastic lesions less likely to produce fracture are noted only incidentally in routine films, leading to a work-up discovering both the primary and metastatic sites (typically prostatic metastases).

Infectious Disorders

Osteomyelitis of the vertebral column or discitis (often postoperative) are relatively infrequent events. In severe cases, particularly in debilitated individuals, bacterial or tuberculous infections may result in large, purulent paravertebral collections which may require drainage. Patients may have an unrelenting pain, relatively unaffected by activity or recumbency, but increased at night and sometimes accompanied by either low or spiking fevers (suggesting abscess). X rays or tomograms may be helpful in identifying bone lesions or paravertebral collections, but the sedimentation rate is probably the most sensitive test. Bone scanning or biopsy may also be helpful. Appropriate antibiotics are usually sufficient treatment, but surgical drainage may prove necessary.

Spondyloarthropathy

Ankylosing spondylitis is felt to be an autoimmune disorder occurring primarily in a male population in the 3rd to 5th decades. It involves a clinical syndrome of back pain and stiffness with typical examination findings of restricted spine mobility and chest expansion (less than 2.5 cm). Laboratory workup usually reveals an elevated sedimentation rate, and the HLA-B27 antigen test may be positive. X rays may initially demonstrate erosive changes and sclerosis in the sacroiliac joints, followed by peripheral disc space calcification and leading ultimately to a "bamboo spine" in more severe chronic

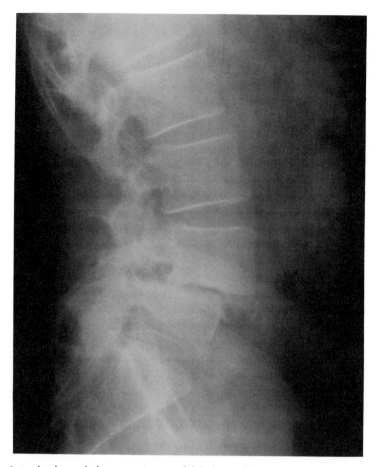

Fig. 3–8.   Lateral radiograph demonstrating spondylolisthesis of L4 on L5.

cases. The process is usually self-limiting, but in severe cases the spine may progress to complete immobility. This is often associated with extreme cervicothoracic kyphosis which may prevent the patient from seeing the horizon, and may also involve other large para-axial joints such as hips and shoulders. However, in end-stages, pain usually disappears. Treatment generally involves use of nonsteroidal anti-inflammatory medications and physical therapy to maintain spine mobility and an erect posture. Other related systemic processes, such as ulcerative colitis, Reiter's syndrome and psoriasis, may have a similar presentation.

Metabolic Disorders

Osteoporosis is the most important of the myriad metabolic disorders which affect the spine. It is particularly prevalent in the postmenopausal female, especially when exacerbated by disuse or use of immunosuppressive drugs. While radiographs can identify loss of bone mineral and coarsening of trabeculae (signaling loss of collagenous substrate) in more than half of the female population over age 50, disturbing symptoms usually occur only when compression fracture develops spontaneously or with minimal trauma. Multiple fractures in the 6th to 9th decades may lead to substantial loss of height, spinal deformity, and immobility. Estrogen replacement may be helpful for the first 15 years following the menopause, but considerable controversy exists over use of calcium, vitamin D compounds, or fluoride, though some evidence suggests sufficient usefulness to warrant their use under medical supervision and repeated scanning under certain circumstances.

Congenital Disorders

Symmetric congenital disorders of the lumbar spine are almost never associated with symptoms, but are of note only because they are accessible to radiographic visualization and are thus frequently noted on routine x rays. Segmentation disorders such as lumbarization of the first sacral segment, "extra" lumbar vertebrae, or sacralization of the last lumbar vertebra are of no clinical significance. Similarly, *spina bifida occulta* involves a break in the bony arch over the spinal canal which is generally stable and is also of no clinical significance. The relatively uncommon neurologic sequelae of a complete neural tube defect (meningomyelocele) are usually apparent and produce extremity, bowel/bladder, motor and sensory deficits rather than a low back pain syndrome. Spinal deformities, both paralytic and nonparalytic, may result. Common spina bifida occulta may have an incidence as high as 15 to 30% of the general population.

The only congenital disorders worthy of consideration of *possible significance* as sources of pain and dysfunction are those which are asymmetrical. A lumbar vertebra that is unilaterally sacralized may produce a pseudoarthrosis between the L5 transverse process and sacral ala on the contralateral side leading to symptoms, possibly necessitating surgical intervention. Hemihypertrophy of a lumbar facet joint may produce asymmetric loading, leading, in time, to degenerative disease. However, in spite of these potential biomechanical disorders, it is important to keep in mind that, historically, there has been a great deal of harm done by the overuse of radiographs to exclude perfectly capable workers from jobs on pre-employment examinations in a misguided attempt to avoid back injury. No study has demonstrated that these common radiographic entities have any predictive value for identifying individuals at risk of low back injury, and the use of x rays for this purpose is falling into well-deserved disrepute.

SUMMARY OF STRUCTURAL SOURCES OF LOW BACK PAIN

We have surveyed the many *potential* sources of pain in the back. The most common sources of acute low back pain are unvisualizable and, therefore, unverifiable as an etiology by any known technique. Conversely, the structural derangements whose presence can be verified by diagnostic testing and correlated with clinical symptoms probably occur in less than 10% of the cases. Thus, they may have only a minor impact on our understanding of the entire problem. While we may speculate on what the future may bring, at present in the vast majority of patients complaining of low back pain, we are merely guessing when we make a structural diagnosis, and we are unlikely to be able to improve our acumen regardless of the intensity of our efforts. Even more disturbing, despite the wide prevalence of popular misconception, is that what we see on a wide variety of structural tests may be totally irrelevant to the source of pain. While this may seem to be a bleak conclusion, it is certainly better to be aware of our ignorance and accept it, rather than deluding ourselves into making decisions based on greater wisdom than we possess. In the next chapter, we shall see how a variety of psychologic factors can directly impact on the pain perception process, quite independent of any precisely diagnosed structural underpinning.

CHAPTER REFERENCES

Allen M, Lindm M: Significant roentgen findings in routine pre-employment examination of the lumbosacral spine: a preliminary report. Am J Surg *80*:762–766, 1950.

Bergquist-Ullman M, Larsson U: Acute low back pain in industry, Acta Orthop Scand (Suppl.) *170*:1–117, 1977.

Bigos S, Spengler D, Martin N, Zeh J, Fisher L, Nachemson A, Wang M: Back injuries in industry: a retrospective study II. Injury factors. Spine *11*:246–251, 1986.

Bigos S, Spengler D, Martin N, Zeh J, Fisher L, Nachemson A, Wang M: Back injuries in industry: a retrospective study III. Employee-related factors. Spine *11*:252–256, 1986.

Crock H: A re-appraisal of intervertebral disk lesions. Med J Aust *1*:983–989, 1970.

Dzioba R, Doxey N: A prospective investigation into the orthopeadic and psychologic predictors of outcome of first lumbar surgery following industrial injury. Spine *9*:614–623, 1984.

Hakelius A, Hindmarsh J: The significance of neurological signs and myelographic findings in the diagnosis of lumbar root compression. Acta Orthop Scand *44*:239–246, 1974.

Jackson R, Montesano P, Jacobs R: Facet joint injections in mechanical low back pain patients: a prospective statistical study. Proceedings of Int'l Soc for the Study of the Lumbar Spine. Orthop Trans *10*:509, 1986.

Kellgren J, Lawrence J: Osteoarthrosis and disc degeneration in an urban population. Ann Rheum Dis *17*:388–397, 1958.

Kettelkamp D, Wright D: Spondylolysis in the Alaskan Eskimo, J Bone Joint Surg *53*A:563–568, 1971.

LaRocca, H. (Ed.) *Finnenson's Low Back Pain*, 3rd ed. Philadelphia, J.B. Lippincott Co. (In press).

Mayer T, Gatchel R, Kishino N, Keeley J, Capra P, Mayer H, Barnett J, Mooney V: Objective assessment of spine function following industrial injury: a prospective study with comparison group and one-year follow-up; Volvo Award In Clinical Sciences, 1985. Spine *10*:482–493, 1985.

Mayer T, Kishino N, Keeley J, Mayer S, Mooney V: Using physical measurements to assess low back pain. J Musc Med *2*:44–59, 1985.

Mixter W, Barr J: Rupture of the intervertebral disc with involvement of the spinal canal, N Engl J Med *211*:210–215, 1934.

Mooney V, Robertson J: The facet syndrome. Clin Orthop *115*:149–156, 1976.

Pope M, Frymoyer J, Andersson G (eds.): Occupational Low Back Pain. New York, Praeger Publishers, 1984.

Rockey P, Fantel J, Omenn G: Discriminatory aspects of pre-employment screening: low back x-ray examinations in the railroad industry. Amer J Law and Med *5*:197–214, 1979.

Splithoff C: Lumbosacral Junction: Roentgenographic comparison of patients with and without backaches. JAMA *152*:1610–1613, 1953.

Troup J: Driver's back pain and its prevention: a review of the postural, vibratory and muscular factors, together with the problem of transmitted road-shock. Appl Ergonom *9*:207–214, 1978.

Verbiest H: A radicular syndrome from developmental narrowing of the lumbar vertebral canal. J Bone Joint Surg *36*B:230–237, 1954.

Waddell G, Kummel E, Lotto W, Graham J, Hall H, McCulloch J: Failed lumbar disc surgery and repeat surgery following industrial injuries. J Bone Joint Surg *61*A:201–207, 1979.

Weber H: Lumbar disc herniation: a controlled prospective with 10 years of observation. Spine *8*:131–140, 1983.

Wiltse L, Newman P, MacNab I: Classification of spondylolysis and spondylolisthesis. Clin Orthop *117*:23–29, 1976.

Wiltse L, Widell E, Jackson D: Fatigue fracture: the basic lesion in isthmic spondylolisthesis. J Bone Joint Surg *57*A:17–22, 1979.

Wiltse L: Chemonucleolysis in the treatment of lumbar disc disease. Orthop Clin N Amer *14*:605–622, 1983.

ADDITIONAL REFERENCES

Beals R: Compensation and recovery from injury. West J Med *140*:233–237, 1984.

Bistrom O: Need degenerative changes in the spinal column entail back pain. Ann Chir Gynecol Fenn *43*:29–44, 1954.

Cady L, Bischoff D, et al.: Strength and fitness and subsequent back injuries in firefighters. J Occup Med *21*:269–272, 1979.

Chrisman O, Mittnacht A, Snook G: A study of the results following rotatory manipulation in the lumbar intervertebral-disc syndrome. J Bone Joint Surg *46*-A:517–524, 1964.

Clinical Biomechanics of the Spine. White A, Panjabi M (eds.), Philadelphia, J.B. Lippincott Co., 1978.

Frymoyer J, Donaghy R: The ruptured interverteral disc: Follow-up report on the first case 50 years after recognition of the syndrome and its surgical significance. J Bone Joint Surg *67*-A:1113–1116, 1985.

Hussar A, Guller E: Correlation of pain and the roentgenographic findings of spondylosis of the cervical and lumbar spine. Am J Med Sci *232*:518–527, 1956.

Lawrence J: Disc degeneration. Its frequency and relationship to symptoms. Ann Rheum Dis *28*:121–137, 1969.

Magora A, Schwartz A: Relation between the low back pain syndrome and x-ray findings. 1. Degenerative osteoarthritis. Scand J Rehabil Med *8*:115–125, 1976.

Mayer T, Smith S, Keeley J, Mooney V: Quantification of lumbar function Part 2: Sagittal plane trunk strength in chronic low back pain patients. Spine *10*:765–772, 1985.

Mayer T, Smith S, Kondraske G, Gatchel R, Carmichael T, Mooney V: Quantification of lumbar function Part 3: Preliminary data on isokinetic torso rotation testing with myoelectric spectral analysis in normal and low back pain subjects. Spine *10*:912–920, 1985.

McKenzie R: Lumbar Spine Mechanical Diagnosis and Therapy. Waikanae, New Zealand, Spinal Publications, Ltd., 1981.

Morris J: Low back bracing. Clin Orthop *102*:126–132, 1974.

Nachemson A: Lumbar spine instability: a critical update and symposium summary. Spine *10*:290–219, 1985.

Nachemson A, Andersson G: Classification of low back pain. Scand J Work Environ Health *8*:134–136, 1982.

Nordby E: Epidemiology and diagnosis in low back injury. Occup health safety *50*:38–24, 1981.

North P, Brown T: The immobilizing efficiency of back braces: their effect on the posture and motion of the lumbosacral spine. J Bone Joint Surg *39*-A:111–139, 1957.

Peck D, Nichols P, Beard C, Allen J: Are there compartment syndromes in some patients with idiopathic back pain? Spine *11:*468–475, 1986.

Ransford A, Cairns D, Mooney V: The pain drawing as an aid to the psychologic evaluation of patients with low back pain. Spine *1*:127–134, 1976.

Rothman R: Patterns in lumbar disc degeneration. Clin Orthop *99*:18–29, 1974.

Sander R, Meyers J: The relationship of disability to compensation status in railroad workers. Spine *11*:141–143, 1986.

Spengler D, Bigos S, Martin M, Zeh J, Fisher L, Nachemson A: Back injuries in industry: a retrospective study I. Overview and cost analysis. Spine *11*:241–245, 1986.

Spinal Disorders: Diagnosis and Treatment. Ruge D, Wiltse L (eds.), Philadelphia, Lea & Febiger, 1977.

Weber H: Lumbar disc herniation: a prospective study of prognostic factors including a controlled trial. Part I. J Oslo City Hosp *28*:33–64, 1978.

Weber H: Lumbar disc herniation: a prospective study of prognostic factors including a controlled trial, Part II. J Oslo City Hosp *28*:33–64, 1978.

Wiesel S, Cuckler J, DeLuca F, Jones F, Zeide M, Rothman R: Acute Low-Back Pain: An objective analysis of conservation therapy. Spine *5*:324–330, 1980.

Chapter 4

The Process of Pain Perception

As we reviewed in the previous chapter, there has been great difficulty isolating specific structural entities that cause low back pain. Traditionally, however, one of the contributing factors to the poor success rate of many medical approaches to pain has been the way medicine has tried to dichotomize pain complaints as either "organic" or "psychogenic" in nature. This overly simplistic and naive conceptualization seriously interfered with the physician's ability to fully understand the patient and his or her pain. Indeed, a recent report by the National Institutes of Health calls for a major effort to upgrade pain education programs in medical and nursing schools. This report raises concerns that the education and training of many health care professionals do not place enough emphasis on contemporary methods of pain assessment and management. Communication among physicians, nurses, other health-care professionals and patients regarding pain is still less than adequate. As will be discussed in this chapter, pain is a complex phenomenon which involves not only physiologic sensations and mechanisms, but also significant behaviorial/psychologic components as well. An orientation or model of chronic pain that integrates both the physiologic and psychologic components has the best chance of allowing a comprehensive understanding of the pain process. It also has important implications and clinical applications for the assessment and treatment of patients with chronic low back pain.

EARLY PHYSIOLOGIC MODELS OF PAIN

The earliest model of pain conceptualized it as some specific type of activity in the sensory nervous system. As Melzack (1973) has noted, "The best classical description of the theory was provided by Descartes in 1644, who conceived of the pain system as a straight-through channel from the skin to the brain. He suggested that the system is like the bell-ringing mechanism in a church: a man pulls the rope at the bottom of the tower, and the bell rings in the belfry. So too, he proposed, a flame sets particles in the foot into activity and the motion is transmitted up the leg and back into the head where, presumably, something like an alarm system is set off. The person feels pain and responds to it."

Two centuries later, in 1894, a more formal model of pain was proposed by Von Frey (Melzack, Wall, 1965). It was referred to as the *specificity theory of pain.* Its basic assumption was that there are specific sensory receptors which are responsible for the transmission of sensations such as touch, warmth, pain, etc. These sensory receptors differ in their structure with the differences rendering them sensitive to specific kinds of stimulation. The nociceptors believed to be associated with the sensation of pain were assumed to be free nerve endings. Pain, therefore, was viewed to have *specific* central and peripheral mechanisms similar to those of other bodily senses. Pain was viewed as a simple neurophysiologic event in which nociception is transmitted along nerve pathways through a specific afferent system to a "pain center" in the brain.

At about this same point in time that Von Frey was proposing his specificity theory of pain, Goldschneider presented an alternative conceptualization which he labeled the *pattern theory of pain* (Melzack, Wall, 1965). This model attempted to account for some of the more complex phenomena such as differences in the quality and quantity of pain. Goldschneider suggested that pain sensations were the result of the transmission of nerve impulse *patterns* originating from, and coded at, the peripheral stimulation site. Differences in the patterning and quantity of peripheral nerve fiber discharge were viewed as producing differences in the quality of sensation. Thus, a minimal tactile stimulus to an area may cause a feeling of touch, whereas stronger tactile stimuli cause pain. If the same nerve fibers are being stimulated and discharged, then the difference in sensation was viewed as due to an increased discharge and spatial summation. It was assumed that this pattern of stimulation produced by a specific stimulus had to be coded by the central nervous system. Therefore, the experience of pain was the result of central nervous system coding of nerve impulse patterns, and was not simply due to a specific and direct connection between pain receptors and pain sites.

Over the years, there has been partial support for portions of both of these above two early simplistic models of pain. In support of the specificity theory, for example, Bonica (1953) reported that there is a unique, specific, and immediate experience of pain originating in the skin when appropriate stimulation is administered. Moreover, he also identified two sets of sensory fibers, which have stimulus-specific conducting properties, that were clearly involved in the transmission of pain. Likewise, in partial support of the pattern theory, it has been demonstrated by Melzack and Wall (1982) that skin receptors have some specialized properties by which they can transmit specific types and ranges of stimulation in the form of *patterns* of impulses.

In spite of such partial support for these two models, there have been a number of reported findings which cannot be adequately accounted for by them. For example, as will be discussed in a later section of this chapter, research has demonstrated that psychologic factors, such as the anxiety level of an individual, can significantly affect and modify the pain experienced from the same noxious stimulus. This intervening psychologic mechanism was not taken into account by the specificity theory which proposed a specific and direct stimulus-response pathway or chain. Another inadequacy of this specificity theory becomes obvious when one realizes that surgical intervention techniques directed at breaking the specific connection between the peripheral body damage site producing the noxious stimulation and the assumed central pain mechanism (e.g., through neural rhizotomy) have not produced widespread therapeutic effects in alleviating chronic pain.

There are similar inadequacies when considering the pattern theory of pain. For example, it does not account for the physiologic evidence of nerve fiber specialization which Bonica (1953) originally reported. Thus, although both the specificity and pattern theories do account for certain physiologic mechanisms of pain perception, neither of them can *comprehensively* deal with the complex mechanism of pain perception. Moreover, the ever-evolving field of neurotransmitter mechanisms and the enkephalin compounds have introduced additional complexities that these models cannot effectively incorporate. Pain is no longer viewed as the result of a straight-through transmission of impulse from the skin to the brain.

NOCICEPTION

Recent physiologic research has demonstrated a number of structures within the nervous system that contribute to pain. The term *nociceptor* has replaced the older term *pain receptor* in order to highlight the fact that these sensory units contribute to the pain experience rather than creating it. Peripheral nociceptors are specialized transducer-like units and bare nerve endings that have terminations in the skin, deep somatic tissues, and the viscera. There are two major groups of these peripheral nerve fibers that are involved in nociception: (1) *A-delta* fibers, which are small myelinated fibers that appear to mediate immediate or sharp pain. It is estimated that nearly 25% of these fibers are nociceptors. (2) *C fibers,* which are even smaller fibers that are unmyelinated. These appear to mediate diffuse and dull or aching pain. It is estimated that approximately 50% of C fibers are nociceptors. There are also other fibers (*A-alpha-beta* fibers) that transmit other sensory modalities of a more innocuous nature.

There are two basic classes of these *A-delta* and *C* fibers. One class of these fibers is called *mechanical nociceptors* because they respond maximally to intense mechanical stimulation. Another class of fibers is called *polymodal nociceptors* because they respond maximally to mechanical and temperature stimulation. They may also be activiated in tissue damage by various endogenous biochemicals such as serotonin, histamine, and prostaglandins.

These peripheral nerve fibers enter the spinal cord through the dorsal horn, where they undergo considerable modulation from within the dorsal horn as well as descending impulses from higher brain centers (this modulation is quite complex and its scientific understanding is continually undergoing elucidation) (Fig. 4–1). The afferent pathway from the dorsal horn crosses to the opposite anterolateral segment of the spinal cord and then ascends in the spinothalamic tract. It ascends to the sensory cortex via the thalamus, and also by alternative pathways to the reticular activating system with widespread subsequent radiation to lower and higher brain centers (the role of many higher centers and their interaction with the lower brain-stem system is still quite poorly understood). Moreover, the spinothalamic tract communicates with other levels in the spinal cord.

Thus, nociceptive stimuli travel from the periphery to the cerebral cortex via specific afferent pathways to specific brain sites. However, these pathways are subject to modulation at various sites in the dorsal horn, the spinothalamic tract, and lower and higher brain centers. This helps to explain why an incoming peripheral pain signal can be modulated by downward afferent processes. As we shall see next, the role of such higher central modulation effects has been taken into account by recent conceptualizations of pain.

THE GATE CONTROL THEORY OF PAIN

In 1965, Melzack and Wall introduced the *gate control theory of pain* in an attempt to more adequately take into account many of the diverse psycho-

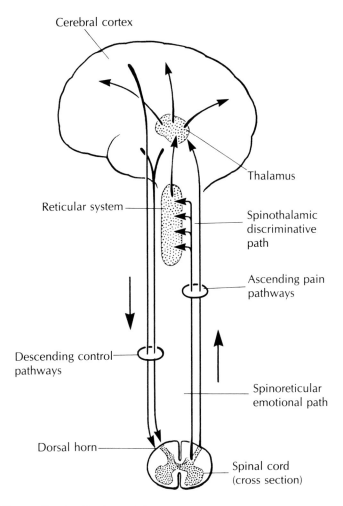

Fig. 4–1. Pathways of nociceptive transmission.

physiologic mechanisms that appear to be involved in the pain perception process. Although there are limitations of this theory, it did for the first time introduce to the scientific community the importance of central, psychologic factors in the pain perception process. It gave credence to the potentially significant role that such psychologic factors play.

This theory assumes that there are a number of structures within the central nervous system that contribute to pain. It is the interplay between these structures that is critical in determining if, and to what extent, a specific stimulus leads to pain. Thus, pain is not viewed as the result of "straight-through" transmission of impulses from the skin to the brain. Rather, the pathway is far more complex, involving considerable opportunities for modulating the incoming pain signal by other afferent sensations and even by descending inhibiting impulses from higher centers.

In basic terms, this gate-control theory proposes the presence of a neurophysiologic mechanism in the dorsal horn of the spinal cord which serves as a *gate* that can increase or decrease the flow and transmission of nerve impulses from peripheral fibers to the central nervous system. Thus, sensory input is subjected to the possible modulating influence of the gate before it evokes any pain perception. It is further proposed that the degree to which this gate increases or decreases sensory transmission is determined by the relative activity in large-diameter fibers (*A-beta* fibers) and the small-diameter *A-delta* and *C* fibers, as well as by descending efferent influences from the brain. As we indicated earlier, the A-delta fibers tend to transmit the faster pain signals that help us localize the site of the pain, whereas the C fibers tend to be more active in the ongoing deep, and more diffuse, residual pain that remains after the initial injury. Figure 4–2 presents a schematic of this gate-control theory.

A summary of the more specific propositions of this theory has been presented by Gatchel and Baum (1983), and is as follows:

1. The substantia gelatinosa functions as a gate-control system which modulates the amount of input transmitted from the peripheral fibers to the dorsal horn transmission (T) cells.

2. The gate-control mechanism is influenced by the relative degree of activity in the large-diameter A-beta fibers and the small-diameter A-delta and C fibers. Activity in the large fibers closes the gate, tending to inhibit transmission; small-fiber activity opens the gate and tends to facilitate transmission.

3. This spinal-gating mechanism is influenced by efferent nerve impulses that descend from the brain. As a result, psychologic processes such as anxiety, depression, attention, and past experience can exert their influence directly on the pain perception process. Melzack and Wall refer to this as the *central control mechanism.* This mechanism is assumed to play a major role in identifying sensory impulses from the periphery, assessing these signals in terms of past experience, and ultimately modulating properties of the gate control system.

4. When the output of the spinal cord T cells, determined by the interaction of the spinal-gating mechanism and the central control mechanism, exceeds a critical threshold level, it activates neuromechanisms that con-

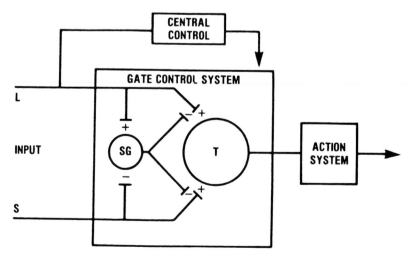

Fig. 4–2. The Melzack and Wall theory of pain. (From Melzack, R., Wall, PD: Pain mechanisms: A new theory. Science, *150*:971–979, November 19, 1965. Copyright 1965 by the AAAS.)

stitute the action system responsible for both pain perception and behavior.

This particular theory represented a significant advance in our conceptualization of pain. It is comprehensive enough to account for the evidence suggesting specific types of pain receptors, as well as allowing for the possibility that pain stimulation and transmission may occur in patterns of sensations. In addition, it allows for the significant role that downward central nervous system mediation can play in pain perception. It also can partially account for different types of pain as well as the differential effects of time variables upon the pain process (Fordyce, Steger, 1979). Finally, it views pain as a complex set of phenomena rather than a simple specific or discrete entity. Of course, as new understanding of pain neurophysiology, neurotransmission, and endogenous opiate-like enkephalin substances develops, a more refined model will evolve.

It should also be noted that this theory has led to the development of a procedure for artifically stimulating the nervous system in order to relieve pain. Electrical stimulators have been developed which can be used on or beneath the surface of the skin, or implanted near the spinal cord. Electrical pulses can then be administered in the vicinity of areas where pain is reported or in the region of the major nerves serving these areas. This method is based on the assumption that electrical stimulation activates the large-diameter fibers and thereby "close the gate." Stimulation of activity in these large fibers is believed to activate cells of the substantia gelatinosa and thus inhibit the activity of T cells, which affect the action system responsible for pain response and perception. This electrical stimulation procedure often produces relief from pain during the stimulation as well as time durations that outlast the period of stimulation. It should be noted that not all individuals benefit from this type of treatment; moreover, when effective, the relief from pain is usually only temporary (Long, 1976; Melzack, 1975).

NEUROCHEMICAL BASES OF PAIN

There has been an increasing amount of interest in recent years in endogenous opiate-like substances that constitute a neurochemically-based internal pain-regulation system. These *opioids* are produced in many parts of the brain and glands of the body, and have been presumed to play a significant role in pain reduction. The first major endogenous opioid to be clearly isolated was *enkephalin.* Since then, numerous similar substances have been identified. Three basic families of these opioids are now usually considered (Akil, Watson, Young, Lewis, Khachaturian, Walker, 1984): *beta-endorphin,* which produces peptides that appear to project primarily to the limbic system and brain stem; *proenkephalin,* which produces peptides that are widely distributed to the neuronal, endocrine, and central nervous systems; and *prodynorphin,* which is distributed to the brain, gut, and pituitary. This overall system of opioids is highly complex, with each family having a variety of forms, different potencies, and different active receptor sites.

Investigators still do not know all of the functions of the endogenous opioids and what factors are important in triggering their arousal. One particularly interesting mechanism is beta-endorphin mediation of the *placebo effect* involved in the reduction of pain. In a number of painful conditions, it is commonly found that one-third of the patients experience significant relief from pain following the administration of a placebo (Beecher, 1956). The exact mechanism involved in this placebo analgesia effect is presently not entirely understood. However, the analgesic placebo effect and the analgesia produced by active narcotics appear to have similar effects. For example, with repeated use over a long period of time, placebo analgesia becomes less effective (i.e., tolerance develops), there is an urge to continue taking the placebo with a tendency to increase the "dosage" over time, and an abstinence-withdrawal syndrome appears when use is suddenly discontinued. Also, a placebo may partially decrease or reverse withdrawal symptoms in narcotic addicts, and individuals who react to placebos experienced significantly greater relief from postoperative pain after receiving narcotic analgesias (cf. Levine, Gordon, Fields, 1978). Thus, placebos appear to have a significant effect on reducing pain.

A study by Levine, Gordon, and Fields (1978) has demonstrated how beta-endorphins may be involved in this phenomenon. In this study, which was a double-blind investigation, the effects of placebo medication and a drug called *naloxone* on postoperative dental pain (produced by a major tooth extraction) were evaluated. Naloxone is a pure opiate antagonist. It was assumed that if placebo-induced analgesia is mediated by the endogenous beta-endorphins, then naloxone, the opiate antagonist, would possibly block their effects. Three hours after the surgical procedure, half of the patients received the placebo medication; the other half of the patients received naloxone. Four hours after the surgical procedure, patients received the other medication. Patients were requested to report their degree of pain on two pain-rating scales after receiving their medications.

Results of this study indicated the following: (1) Patients given naloxone experienced, as expected, significantly greater pain than when the placebo was administered. Since naloxone is an opiate antagonist, it would not be expected to reduce pain. (2) Patients given the placebo were found to be either placebo responders whose pain was reduced or unchanged (39% of the patients were found to be placebo responders), or placebo nonresponders whose pain increased (61% of the patients were found to be placebo nonresponders). It should be noted that this percentage of responders to nonresponders is similar to the one-third/two-thirds placebo responder-nonresponder percentage normally found in the research literature. (3) When naloxone was given as the second drug, it produced no additional increase in pain level in the nonresponders, but it did increase the pain levels of the placebo responders. Naloxone therefore appeared to block the beta-endorphins that were producing the pain reduction in the placebo responders. Thus, the enhancement of reported pain produced by naloxone could be entirely accounted for by its effects on placebo responders. The results from this study by Levine and colleagues demonstrate that beta-endorphin release mediates placebo analgesia for dental postoperative pain. When beta-endorphins are blocked by naloxone, pain reduction no longer occurs.

Future research will hopefully more clearly delineate the variables actually involved in affecting beta-endorphin activity. Such research on these opioid substances also suggests additional mechanisms for the downward efferent pain-inhibiting mechanisms which are currently not adequately accounted for by the gate-control theory (Snyder, 1977). It also again indicates the importance of psychologic processes in the pain perception process. In the next section, we will discuss, at greater length, the influence of psychologic processes on pain perception.

PSYCHOLOGIC INFLUENCES ON PAIN PERCEPTION

The gate-control theory of Melzack and Wall allowed for the significant role that downward central nervous system mediation could play in the pain perception process. Indeed, over the years, there were a number of studies that highlighted the important impact that psychologic factors can exert on pain perception. For example, Beecher (1956) was the first influential writer to emphasize the importance of the psychologic status of an individual in determining his or her response to pain. Beecher's belief initially stemmed from his observation of wounded soldiers returning from battle during World War II. In his classic investigation, Beecher (1956) compared the requests for pain-killing medication made by soldiers taken to combat hospitals following wounds received in combat at Anzio, Italy to those requests made by civilians with comparable *surgical* wounds. It was found that only 25% of the combat-wounded soldiers requested medication. Most of the soldiers either denied having pain from their extensive wounds or had so little that they did not think medication was necessary. In marked contrast, the civilians with similar wounds obtained during surgery experienced much more pain, with greater than 80% of these patients requesting pain medication. Beecher interpreted these results as suggesting that psychologic factors such as an individual's emotional state and secondary gain/relief (most likely experienced by soldiers who were allowed to leave the aversive life-threatening combat zone due to their wounds, and probably would eventually be sent home) can significantly affect the experience of pain. Such factors would not be expected to be operating with a civilian population.

There have been other studies demonstrating the importance of the psychologic state of an individual on pain perception. For example, Sternbach (1974) has reported that pain tends to increase as the anxiety level of the individual increases. In an earlier study, Hill, Kornetsky, Flanguy, and Wilder (1952) demonstrated that induced-anxiety conditions were associated with higher intensities of self-reported pain relative to no anxiety conditions. Another interesting finding of this study was that morphine was much more effective in decreasing pain when the patient's anxiety level was high, and had little or no effect if that individual's anxiety level was low. Thus, the emotional state of the individual can play an important role in the pain perception process. Indeed, as will be discussed later in Chapter 12, there is a strong association between pain and depression.

Cultural and social factors have also been shown to greatly influence the perception of pain (cf. Weisenberg, 1977a, b). For example, Zborowski (1952) noted that members of some cultures report pain sooner and react to it more intensely than members of other cultures. Italian patients were more likely to respond to pain or discomfort they were experiencing, and to be comforted by anything that might make the pain go away. In contrast, Jewish patients reacted to the potential medical significance of the pain, and were comforted when they received an appropriate explanation for the pain.

In related laboratory-conducted studies, Tursky and Sternbach (1967) and

Sternbach and Tursky (1965) have demonstrated significant differences in re-actions to pain (in this case to electric shock) among ethnic groups: "Yankees" (protestants of British descent) had a "matter of fact" orientation toward pain and assumed it was a common experience; Irish subjects tended to inhibit their pain expressions and suffering; Italians demonstrated an immediacy of pain experience, and emotionally exaggerated their pain, demanding fast relief; Jews also emotionally exaggerated their pain, and had great concerns about the meaning and any future implications of the pain. Christopherson (1966) has also demonstrated that there are significant differences in the magnitude of pain responding to identical pain stimulation as a function of the cultural background of an individual. Thus, social-cultural factors can play a significant role on how pain is perceived and expressed.

LEARNING INFLUENCES ON PAIN PERCEPTION

These social-cultural differences in attitudes and responses to pain appear to be learned. There are three basic types of learning—observational learning, classical conditioning, and operant conditioning. We will review these three types and discuss how they relate to pain. In so doing, it will be important to keep in mind that they can occur separately, or in various combinations, in helping to produce and/or maintain chronic pain behavior.

Observational Learning

Observational learning is defined simply as that learning which occurs with-out any apparent direct reinforcement (Bandura, 1969). Many behaviors can be acquired if an individual merely sees the particular behavior displayed or modeled by another person. Examples of behaviors acquired by observational learning abound. For example, investigations of dental fears in children have revealed that the attitudes and feelings of a child's family toward dental treat-ment are important in determining that child's own anxiety toward dental treatment. In one such study, it was found that children with anxious mothers showed significantly more emotionally negative behavior during a tooth ex-traction than did children of mothers with low anxiety (Weisenberg, 1977b).

Classical Conditioning

A second major type of learning is *classical conditioning.* In a rather dramatic demonstration of how pain perception and response can be modified through learning, Pavlov (1927) used a classical conditioning procedure. Classical con-ditioning is one of the most basic forms of learning in which a learned asso-ciation or connection develops between two stimuli. In a series of well-known studies, Pavlov demonstrated that if a neutral stimulus or event such as a bell was presented to a dog just prior to the presentation of food (an *unconditioned* stimulus which normally elicits an automatic unconditioned reflex of saliva-tion), after a number of such presentations, the bell would elicit a conditioned or learned salivation response when presented by itself in the absence of food.

Pavlov subsequently observed what would happen if a slight change was made in this classical conditioning procedure. Instead of preceding food with the sound of the bell, it was preceded by aversive stimuli such as electric shock or a skin prick. Normally, such stimuli presented alone will produce a variety of negative emotional responses. What Pavlov found was that after this conditioning, the dogs subsequently failed to demonstrate any emotional responses to the aversive stimuli. Instead, these dogs began perceiving these painful stimuli as signals that food was on the way. The electric shock now actually elicited salivation and approach behaviors!

Operant Conditioning

Finally, the third major type of learning is called *operant conditioning.* Table 4–1 presents differences between classical and operant conditioning. Operant conditioning refers to the strengthening of a response and behavior through reward or "reinforcement." That is to say, the probability that a behavior will be performed again is increased if it is followed by some form of reinforcement. Behavior is controlled by its consequences. If a behavior is followed by a reward, it has a high probability of recurring; if it is ignored or punished, it has a low probability of recurring. Obviously, a great deal of our everyday behavior is learned and maintained through operant conditioning. For example, most of us work because of the rewards (both tangible, such as money, and intangible, such as a pleasant work environment) that it produces.

In terms of pain, many times a person in pain will elicit a great deal of sympathy and attention (both of which are rewarding). In addition, suggestions are usually made by others to rest and stay inactive; "pain-relieving" medications are usually administered; and often financial compensation is provided. The longer these reinforcing consequences continue, the longer the patient is likely to display the maladaptive pain behaviors such as inactivity and avoidance of work. Thus, this type of learning or conditioning can significantly contribute to the maintenance of pain behavior.

This operant conditioning conceptualization of pain was systematically employed in the operant pain treatment program originally developed at the University of Washington's Department of Rehabilitation Medicine by Fordyce and colleagues (Fordyce, Fowler, Lehmann, DeLateur, 1968). This program involved a 4- to 8-week inpatient period designed to gradually increase the general activity level of the patient, and to decrease medication usage. The program is based on the assumption that, although pain may initially result from some underlying organic pathologic condition, environmental reinforcement con-

Table 4–1.   Differences Between Classical and Operant Conditioning

	Classical Conditioning	Operating Conditioning
Type of response	Involuntary, related to biological survival; produces change in organism; elicited by a stimulus	Voluntary; operates on the environment; elicited by the organism
Temporal relation of response to reinforcer during acquisition	Response follows	Response precedes
Functional relation of response to reinforcer	Presence of reinforcer independent of response	Presence of reinforcer contingent on response and changes probability of response

sequences (such as attention of the patient's family and the rehabilitation staff) can modify and further maintain various aspects of "pain behavior," such as complaining, grimacing, slow and cautious body movements, requesting pain medication, and so on. Viewing pain as an operantly conditioned behavior, Fordyce assumes that the potentially reinforcing consequences such as the concern and attention from others, rest, medication, avoiding unpleasant responsibilities and duties, as well as other events, frequently follow and reinforce the maladaptive pain behavior and, as a consequence, hinder the patient's progress in treatment.

In their treatment program, Fordyce and colleagues systematically controlled environmental events (e.g., attention, rest, medication) and made them occur contingent on adaptive behaviors. A major goal of the program is to increase behaviors such as participation in therapy and activity level while simultaneously decreasing or eliminiating pain behaviors. It should also be noted that members of the patient's family are actively involved in the treatment program and work closely with the rehabilitation staff. They are taught how to react to the patient's behavior in a manner that will reduce pain, and to maximize the patient's compliance with, and performance in, the rehabilitation program. Using this operant approach, the patient is basically taught to reinterpret the sensation of pain and tolerate it, while performing more adaptive behaviors that will gain the attention and approval of others. Such a program is initially conducted in the hospital, and can later be continued on an outpatient basis.

Of course, such examples do not imply that all pain is learned. The point being made is that our pain perceptions and responses often have a significant psychologic learning component that directly and significantly contributes to these experiences of pain. Thus, psychologic variables play a direct role in the pain experience. How one reacts to pain sensations is as important an issue as the specific physiologic mechanisms involved in transmitting and generating pain experiences. Pain is a complex *behavior* and not simply a sensory effect.

PAIN BEHAVIOR

With the above view in mind, it is clear that one must conceptualize pain like any other form of complex behavior, consisting of multiple behavioral components. As Fordyce and Steger (1979) have indicated, in order to describe pain:

" . . . there must be some form of pain behavior by which diagnostic inferences and treatment judgments can be made. A patient will signal the type of pain he or she is experiencing by describing the intensity, frequency, location, and type of pain experienced. In addition to these verbal cues available to the patient's environment as an indication of his or her pain, there is a myriad of nonverbal signs used to communicate pain experiences. These include grimaces, sighs, moans, limps, awkward or strained body positions, the use of a cane or crutch, and many other symbols associated in our society with discomfort or physical problems."

Traditionally, in attempts to describe pain, the focus was only on the physiologic or structural mechanisms underlying the report of pain, and not on other components such as behavioral indices and self-report. The reliance on strictly one component, such as structural measures, does not yield a valid or precise measure of an individual's pain. Again, pain is a complex behavior and not purely a sensory event. One needs to consider multiple behavioral components in the assessment and treatment of this behavior.

ORGANIC VERSUS PSYCHOGENIC PAIN

Together with the traditional attempt to describe pain in terms of the physiologic or structural mechanisms underlying the report of pain, there was a tendency to view *organic pain* as one type of pain and *psychogenic pain* as another kind of pain. The term *psychogenic* or *psychosomatic* was used to imply that the pain was due to purely psychologic causes, or that it was all "in the patient's mind," or that it was not "real" pain because an organic basis for it could not be found. This is an unfortunate myth. "Psychogenic" pain is not experienced any differently from that pain arising form some clearly delineated injury or physical disease. Moreover, the diagnosis of organically caused pain does not rule out the important role that psychologic variables play for any particular patient. Indeed, in our earlier discussion of the gate-control theory of pain, we saw how the experience of pain may be produced by psychologic factors through the hypothesized central-control trigger mechanism.

ACUTE VERSUS CHRONIC PAIN

It is also important to discriminate among three major categories of pain: acute pain, chronic malignant pain, and chronic benign pain. Chronic malignant pain is experienced by cancer patients and those with other progressive disorders. Acute pain is often the result of some specific and readily identifiable tissue damage (e.g., a broken leg, surgical lesion, etc.). With this type of pain, a physician usually prescribes a specific treatment which helps relieve the pain and results in its not persisting beyond the expected period of recovery. In contrast, while chronic benign pain, such as chronic back pain, usually begins with some specific acute episode, prescribed treatments have not resulted in any significant reduction of the pain. Traditional medical treatment has failed to solve the patient's problem, and as a result chronicity begins to set in.

Fordyce and Steger (1979) have also noted that besides the time duration factor, an additional variable which differentiates acute from chronic benign pain concerns the type of anxiety experienced by the patient. In acute pain experiences, there is usually an increase in anxiety as pain intensity increases, which is then followed by a reduction in this anxiety once treatment begins. As we discussed earlier, a reduction in anxiety generally results in a decrease in pain sensation. Thus, there is a cycle of pain reduction, followed by anxiety reduction, resulting is still more pain reduction, etc. This cycle, however, is quite different for chronic pain patients. For these patients, the initial anxiety associated with the pain persists and may eventually result in the development of feelings of greater anxiety, despair, and helplessness because of the failure of the health system's attempts to alleviate it.

There is evidence to suggest that chronic-pain patients develop specific psychologic problems, because of the failure of attempts to alleviate their pain, that distinguish them from acute-pain patients. For example, Sternach, Wolf, Murphy, and Akeson (1973) compared the MMPI profiles of a group of acute low back pain patients (pain present for less than 6 months) to those of a group of chronic low back pain patients (more than 6 months). Results indicated significant differences between the two groups on the first three clinical scales (*Hypochrondriasis, Depression, and Hysteria*). A sample MMPI profile will be presented in Chapter 12. The combined elevation of these three scales is often referred to as the *neurotic triad*, since it is commonly found in neurotic individuals who are experiencing a great deal of anxiety. These results indicate that during the early acute stages of pain, there are no major psychologic problems produced by it. However, as the pain becomes chronic in nature, psychologic changes begin to occur. These changes are most likely due to the constant discomfort, despair, and preoccupation with the pain which comes to dominate the lives of these patients. As Sternbach (1974) has noted in his description of chronic-pain sufferers:

"Pain patients frequently say that they could stand their pain much better if they could only get a good night's sleep. They feel as though their resistance is weakened by their lack of sleep. They never feel rested. They feel worn down, worn out, exhausted. They find themselves getting more and more irritable with their families, they have fewer and fewer friends, and fewer and fewer interests. Gradually as time goes on, the boundaries of their world seem to shrink. They become more and more preoccupied with the pain, less and less interested in the world around them. Their world begins to center around home, doctor's office, and pharmacy." (p. 7)

We have also found similar results from research conducted with patients participating in the PRIDE program. Barnett (1986) found significant elevations on a variety of MMPI scales before the start of the treatment program in the chronic low back pain patients. The interesting additional finding was that at a 6-month follow-up period after successfully completing this treatment program, there was a significant *decrease* in these scales to normal levels. Thus, these results suggest that the elevations of scores on psychologic tests such as the MMPI seen in chronic low-back pain patients are most likely due to the trauma and stress associated with the chronic condition and not due to some stable psychologic traits. When successfully treated, these elevations disappear.

The importance of the different consequences of acute versus chronic pain is further illustrated in a study by Shealy and Maurer (1974). These investigators evaluated the relative effectiveness of transcutaneous nerve stimulation as a treatment method for acute and chronic pain. It was found that this particular treatment was 80% effective for alleviating pain in the acute patients, but only 25% effective for the chronic patients. Thus, response to treatment is a factor which is significantly affected by this acute-chronic pain dimension.

It is therefore obvious that the treatment of the chronic back pain sufferer will often have to deal not only with the pain experience, but also with the psychologic consequences such as anxiety and dysphoria produced by the long-term "wearing down" effects which may produce a "layer" of behavioral-psychologic problems over the original pain experience itself. Chronic low back pain is a complex behavior which is not due merely to some specific structural cause! As will be discussed when reviewing the functional restoration treatment approach, a number of cognitive-behavioral techniques are employed to deal with such problems as part of a comprehensive treatment program.

CHAPTER REFERENCES

Akil H, Watson SJ, Young E, Lewis ME, Khachaturian H, Walker JM: Endogenous opioids: Biology and function. Annual Review of Neuroscience, *7*:223–255, 1984.
Bandura A: Principles of Behavior Modification. New York, Holt, Rinehart & Winston, 1969.

Barnett J: The Millon Behavioral Health Inventory and the Minnesota Multiphasic Personality Inventory Compared as Predictors of Treatment Outcome in a Rehabilitation Program for Chronic Low Back Pain. Unpublished dissertation. University of Texas Health Science Center, 1986.

Beecher HK: Relationship of significance of wound to the pain experienced JAMA, *161*:1609–1613, 1956.

Bonica JJ: The Management of Pain. Philadelphia, Lea & Febiger, 1953.

Christopherson V: Socio-cultural correlates of pain response. Final report of Project #1390, Vocational Rehabilitation Administration, Washington, D.C.: United States Department of Health, Education, and Welfare, 1966.

Fordyce WE, Steger JC: Chronic pain. In OF Pomerlau and JP Brady (Eds.), Behavioral Medicine: Theory and Practice. Baltimore, Williams & Wilkins, 1979.

Fordyce WE, Fowler RS, Lehmann JF, DeLateur BJ: Some implications of learning in problems of chronic pain. J Chronic Dis, *21*:179–190, 1968.

Gatchel RJ, Baum A: Introduction to Health Psychology. New York, Random House, 1983.

Hill HE, Kornetsky CG, Flanguy HG, Wilder A: Effects of anxiety and morphine on the discrimination of intensities of pain. Clin Invest, *31*:473–480, 1952.

Levine JD, Gordon NC, Fields HL: The mechanism of placebo analgesia. Lancet, *2*:654–657, 1978.

Long DM: Use of peripheral and spinal cord stimulation in the relief of chronic pain. In JJ Bonica and D Albe-Fessard (Eds.), Advances in Pain Research Therapy (Vol. 1). New York, Raven, 1976.

Melzack R: The Puzzle of Pain. Harmondsworth, Penguin, 1973.

Melzack R: Prolonged relief of pain by brief, intense, transcutaneous somatic stimulation. Pain, *1*:357–373, 1975.

Melzack R, Wall PD: Pain mechanisms: A new theory. Science, *150*:971–979, 1965.

Malzack R, Wall PD: The Challenge of Pain. New York; Basic Books, 1982.

Pavlov IP: Conditioned Reflexes. New York, Dover Publications, 1927.

Sheahy C, Maurer D: Transcutaneous nerve stimulation for control of pain. Surg Neurosurg, *2*:45–47, 1974.

Snyder S: Opiate receptors and internal opiates. Scient Amer, *236*:44–56, 1977.

Sternbach RA: Pain Patients: Traits and Treatment. New York, Academic Press, 1974.

Sternbach RA, Tursky B: Ethnic differences among housewives in psychophysical and skin potential responses to electric shock. Psychophysiol, *1*:241–246, 1965.

Sternbach RA, Wolf SR, Murphy RW, Akeson WH: Traits of pain patients: The low-back "loser." Psychosomatics, *14*:226–229, 1973.

Tursky B, Sternbach RA: Further physiological correlates of ethnic differences in responses to shock. Psychopysiol, *4*:67–74, 1967.

Weisenberg M: Cultural and racial reactions to pain. In M. Weisenberg (Ed.), The Control of Pain. New York, Psychological Dimensions, 1977, (a).

Weisenberg M: Pain and pain control. Psychol Bull, *84*:1004–1008, 1977, (b).

Zborowski M: Cultural components in responses to pain. J Social Issues, *8*:16–30, 1952.

Chapter 5

Pain Versus Function

As was highlighted in the last chapter, chronic pain is a complex phenomenon which involves behavioral-psychologic factors in addition to physical ones. This complexity can obviously create an assessment nightmare. Moreover, because of neurophysiologic aspects of individual pain perception, it is often not therapeutically productive to rely solely on self-reported pain as a means of determining degree of severity of the problem or to gauge treatment progress. Unfortunately, in past pain clinic approaches, there was often an excessive dependence on such self-report data.

An alternative to reliance solely on self-report data is the use of actual behavioral-physical *function* as a means of gauging severity and monitoring treatment progress. Such function, as we shall discuss later in this book, can be objectively and reliably measured. This objective, quantified assessment of function serves as the backbone of the functional restoration approach.

By no means, though, does one ignore self-reported pain. Rather, such self-report data are interpreted only in the context of *overall* functioning. Adaptive, positive functioning is sometimes initially associated with an increase in pain complaints. Indeed, the phrase "No pain, no gain" is appropriately stressed to patients undergoing functional restoration. Rather than terminating and delaying further physical training because of these pain complaints, the patient may have to learn to "work through" the pain. Such issues will be discussed further when reviewing details of the actual functional restoration treatment approach.

This orientation emphasizing *function* is not a totally radical or new one. Fordyce, Roberts and Sternbach (1985), who have been leading investigators in the field involving the behavioral assessment and treatment of chronic pain, have cogently noted that it is not enough to simply evaluate and attempt to modify an individual's subjective experience of pain. One must comprehensively evaluate *pain behavior* (a concept discussed in the last chapter) which involves not only what the patient is verbalizing, but also his or her actual functioning. As they emphasize:

" . . . behavioral methods for treating pain problems (chronic pain behaviors) are not intended to "treat pain" in the traditional sense in which this implies directing attention to sources and mechanisms of noxious stimuli generating injury signals which lead to "pain." Behavioral pain methods do *not* have as their principal objective the modification of nociception, nor the direct modification of the experience of pain, although it very frequently happens that both are influenced by these methods. Rather, *behavioral methods* in pain treatment programs *are intended to treat excess disability and expressions of suffering* . . . The goal is to render chronic pain patients functional again and as normal in behavior as possible." (p. 115).

Indeed, these investigators note that one of the major problems with past treatment and theoretical approaches to chronic pain, including some alleged behavioral ones, was focusing too greatly on merely the subjective experience of pain. A distinction needs to be made between "pain" (the subjective experience) and *pain behavior* or behavioral functioning. This is an extremely important point: we believe, and the scientific literature tends to support the fact, that the most appropriate goal is to modify excessive disability by focusing on *function.* The subjective component of pain (however it is assessed) also is often concurrently changed when functioning is changed. However, we have found that there usually will be no major change in the subjective expression of "pain" without an improvement in functional activity and disability. This is the hallmark of the functional restoration approach. *One must focus on observable and objectively evaluated functioning along with self-report in order to comprehensively assess chronic pain behavior.*

In this chapter, we will discuss the general concept of function. It will become more apparent how this concept is a vital component of the sports medicine orientation involved in functional restoration.

FUNCTION: AN OVERVIEW

Function refers to the organism's ability to perform tasks involving homeostasis or manipulation of the environment. In terms of regulating its internal environment, the organism, no matter how simple or complex, must regulate its internal temperature, provide nutrition to cells, eliminate waste, maintain surface defenses and sensory organ information transmission, and replace dying cells. From the point of view of external tasks, the organism manipulates its environment for a multitude of purposes, such as acquiring nutrition, defending itself, protecting itself from harsh environments, and reproducing itself. In order to achieve these survival goals, certain specific bodily functions, oriented externally, are available to the human: ambulation, manual manipulation, sexual encounter, feeding, eliminating waste, breathing, and the variety of cognitive/sensory/communicative skills.

By far, the largest system in humans, in terms of body mass, is the musculoskeletal system. While it has important homeostatic mechanisms related to it, such as calcium storage in bone and shivering as a muscular mechanism for temperature regulation, the evolution of the human musculoskeletal system is most related to interaction with the external environment. The most critical aspect of this external manipulation is, of course, the cognitive and instinctual skills developed through evolution, which is neatly catalogued by the progression of brain elements from brainstem to neocortex. In order to accomplish its planned actions, the brain must have a musculoskeletal system at its disposal. The most important feature of this system characterizing human performance is the ability for manual manipulation or handling (these two words being redundant, originating from *manus,* the Latin root for hand). A variety of other bodily tasks are utilized to increase the effectiveness of manual tasks, many of which involve the lumbar spine. There are a number of important functional principles associated with the performance of such tasks.

Function and Performance

Comprehensive terminology has been proposed by Kondraske (Kondraske, 1986; Kondraske, in press) for describing these function-performance relationships. This author views the human as a defined architectural structure composed of a finite set of inter-connected functional units which possess the capacity to operate along specific dimensions of performance (strength, range of motion, speed, etc.). Considering all functional units collectively results in the realization of a *finite set* of distinct *basic elements of performance* (BEP). Human functional units are either a single or collective set of anatomic structures which work together (function) to realize the respective dimensions of performance. Each functional unit maps into its own performance space, and is responsible for contributing a fraction to the totality of human BEPs. Thus, in order to specify a BEP, one must delineate both the functional unit and dimensions of performance. BEPs are viewed operationally in a steady-state sense and as being independent. At their present state of conceptualization, human BEPs are organized into three primary domains: (1) central processing, (2) physical environmental interface, and (3) physical, life-sustaining.

In the *central processing* domain, BEPs are mediated by neuroanatomic functional units (information processors and associated communication network structures). This functional unit subset does not interface with the environment directly. However, units often operate on the basis of input from, or exercise control over, units in the other two domains. Thus, processors associated with sensory and motor, as well as life-sustaining functional units, are included. Attention and multiple memory resources represent several of the more obvious BEP candidates in this category.

Life-sustaining BEPs are those, as the name implies, which pertain to functions essential to the support of life. The most noticeable components, because of their potential for more immediate impact on observable performance, are mediated primarily by cardiovascular and respiratory anatomic systems with associated peripheral neuroanatomy. Cardiac stroke volume, heart rate, and respiratory rate are potential BEPs in this domain. Renal, digestive and endocrine subdivisions are also included, although they are difficult to measure with many functions not directly perceived and customarily considered non-limiting in activities of daily living.

Physical environmental interface BEPs are those pertaining to the capacity to directly affect or monitor the external environment. These sensory and motor elements are generally mediated by neuromusculoskeletal functional units. Neurologic connections are essential for understanding the dimensions of the musculoskeletal domain, and include sensors with support structures and afferent communication pads, and efferent communication pads associated with musculoskeletal structures. Bilaterality forces consideration of left and right body components as separate resources which contribute to the BEP pool.

The human draws upon these BEP resources in differing amounts to accomplish virtually an *infinite* number and variety of tasks where the amount of performance resource required from each linked functional unit, dimension, and domain is determined by the task. The multi-dimensionality of high level tasks precludes a valid single measurement of performance. A *set* of measurements, representing the multiple dimensions of the task, must be used as a basis for assessment. Functional capacity assessment requires the ability to evaluate these multiple dimensions.

IMPORTANT FUNCTIONAL PRINCIPLES

Conservation of Energy

With the human in a stationary position, the hands are initially limited by reach and the mobility characteristics of the upper extremities that place the hand in a variety of positions. In most postures, however, the lumbar spine is necessary to support the loads manipulated by the hands and transmit them to ground contact. Certain tasks are beyond normal reach and require a decision on the part of the subject as to how best to bring manipulative skills to bear. This is usually done on the basis of the most efficient task performance; that is, the technique that best *conserves energy*. This principle of limiting energy expenditures is a critical factor in this decision. Thus, if the object to be manipulated is directly behind one, the efficient choice would usually be to shift the direction of one's feet and turn the entire body around to face the object. On the other hand, if the task is to move an object from directly in front of a subject through a 180-degree arc, then there are alternate methods requiring a cognitive selection. The individual may decide to turn the entire body by constantly changing foot/floor contact and rotating the feet, or he or she may choose to maintain a steady foot/floor contact approximately midway (90 degree arc) between the two points in question, and twist the trunk in both directions. If additional reach is required, the individual may bend the trunk, or use some combination of twisting, stepping, reaching and bending. However, in any type of repetitive tasks, involving selection among options, conservation of energy is a critical principle (Fig. 5–1).

Safety

Another important functional principle is that a safe method be chosen. There are a variety of feedback mechanisms and reflexes inherent in every complex organism, specifically designed to prevent overload. The overload may be presented in terms of forces, torque, or accelerations. An individual will modify his or her mechanism of performing a task in the presence of perceived overload strictly on the basis of conservation of energy. Thus, a small individual, presented with the task of moving a large number of 50-pound sacks, may move them one sack at a time. By contrast, a larger and more muscular individual may choose to move sacks two or three at a time (Fig. 5–2). If the smaller individual wishes to attempt to perform the task using techniques similar to those of the larger man, he must either: (*a*) override his safety mechanisms; (*b*) have lost his acuity of feedback through a blunting of neuromuscular or cognitive function, failing to perceive risk of injury; or (*c*) train himself to achieve supernormal strength and agility in order to increase the "safety threshold" by improving physical capacity. Conversely, the larger man, if forced by regulations to lift only one sack at a time, may become impatient because he is being forced to use more energy. By using only limited strength, he may become "detuned," actually losing some degree of physical capacity. The interaction of energy and safety principles is dynamic and multivariate. Individual variation may be great, making formulation of regulations extremely difficult.

Modifiers of Performance

Substitution Among Functional Units

The first modifier of functional activity is the process of *substitution*. There may be more than one way of performing similar tasks, and the two cardinal principles of energy conservation and safety will generally dictate which method is chosen. As we discussed before, the size and muscle bulk of the individual may be a critical factor in this choice. Other major factors may be anthropomorphometry and injury status. Thus, in a task involving moving objects from floor to a low shelf, in which bending may be the most efficient

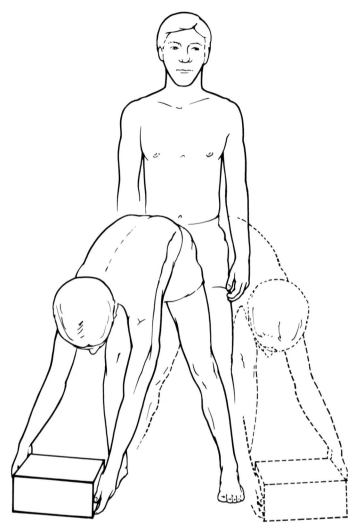

Fig. 5–1. The principle of "conservation of energy." The subject maintains a stable foot/ground contact and "hangs on his ligaments" in maneuvering light to medium loads in an arc.

technique, a smaller individual may be able to perform a task in this way while a taller one may be forced to squat because of the dimensions of the work area. Injury status, particularly insofar as it affects physical capacity, may also be a critical feature. In the same sample, loss of trunk mobility or strength may similarly force the individual to perform the task in a less efficient squatting position. This concept of substitution will be discussed more completely in other parts of this book.

Substitution Within a Functional Unit

In addition to *substitution of tasks,* there may also be *substitution of mesothelial elements,* specifically alternating active muscular and passive ligamentous loading. As we discussed in Chapter 2, the position of the spine may be critical in terms of its mechanism for resisting bending moments. When the

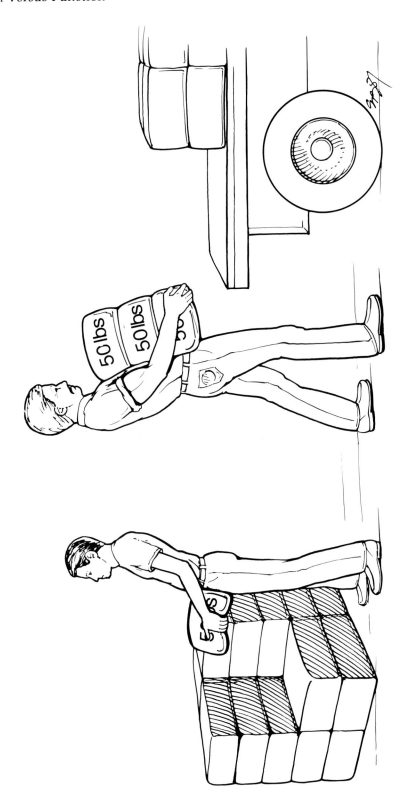

Fig. 5-2. Safety principle of "prevention of overload." Each individual self-selects a "safe limit" based on feedback of physical capacity. The "safe limit" may be considerably greater for one individual than for another. In this example, both individuals utilize their own perception of overload to modify the energy conservation principle.

spine is fully flexed, EMGs show a "silent period" for muscular activity because the spine is literally "hanging on its ligaments" (Basmajian, 1978). While this is an efficient position, the ligaments are subject to "creep" or progressive elastic elongation, and ultimate plastic deformation. Homeostatic feedback mechanisms can sense these changes and alter the posture before overload stresses are applied. In addition, large bending movements applied purely to the ligamentous system may threaten total disruption, causing the person to simply drop the weight or assume a different posture under those circumstances. This may help to explain the reason why weight lifters generally prefer to manipulate extremely heavy loads in postures other than full flexion.

By contrast, the neutral posture probably represents the peak of the length/tension curve for the spinal extensor muscle mass. Contraction of the spinal musculature is less efficient, but provides greater safety from overload. Use of the spine extended posture does not necessarily limit bending, as a good deal of forward bending can occur exclusively from the hips, with muscular support coming primarily from the gluteals, and secondarily from hamstrings stabilizing the pelvis. To get the feel of these two mechanisms of spinal support, try this simple experiment. To "hang from your ligaments," let your spine curve into a fully flexed position, doubling over from the waist, before beginning to bend from the hips. Alternately lock your spine in extension by tightening your back muscles and then allow yourself to flex forward from the hips without bending the spine. In most cases, the first method will feel most comfortable and natural. However, for performing the same actions while lowering an extremely heavy load, or doing repetitive heavy lifting, the second method may prove necessary on occasion.

Resistance

A third mechanism of support is resistance, essentially implying an antagonist effect produced by antagonist muscles. This involves utilizing the abdominal oblique and transverse musculature acting through the lumbodorsal fascia which provide extension through resistance of spine flexion. In any bending situation, the three basic biomechanical principles may be used independently or in combination to provide the most efficient and safe manual handling techniques. Pressuring the abdomen to "float" the upper torso does not appear to be a viable mechanism (Bogduk, Macintosh, 1984; Nachemson, 1985; Gracovetsky, Farfan, Helleur, 1985; Bartelink, 1985). However, it may be possible that greater efficiency imparted to the abdominal musculature and lumbodorsal fascia may improve spine stablization. This encapsulation can be provided either internally or externally; i.e., by a Valsalva maneuver or use of a compressing "weight-lifter's belt."

IMPORTANT FUNCTIONAL MECHANISMS

Ambulation

Ambulation is a critical factor in assisting the individual in manipulating the environment. Walking, running, carrying, and climbing up or down enable the individual to extend his manual influence over ever-wider territory. However, there is a significant cost in energy consumption since ambulation produces considerable caloric expenditure in addition to whatever work is being performed by the upper extremities. The concept of the "spinal engine" demonstrates the importance of lateral bend in the lumbar spine, and counterrotation of the shoulders in propelling the hips forward alternately for locomotion.

Gracovetsky and Farfan (1986) have suggested in a controversial new theory that lumbar lordosis is most important biomechanically for its coupling effect of the spinal articulations on transmitting axial torques from the trunk to the pelvis. They liken the lordotic lumbar spine to a flexible curved rod in which force generated in one plane at one end of the rod may be converted into forces generated in a second plane at the other end. In the case of the spine, lateral bend (coronal plane) through the lumbar spine may be transformed through articular coupled motion to produce axial torques transmitted to the pelvis, propelling the hips forward (Figure 5–3). According to the theory, it is the complex interaction of spinal joints, muscles, and supporting ligaments that provides power to produce locomotion to the bipedal human. However, lest we become too enamored of a seemingly logical theory, we must note that Stokes and his colleagues (1987) have challenged many of its basic tenets. It is unfortunate that both theoretical and experimental underpinnings of spine biomechanics remain controversial and often inconsistently correlated with clinical observations.

A corollary proposes a safety mechanism to prevent spinal overload for ambulation. For simplicity, we may call this the "Chinese coolie posture," in which the pelvis is tucked forward, the knees are bent slightly, and the gait becomes a shuffling, total body rotation without shoulder counterrotation. In fact, this method of ambulation is similar to that utilized by other primates (who lack a lumbar lordosis), and appears to be contingent on the fact that the lordosis is eliminated by this technique. In straightening the spine, coupled lateral bend and rotation, which might produce injury in discs or facet joints, is eliminated in favor of converting the spine temporarily to a relatively rigid rod. The safety thus provided for carrying extremely heavy loads exacts a price in terms of the awkward, rambling gait necessitated by the loss of power of the "spinal engine."

Obviously, the conservation of energy principle would dictate that if a task can be performed *without* ambulation, this method will generally be selected. Not only is there efficiency built into avoiding moving the lower extremities, but a stable foot/floor contact permits other muscular and ligamentous groups to "set themselves" in a more stable way, providing additional energy savings. In this way, the various postural mechanisms, including bending, sitting, squatting, kneeling and twisting, are utilized whenever they can be to avoid walking. Some of these tasks may have important implications for low back function.

Twisting

Twisting is another critical task involving spine biomechanics. It has been shown that the intervertebral disc is particularly sensitive to a combination of compressive and torsional loading (Gracovetsky, Farfan, 1986). The higher the compressive loads, the less the torsional stress resistance of the disc anulus. In fact, the heavier the lifted load, or the more bending that is required as part of the task, the less likely it is that pure trunk twisting will be used to move the load from side to side. Instead, the safety principle will dictate that the task be performed with more lower extremity rotation than trunk rotation as load increases. Finally, under extremely heavy loads, the pelvis will be tucked,

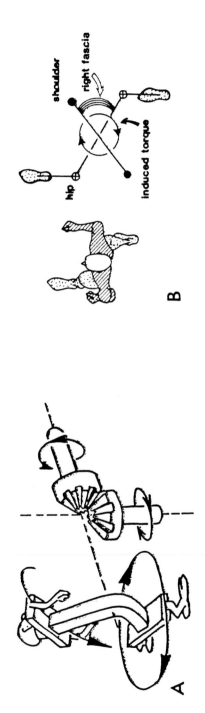

Fig. 5–3. A, B. A curved rod (simulating the lumbar lordosis) can translate forces from one plane to another. This may provide an explanation for the lumbar lateral bend that produces axial torsion at the hips to provide lower extremity propulsion. (From Gracovetsky, S., and Farfan, H.: The optimum spine. Spine, *11*(6):543, 1986.)

and movement of the feet to turn the whole body will be preferentially employed for safety in spite of high energy expenditures.

Kneeling

Kneeling is another static posture for performing manipulation at constant low elevations. In this instance, we may choose to sacrifice mobility in exchange for a stable floor contact which conserves energy and reduces fatigue. Generally, kneeling activities are those performed at or near ground level where the reach permits manipulation of relatively light objects. If frequent changes in elevation are required, the individual will generally choose a squatting rather than a kneeling position. This is also true if manipulation in a wide arc is required, since kneeling produces greater restriction of torsion. The universal use of kneeling for prayer or supplication attests to its being viewed as a stable, restful, and undefended posture. With leg motion impeded in every plane, trunk bending and torsion provide the only options for increasing reach.

"FUNCTIONAL UNITS" AND TASK PERFORMANCE

In analyzing postures, we are immediately confronted with the complexity of multiple segment-links in the body used to perform such tasks. A vast body of ergonomic knowledge has been developed, often using complex modeling systems relying on measurement of the physical properties of body segments. Empirical measures of physical dimensions lead to anthropometric data which ultimately can be utilized to predict physical demands of various tasks. These may include measures of the length, weight, volume, mass center, and moments of inertia of various body segments. For analysis and decision-making, complex systems must be broken down to simpler ones. The same is true for our analysis of function. However, rather than breaking our human system down into anatomic segment links such as hand, wrist, forearm, and upper arm, we will look at *functional units* that may overlap, but which provide a physiologic unit. Examples of human functional units are given in Table 5–1.

The division of the body into a series of functional units helps to focus our attention on elements of function which work together to provide specific capabilities, rather than on individual joints or muscles. The conundrum of whether to split and subdivide every anatomic unit for descriptive purposes, or to lump some together based on complementary actions, has divided anatomists for hundreds of years. It is therefore doubtful whether general agreement will be obtained on our choice of functional units in separating structure from function. What is clear, however, is that some simplification is required in order to provide meaningful analysis of system performance.

The anatomy and biomechanics of the lumbo-pelvic functional units have been described in Chapter 2. When studying an individual functional unit, we have the luxury of focusing on the specific subunits, including bones, joints, ligaments, muscles, and nerves. In so doing, we can describe some of the basic elements of performance which permit the functional unit to work as an integrated subsystem of the complete organism. In terms of how we view the lumbo-pelvic unit, certain observations should be borne in mind:

1. The lumbar spine portion of the units consists of a segmented rod with complex interconnections, and both an intrinsic and extrinsic set of muscles and ligaments providing three separate systems of support.

Table 5–1.   Human Functional Units of the Biomechanical Chain and Their Purposes

Name of Functional Unit	Anatomic Structures	Performance Characteristics of Functional Unit
1. Hand	Digits, metacarpals	Environmental manipulation: grasping, pinching, etc.
2. Upper extremity	Wrist, forearm, elbow, upper arm, shoulder	Reach: placing hand in favorable position.
3. Neck	Cervical vertebrae	Supporting and maneuvering head; cognitive/sensory controller for optimum performance.
4. Shoulder girdle/thoracic	Shoulder girdle, ribs, lower cervical and thoracic spine	Linking head and upper extremities to axial skeleton.
5. Lumbo-pelvic	Lumbar spine, sacrum, pelvis, hips	Transmission of loads, locomotion, bending.
6. Lower extremity	Hips, thighs, knees, lower leg, ankles, feet	Providing stable base for loading, changing elevation, locomotion.

2. Hips and spine move in tandem, particularly in forward flexion.
3. Gluteal muscles provide the "power pack" for forward bending, by lowering the torso through the hips as a segmented crane might be lowered at its base.
4. Hamstrings, by attaching on the ischium, provide a pelvic stabilizing and counterbalancing effect around the hip fulcrum, and thus are part of the lumbo-pelvic functional unit.
5. Visual feedback to the spinal portion of the unit is impeded by deep placement and inaccessibility of spinal structures, as well as multiple small, complex interconnections (18 joints from T12-S1).
6. Visual feedback is impaired in the spinal portion of the lumbo-pelvic unit by lack of recognizable bilaterality, thus eliminating visualization of a comparison side as is present in the extremities.

Loss of function implies loss of mobility and strength. The beneficial effects of motion on both joints and soft tissue have been well established (Akeson, Amiel, Abel, Garfin, Woo, 1987; Woo, Buckwalter, 1988). In addition, muscles respond well to exercise and degree of fitness in both normal processes and healing (Bortz, 1984; Radin, 1985; Woo, Buckwalter, 1988). Evidence also supports the positive effect of physical activity on connective tissue tensile strength and collagen maturation (Tipton, Vailas, Matthes, 1985; Videman, 1987), with healing expedited by early motion. In contrast, immobilization produces multiple detrimental effects on all soft tissues, including joints, tendons, muscles, ligaments, and discs (Booth, 1987; Bortz, 1984; Tipton, Vailas, Matthes, 1985; Woo, Buckwalter, 1988; Holm, Nachemson, 1982). Thus, there is abundant evidence that maintenance of function is a powerful homeostatic mechanism, with decrease in activity associated with adverse effects on all mesothelial tissues. Resumption of activity following injury maintains residual structure and promotes more rapid healing.

A sports medicine approach to overcoming physical capacity deficits in the lumbo-pelvic unit must, of necessity, treat the loss of function in *each* basic element of performance before overall improvement of the functional unit can be anticipated. This approach is greatly facilitated by the ability to measure performance in these elements. Indeed, the objective, quantified assessment of these elements serves a vital role in functional restoration. In Part II of this text, we will discuss techniques utilized for quantifying range of motion, strength, endurance, and the ability to perform a variety of specific tasks. Again, as noted earlier, assessment of such function is an important method of gauging severity and monitoring treatment progress. Self-reported pain is used only in the context of overall functioning.

CHAPTER REFERENCES

Akeson W, Amiel D, Abel M, Garfin S, Woo S: Effects of immobilization on joints. Clin Orthop *219*:28–57, 1987.

Bartelink D: The role of abdominal pressure in relieving the pressure on the lumbar intervertebral discs. J Bone Joint Surg *39*B:718–725, 1985.

Basmajian J: Muscles alive: Their Functions Revealed by Electromyography. 4th Ed. Baltimore, Williams & Wilkins, 1978.

Bogduk N, Macintosh J: The applied anatomy of the thoracolumbar fascia. Spine *9*:164–170, 1984.

Booth F: Physiologic and biochemical effects of immobilization on muscle. Clin Orthop *219*:15–20, 1987.

Bortz W: The disuse syndrome. West J Med *141*:691–694, 1984.

Fordyce W, Roberts A, Sternbach R: The behavioral management of chronic pain. A response to critics. Pain *22*:113–125, 1985.

Gracovetsky S, Farfan H: The optimum spine. Spine *11*:543–573, 1986.

Gracovetsky S, Farfan H, Helleur C: The abdominal mechanism. Spine *10*:317–324, 1985.

Holm F, Nachemson A: Nutritional changes in the canine intervertebral disc after spinal fusion. Clin Orthop *169*:234–258, 1982.

Kondraske G: Human performance: measurement, science, concepts and computerized methodology. Neurology (in press).

Kondraske G: Towards a standard clinical measure of postural stability. *In* Proceedings of the 8th Annual Conference of the IEEE Engineering in Medicine and Biology Society (Kondraske G, Robinson C, Eds.), *3*:1579–1582, 1986.

LeVeau B: Biomechanics of Human motion. 2nd Ed., Philadelphia, W.B. Saunders Co., 1977.

Macintosh J, Bogduk N, Gracovetsky S: The biomechanics of the thoracolumbar fascia. Clin Biomech *2*:78–83, 1987.

Nachemson A: Lumbar Spine Instability: A critical update and symposium summary. Spine *10*:290–291, 1985.

Radin E: Role of muscles in protecting athletes from injury. Acta Med Scand (Suppl) *711*:143–147, 1985.

Stokes I, Krag M, Wilder D: A critique of "the optimum spine." Spine *12*:511–512, 1987.

Tipton C, Vailas A, Matthes R: Experimental studies on the influences of physical activity on ligaments, tendons and joints: a brief review. Acta Med Scand (Suppl) *711*:157–168, 1985.

Videman T: Connective tissue and immobilization: key factors in musculoskeletal degeneration? Clin Orthop *221*:26–32, 1987.

Woo S, Buckwalter J: Injury and Repair of the Musculoskeletal Soft Tissue. Park Ridge, IL, AAOS Symposium, 1988.

ADDITIONAL REFERENCES

Cady L, Bischoff D, et al.: Strength and fitness and subsequent back injuries in firefighters. J Occup Med *21*:269–272, 1979.

Chaffin D, Andersson G: Occupational Biomechanics, New York, Wiley-Intersciences, 1984.

Frankel V, Nordin M: Basic biomechanics of the skeletal system. Philadelphia, Lea & Febiger, 1980.

Kondraske G: On human performance. IEEE Trans. Biomed Eng (In Press).

Nachemson A, Andersson G, Schultz A: Valsalva maneuver biomechanics. Effect on lumbar trunk loads of elevated intra-abdominal pressure. Spine *11*:476–479, 1986.

Roebuck J, Kroemer K, Thompson W: Engineering Anthropometry Methods. New York, Wiley-Intersciences, 1975.

Chapter 6

Current Common Evaluation and Treatment Methods for Lumbar Dysfunction

We have emphasized the importance of assessing and treating *function* when dealing with the complex phenomenon of chronic low back pain. Before proceeding to a thorough review of how the functional restoration approach achieves this, a brief overview of traditionally accepted patient management and evaluation techniques that have gained widespread clinical use will be provided in this chapter. Many of these techniques are part of functional restoration. Additional critical information on newly-developed methods utilized in functional restoration rehabilitation is covered in Part II.

PATIENT HISTORY

The patient history, though a subjective statement on the part of the patient of events leading up to the present disability, is still the basic ingredient for determination of initial medical management. This history focuses on a few critical elements:

a. The chief complaint
b. History of the current episode
c. Previous history of spine problems
d. Past medical history

As part of the history of a back problem, certain critical factors must be carefully evaluated. Since the question of injury may have significant medical and/or legal implications, the relationship of the pain to a "traumatic event" must be carefully assessed and documented. Suspicion of a substantial skeletal or visceral injury may predispose the evaluating physician to obtain certain diagnostic tests. On the other hand, a pattern of pain that is unrelenting, unresponsive to recumbency, is present primarily at night, or is related to other systemic manifestations (such as fever, weakness, weight loss, or lassitude) may alert the physician to back pain of neoplastic, metabolic, infectious, or inflammatory etiologies. Furthermore, it is important to evaluate for significant neurologic complaints affecting motor and sensory function in the lower extremities or bowel/bladder function, and any correlation of pain to posture. The history helps the physician make an initial determination of the back pain as possibly requiring invasive as opposed to conservative treatment.

It is also important to assess disability factors initially. Is this a passing, mild episode, or one that disables the patient severely from work and/or recreation?

The disabled individual naturally receives a higher priority for aggressive management than one with minimal loss of productivity. Is the disability related to a particularly heavy job demand or to poor physical fitness? What is the duration of the present episode and that of previous episodes? Has there been compensation or litigation involved in these incidents? This part of the initial assessment may be assisted by a variety of self-report measures that are potentially quantifiable, such as the Pain Drawing, Analogue Disability Questionnaire, and Depression Inventory (see Chapter 12). Is the patient currently taking medication, has he had prior spine surgery, injections or diagnostic tests, and what has been his response to previous treatment? Armed with this information, the physician may then proceed with the physical examination.

INITIAL PHYSICAL EXAMINATION

The initial physical examination is primarily focused on assessing a few critical parameters:
   a. Objective evidence corroborating pain complaints (spasm, deformity, immobility)
   b. Evidence confirming need for possible invasive treatment (neurologic deficits, facet signs)
   c. Evidence of systemic illness (local tenderness, general debility, fever, adenopathy, etc.)
   d. Evidence of symptom magnification (non-organic signs)

Each phase of the physical examination generally involves observation, palpation, and testing. It customarily proceeds from the standing to supine to sitting positions. In the standing position, one observes for posture, deformity (scoliosis, pelvic tilt, list), pelvic asymmetry or muscular asymmetry. Palpation may elicit specific localized tenderness near a single segment, or more often a generalized tenderness and irritability. Muscle spasm may be confirmed, and tenderness over the pelvic region, such as the sacroiliac joint, sciatic notch, greater trochanter, or fibro-fatty nodule may assist the examiner. Observing the pattern of the patient's gait, including toe and heel walking, may indicate a short leg, confirming sciatic involvement, or identify possible motor deficits (Fig. 6–1). A companion test involves performing a squat to assess quadriceps strength. The three tests of toe-heel, standing, and squatting are effective in providing initial suggestion that S1, L5 or L4 nerve roots, respectively, may be compressed on the involved side.

After observing and palpating the spine, the patient's range of motion is traditionally checked in sagittal, axial, and coronal planes. Only if truly asymmetric spine motion in axial and coronal planes is present can a definite mobility deficit be identified, since limitations of motion are generally due to patient pain perception. In a subsequent chapter (Chapter 9), we will discuss the separation of hip from true lumbar motion, and simple observations which can be made by the examiner in an office to detect spine/hip and hip/straight leg raise (SLR) ratio discrepancies, and which can help assess patient effort in performing these tests.

In the supine position, abnormalities of pulse, muscle, circumference, leg lengths, and other disorders of the extremities can be evaluated. Straight leg raising or bowstring tests are followed by a variety of provocative stretch tests

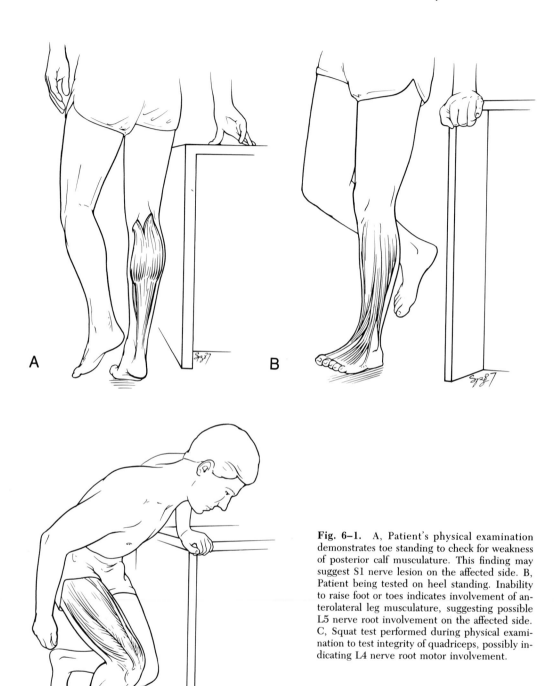

A

B

C

Fig. 6–1. A, Patient's physical examination demonstrates toe standing to check for weakness of posterior calf musculature. This finding may suggest S1 nerve lesion on the affected side. B, Patient being tested on heel standing. Inability to raise foot or toes indicates involvement of anterolateral leg musculature, suggesting possible L5 nerve root involvement on the affected side. C, Squat test performed during physical examination to test integrity of quadriceps, possibly indicating L4 nerve root motor involvement.

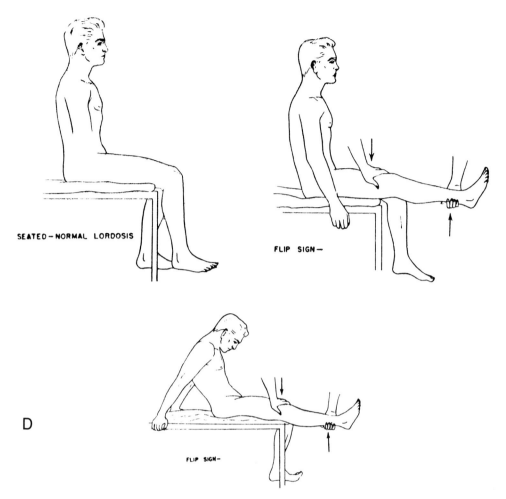

SEATED – NORMAL LORDOSIS

FLIP SIGN –

D

FLIP SIGN –

Fig. 6–1 (cont.). D, The flip test. (From Michele, A.A.: The flip sign in sciatic nerve tension. Surgery, *44*:940, 1958.)

to produce root tension signs that can be evaluated (Table 6–1). Manual resistance can be applied to key muscle groups to further assess motor deficit, particularly looking at toe and foot plantar- and dorsiflexors, hind foot in- and evertors, quadriceps, and hip extensors as the most commmonly involved muscle groups. A careful examination of skin dermatomes is then performed to identify sensory abnormalities in the most commonly involved nerve roots of surgical significance, L5, S1 and L4 (in that order) (Figs. 6–2, 6–3 and 6–4).

It is interesting to note that the sitting leg-raising test is *not* identical to the supine test, so no inferences can be drawn from the relative angles obtained in both positions of knee flexion. This is because, in the supine position, the pelvis is locked into extension by the extended contralateral hip. In the sitting position, the contralateral hip is flexed, allowing the spine to assume a flexed, rather than lordotic, position. Since the pelvic and spine posture is uncontrolled, further straightening of the affected limb may be possible before sciatic stretch occurs and the patient is forced to extend the spine and hips. Thus,

Table 6–1. The Most Important Provocative Root Tension Tests

Test	How to Perform	Patient Report If (+) Test
1. Lasegue's test	Perform classic straight leg raising tests or "bow-string test" initially flexing hip to 90 degrees, then extending lower leg. Pain increased by foot dorsiflexion	Pain radiating at least to calf, usually to foot
2. Sitting leg raising test ("flip test")	The patient sits at edge of table and examiner extends one lower leg at hip	Patient rapidly leans backward with pain to calf or foot: consistent with supine straight leg raising
3. Medial rotation test	Straight leg raising test is performed and further provocation obtained by internally rotating leg	Pain to calf or foot increased by internal rotation maneuver
4. Femoral stretch test	In prone position, buttocks are held down, hip is extended, and knee is flexed. Pelvic flexion must be avoided	Anterior thigh pain is produced in femoral nerve distribution

this is *not* a reliable confirmatory test for supine straight leg raising or "malingering."

In the prone position, the back, buttocks, and extremities can be examined in the unloaded position. Further evidence of local tenderness, discoloration, swelling, or redness may indicate fracture or infection and can lead to appropriate diagnostic testing. Atrophy of buttocks or paravertebral musculature may be most obvious in this position. Femoral stretch tests may be conveniently performed.

In the sitting position, the straight leg raising test noted above is generally performed while examining the patient's foot. This is also a convenient position for checking patellar and ankle reflexes. In equivocal cases, the ankle jerk can best be detected with the patient kneeling on the examination table while applying slight pressure against the examiner's thumb through the flexor hallucis tendons.

Non-organic signs are also particularly important to evaluate. Waddell, McColloch, Kummel and Venner (1979) have identified several of these tests, including head compression, superficial hypersensitivity, non-anatomic tenderness, simultaneous hip/shoulder rotation, distraction tests, over-reaction and non-physiologic responses to motor and sensory tests. When these tests are positive, the disorder is usually also accompanied by significant symptom magnification in a pain-prone individual, and concern about validity of structural tests and the appropriateness of the candidate for invasive treatment must be assessed. It should be stressed here that these tests do not mean that the

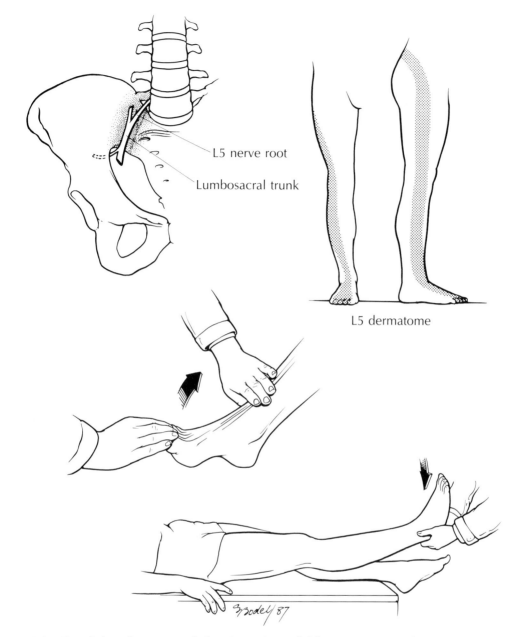

L5 nerve root

Lumbosacral trunk

L5 dermatome

Fig. 6–2.   Typical physical examination findings in a patient with L5 nerve root compression.

patient is "faking" or "malingering," but rather that a psychologic "overlay" may modify the response to pain and must be therefore carefully considered by the physician before entering into a treatment approach.

STRUCTURAL DIAGNOSTIC TESTS

At this point, the physician evaluator is ready for a preliminary diagnosis. As we noted in Chapter 3, the large majority of patients will, at this point, have a nonspecific diagnosis of "sprain," "strain," or "lumbar syndrome." These are

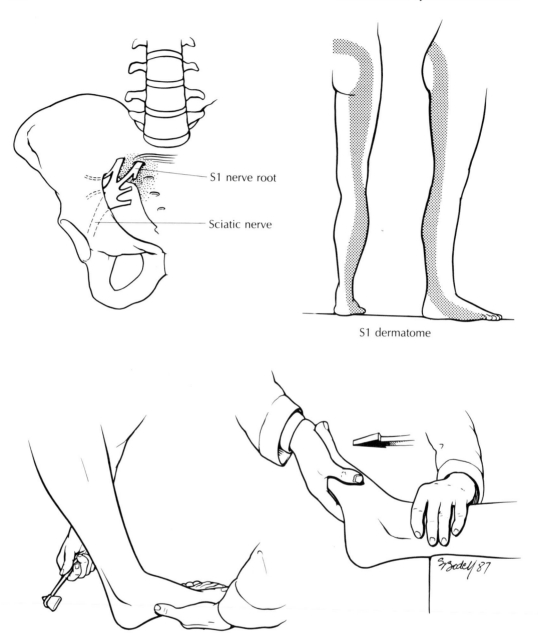

S1 nerve root

Sciatic nerve

S1 dermatome

Fig. 6–3. Typical physical examination findings in a patient with S1 nerve root compression.

the individuals who generally have back pain, with or without leg pain, lacking confirmatory physical findings of nerve root compression or signs of stenosis, tumor, or infection. Also, as previously indicated, soft tissue diagnoses are not subject to pathologic confirmation with any diagnostic study, and may be present with only minimal physical examination findings as a perfectly legitimate injury. In other words, there is no way, at the present time, to definitively "rule in or rule out" such an injury. This large group of individuals generally requires

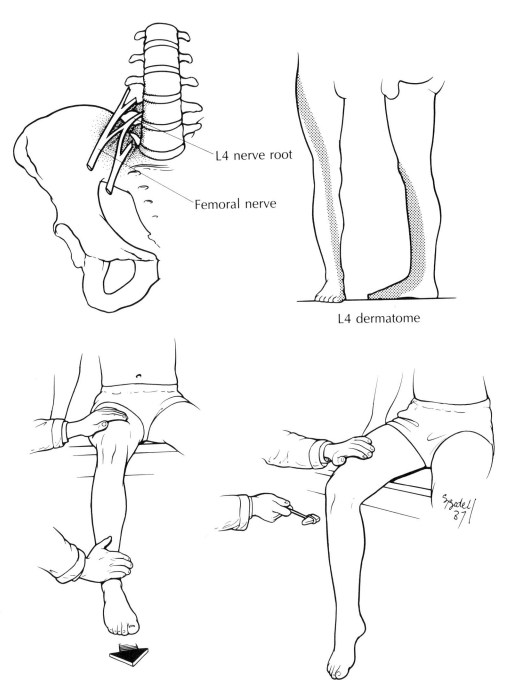

L4 nerve root

Femoral nerve

L4 dermatome

Fig. 6–4. Typical physical examination findings in a patient with L4 nerve root compression including affected dermatome.

very little in the way of diagnostic studies. The present medical/legal environment is frequently used to justify the taking of initial lumbar x rays. Such x rays may possibly include even oblique views to identify the pars interarticularis (with considerable increase in cost and radiation), although these films are rarely helpful. It has been estimated that only 1 in 1000 films taken for this group of patients identifies a pathologic condition that alters the course of medical treatment. On the other hand, the documentation of a degenerative pathologic condition including osteophytes, disc space narrowing, spondylolysis, spondylolisthesis, asymmetric sacralization, or facet hypertrophy, may not alter the treatment program but may merely have significance in "documenting the disorder" or "showing that there is something wrong," for legal purposes. While Chapter 3 would indicate that using x rays for this purpose is scientifically unsound, and also produces high cost and unnecessary radiation exposure, this belief is so firmly grounded in the general population that it is presently unshakable. Thus, diagnostic testing, including tests considerably more invasive than x rays, are, in practice, often performed for legal defensive, rather than purely medical, purposes.

In a minority of cases, more difficult decisions need to be made. First of all, has substantial trauma, with or without neurologic involvement, been sustained? In this case, care in moving the patient, appropriate x rays, and evaluation in a trauma center (for severe cases) may be indicated. Early decompression or stablization may ultimately prove necessary, though these cases will usually be flagged early by a history of high-energy impact and evidence of trauma to other body parts.

Back pain occurring with a questionable traumatic incident and associated with leg pain and neurologic involvement, particularly if accompanied by multi-nerve root signs and effects on bowel/bladder function, may also demand more attention. The rare, but potentially devastating, *cauda equina syndrome* demands immediate recognition, diagnostic testing, and surgical treatment if permanent sequelae are to be avoided. In more common cases of single nerve root compression, the initial level of neurologic dysfunction must be documented and carefully followed for progressive motor involvement. Signs of systemic disease also warrant more prompt attention, as many of these situations are potentially life-threatening, or present the opportunity for a clear-cut diagnosis after confirmatory studies.

The following is a review of the common diagnostic procedures.

Spinal Radiographs

X rays of the lumbar spine are generally indicated only in acute severe trauma, or if pain has failed to respond within several weeks of symptom onset. If films have been taken in the past 2 years, they rarely need to be repeated (Scavone, Latshaw, Rohrer, 1981). The typical spine series consists of standing AP and lateral films, with a spot lateral showing the lumbosacral junction including L4 and L5 discs. Oblique views may be taken to show spondylolysis (Fig. 6–5), and flexion/extension films may be used to demonstrate "segmental instability." Different frames for biplanar radiography have been proposed, but these continue in a research environment only at this time. In some cases, it may be necessary to visualize the sacrum, coccyx, and sacroiliac joints.

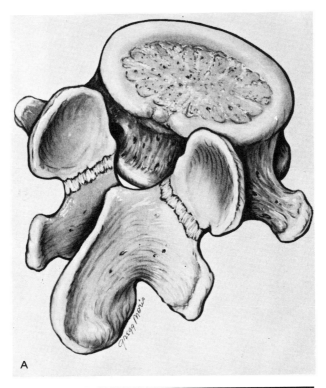

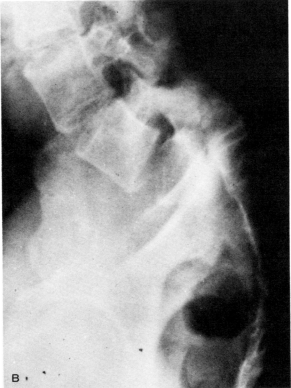

Fig. 6–5. A, Illustration of pars interarticular defect, or spondylolysis producing sagittal destabilization of the posterior elements. B, Radiograph of a high-grade spondylolisthesis following bilateral spondylolysis defects. (From Ruge, D., and Wiltse, L.L.: Spinal Disorders: Diagnosis and Treatment. Philadelphia, Lea & Febiger, 1977.)

Electrodiagnostic Testing

These studies measure physiology and, as such, are differentiated from the majority of other tests which provide images of the anatomy. The electromyogram (EMG) is the most commonly done of these tests, and measures the electrical activity of muscles through needle electrodes. If a pattern of muscle involvement, usually demonstrating fibrillation potentials or positive waves, develops in the paraspinal musculature and involved extremity following a typical myotome pattern, then the EMG may provide confirmatory evidence that nerve root compression exists (Fig. 6–6). The EMG may be most helpful when it is completely normal. The limitation of the testing is that it is subject to both intra- and inter-observer reliability problems, but when a classic pattern is present, correlation with surgical pathology may be as high as 90%.

Nerve conduction studies, measuring the velocity of an artifically induced signal through a peripheral nerve, may help to identify the existence and site of peripheral nerve root compression. This test may occasionally be used to delineate a spinal from a peripheral nerve compression. Finally, there is currently research interest in utilizing somato-sensory evoked potentials (SSEP) to assess the afferent system to identify lesions of nerves that failed to provoke motor involvement. Though currently used for surgical spinal cord monitoring, the SSEP is not commonly used for clinical low back assessment preoperatively.

Computer-Assisted Tomographic (CT) Scanning

The CT scan has become the most commonly performed spinal imaging test, often used as the only presurgical scanning test and replacing the lumbar myelogram. This has been done in spite of controversy surrounding current enthusiasm (Wiesel, Tsourmas, Feffer, Citrin, Patronas, 1984). Basically, the computer manipulates millions of microscopic x ray exposures or "pixelles," taken at various angles, and reformats them into thin "cuts" only 1 to 2 mm thick in axial, sagittal and coronal reconstructions. In so doing, extremely explicit identification of anatomy can be shown, particularly changes in discs, facets, spinal canal dimensions, and neuroforamina. At the present time, there is great risk of overinterpretation of these tests, since almost everyone shows some "significant" degenerative abnormality on CT scan. Indeed, many totally asymptomatic individuals have apparent surgically treatable disorders such as HNP or spinal stenosis revealed on CT scan (Fig. 6–7). The surgeon must cautiously interpret these tests in light of clinical findings. As stated previously, these tests are also frequently used to document an injury-induced abnormality for medical/legal purposes.

Myelography

Lumbar myelography is now performed almost exclusively with water-soluble dyes through a lumbar puncture. The specific features of the newest dyes, such as low viscosity, decreased arachnoid irritation, water-solubility and apparent minimal risk of subsequent arachnoiditis, have made the procedure considerably more palatable to the patient. In spite of the decreased incidents of spinal headache and lowered discomfort during the procedure, it is still significantly invasive and produces considerable anxiety in patients. Seizure complications, particularly in alcoholics, may provide additional complica-

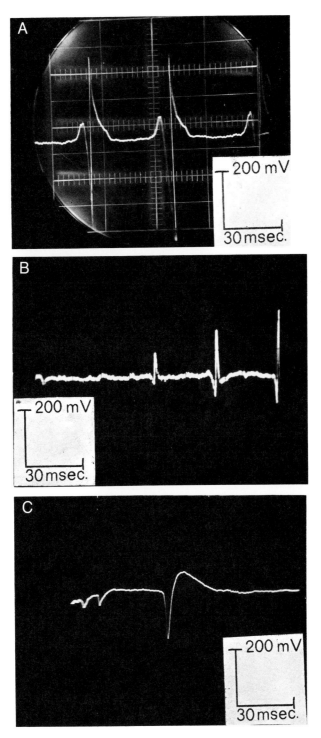

Fig. 6–6. A, Electromyographic recordings of normal potentials. B, Abnormal electromyographic recording showing fibrillation potentials. C, Electromyographic recording of positive Sharp waves. (From Ruge, D., and Wiltse, L.L.: Spinal Disorders: Diagnosis and Treatment. Philadelphia, Lea & Febiger, 1977).

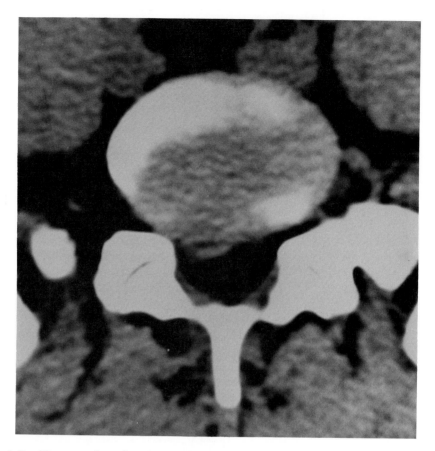

Fig. 6–7.   CT scan, axial cut, demonstrating herniated nucleus pulposus (HNP).

tions. Because of these potential complications, it is generally still performed as an inpatient procedure, increasing both cost and time demands relative to CT scans.

The test is particularly useful for assessing intrathecal neoplasms and extradural compression of the neural canal. However, it is difficult to interpret in the patient whose *cauda equina* fails to reach to the lowest disc level (termed an "insensitive" study), or in the postoperative patient, where myelography may be combined with CT scanning. The dye column can also be "run up" the spine to assess the cervicothoracic cord, identifying extradural stenosis or acute compression, as well as intradural complications (Fig. 6–8).

Magnetic Resonance Imaging (MRI)

This noninvasive test, involving imaging of tissues through the use of extremely powerful magnets, is rapidly gaining acceptance for imaging the spine (Fig. 6–9). Unlike radiography, it appears to have no adverse biologic effect. The technique currently appears superior to CT scanning in identifying soft tissue structures, particularly in the postoperative patient where scar formation may affect the accuracy of radiographic tests. Availability of MRI scanners is rapidly increasing (as is the cost of evaluation). It appears that considerably

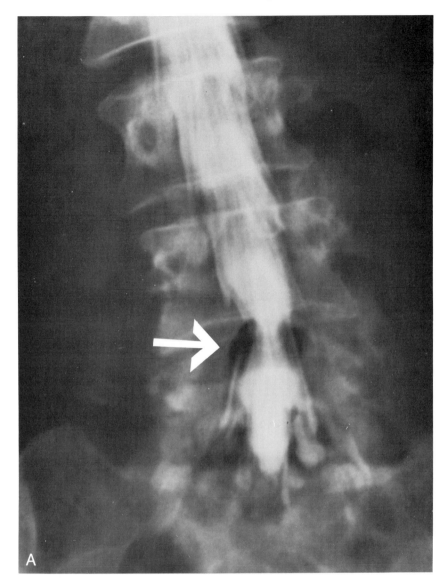

Fig. 6–8. A, Myelogram demonstrating herniated nucleus pulposus, primarily to the left, at L4–L5 (arrow).

more time and research will be required to identify the proper role of this new imaging modality.

Blood Tests

The vast majority of low back pain problems are unassociated with positive blood tests, but the small minority involving infection, systemic arthritis, neoplasm, or metabolic disease may be important to identify. If history and physical examination identify signs and symptoms characteristic of these diseases, appropriate blood tests may be performed including Erythrocyte Sedimentation Rate (ESR), Complete Blood Count (CBC), combination of chemistries (such as

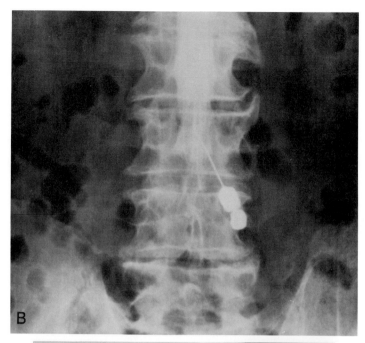

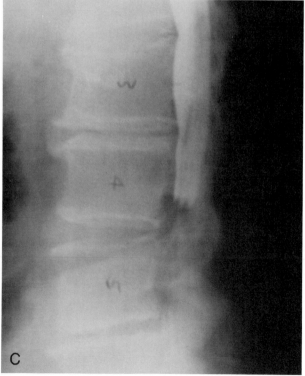

Fig. 6–8 (cont.).   B, Myelogram demonstrating total myelographic block produced by spinal stenosis at the L4 level on AP projection. C, Lateral projection demonstrating total myelographic block at L4 produced by spinal stenosis.

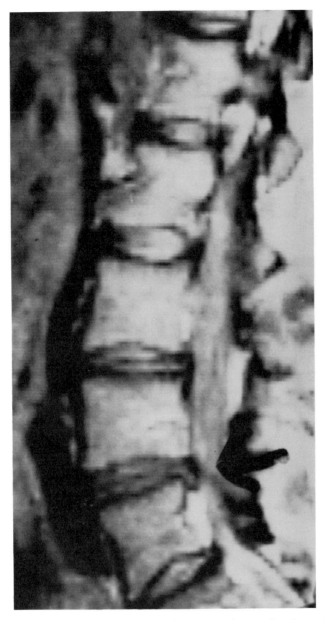

Fig. 6–9.   Magnetic resonance imaging (MRI) scan demonstrates herniated nucleus pulposus (HNP) at L4–L5.

SMAC-20), acid phosphatase, protein electrophoresis, or HLA-B27 antigen test. Symptoms will dictate which test is to be performed, and findings on the test may direct the physician to additional studies.

Bone Scanning

The bone scan involves injection of a radioisotope into the general circulation where it is selectively concentrated in areas of rapid bone turnover. As such, it may be used to identify healing fractures or sites of rapid bone lysis/repair.

Many bone neoplasms, primary or metastatic, and most infections, as well as some metabolic processes, can be identified using the radionuclide scan. Osteoarthritic subchrondral bone changes will likewise create areas of positive uptake.

Discography

The discogram is performed by inserting a needle into the nucleus pulposus, usually under fluoroscopic control from the posterolateral position, and injecting a dye. The test interpretation depends on the radiographic abnormality of degeneration, identifying anular tears, epidural flow, or vertebral flow through vessels transiting the vertebral endplate. The second interpretive factor is the presence of "concordant pain," requiring the alert patient to identify pain produced at the time of injection as pain identical or similar to that experienced when physically active. The test has remained controversial for several reasons: (a) degenerative changes are common and increase dramatically with aging, with prevalence rates in patients and the general age-matched population identical; (b) interpretation of patient pain report is subjective, on the part of both the patient and the clinician, and is affected by wide inter-observer variability; (c) surgical treatment resulting from a positive test is highly invasive without controlled studies corroborating its cost/benefit relationship; and (d) the invasive nature of the test, usually adding cost and disadvantage of an inpatient procedure. While discography has recently become more popular, proponents and critics are no less polarized in their views, and it remains for future investigation to establish its proper role.

Thermography

Thermography is currently an extremely controversial procedure involving the measurement of superficial skin temperatures by liquid crystal or infrared means to identify changes in local blood flow. Proponents of this testing procedure contend that measurement of skin temperature provides a noninvasive measure of neural compression. Acceptance of this method awaits demonstration of controlled studies correlating surgically proven disc lesions with preoperative thermographic predictions.

CONSERVATIVE MANAGEMENT OF ACUTE LOW BACK PAIN

The natural history of low back pain discussed in Chapter 3 is well understood, and the reader is again referred back to this discussion. Because low back pain is a benign, generally self-limited disease, this natural history is extremely important. The fact that 90% of back pain patients resolve their problem spontaneously in 3 months, more or less, suggests that this is not a disease process requiring expenditure of large amounts of funds, effort, or medical attention for the vast majority of patients. In fact, some nihilists would suggest that most low back pain patients get well even without, or often *in spite of,* medical attention.

It is beyond the scope of this chapter to exhaustively discuss conservative management techniques. Only a broad outline and some salient points will be made about the most commonly utilized and best understood modalities for care. The conservative regimen is utilized in almost all cases of low back problems unless immediate surgical intervention is called for. The rather rare circumstances in which surgical procedure proves necessary within the first 6 weeks are: (a) severe trauma necessitating decompression or stablization; (b) cauda equina syndrome; (c) neoplasm necessitating biopsy or resection; (d) infection necessitating biopsy or drainage; (e) rapidly progressive neurologic lesion producing paralysis or bladder/bowel dysfunction. Pain alone, regardless of severity, is *not* an indication for surgical intervention without these other factors, since marked variation of pain perception and display is present in the general population. The clinician who is swayed by severity of pain report is likely to pay the most attention to, and be most therapeutically aggressive with, the manipulative, somatizing patient with whom he or she should actually be most conservative.

Many of the treatments for acute low back pain are performed for purposes of producing patient comfort, rather than for any therapeutic benefit that hastens the conclusion of the acute episode. In fact, no controlled studies have given any experimental evidence of efficacy of one form of treatment over another, even though patients may have strong preferences (Deyo, 1983; Deyo, Diehl, Rosenthal, 1986; Vanharanta, Videman, Mooney, 1986). These preferences may have great socioeconomic significance, as in the widespread use of chiropractors in the United States, whose treatment primarily involves the use of manipulative skills. Similarly, the use of passive electrical modalities and exercise in physical therapy varies widely in acceptance internationally among patients, physicians, and third-party payers.

Treatments Associated with Early Healing

Bedrest

Because most patients with low back pain note a decrease in symptomatology in the recumbent position, bedrest is the oldest and most consistently used modality for acute back pain. Over a short period of time, it appears to speed earlier return to full activity by resting the tissues. However, prolonged bedrest may promote relatively rapid disuse changes in the back, as well as behavioral changes for the pain-prone individual.

Traction

Though traction makes good sense in principle, it has long been known that the forces required to overcome stabilizing forces in the spine and obtaining any meaningful traction are too great to be obtained through pelvic traction in the supine position. In fact, the rationale for applying this treatment has traditionally been to "enforce bedrest." It appears that at least 25% of the total body weight must be applied as a distracting force to overcome inertia and achieve distraction of lumbar vertebrae. There appears to be some evidence, however, that "autotraction" administered through use of forces applied by the patient's extremities may be useful in more rapidly relieving muscle spasm and pain than the use of corsets. Large distraction forces can also be obtained using "gravity traction" through a number of suspension mechanisms, though these produce some risk associated with the inverted position.

Corsets and Braces

These devices, producing rest through "immobilization" of the spine, also have a long history. Their use is justified by the advantage of permitting the patient to remain ambulatory, while "resting" the spine through immobilization. The lack of immobilizing capabilities of a variety of corset devices was demonstrated some 30 years ago, leading to the popularity of soft corsets which supposedly exerted their salutary effect by increasing intra-abdominal pressure, thereby relieving loads on the lumbar spine. This concept has now been disproven both biomechanically and clinically, as the abdominal compression necessary to effect any meaningful decrease in disc pressure would also be sufficiently high to cut off venous return from the extremities through the vena cava. In spite of the loss of the scientific underpinnings for this form of treatment, it remains a popular mode of early therapy.

Physical Modalities

Manipulation

While manipulation is generally equated with chiropractic care in the United States, the technique is frequently also delivered by physicians, osteopaths, or physical therapists. Several clinical trials of this technique have been performed. Although the results have been equivocal, some short-term benefit seems to be derived in a significant number of cases in comparison to diathermy, flexion exercises, or back school. Dramatic, sudden improvement is also obtained in a small number of cases, though recurrence and remanipulation with unpredictable results is commonplace. A major part of the controversy concerning manipulation is the fact that there are few tenable hypotheses concerning the mechanism of action of manipulative treatment. The most reasonable theory involves sudden mobilization of the facet joints, but confirmation of the mechanism of action of the manipulation techniques is unlikely to be forthcoming in the near future.

Exercises

Exercises for acute back pain fall into three categories: (1) a flexion exercise program involving flexion of the spine and hips and some abdominal strengthening, generally credited to Williams (1955); (2) a hyperextension program, following an initial evaluation based on patient report of movements which decrease pain, generally credited to McKenzie (1981); and (3) a general mobilization program in all planes for increasing range of motion. No controlled study, as yet, has demonstrated unequivocal advantages of one type of exercise over another, nor of exercise over other forms of acute treatment. Exercise programs are popular as they can be taught as a remobilization technique to patients who can practice themselves. The potential for demonstrating improved range of motion also exists, thereby making exercise a functional test to better assess the treatment approaches. Unfortunately, the natural history of acute back pain confounds most attempts at scientific study.

TENS/Acupuncture

With the advent of the "gate control theory" of pain by Melzack and Wall (1965), many investigators became intrigued with the potential for blocking pain impulses through imparting a benign superficial stimulus. This research led ultimately to the proliferation of TENS (transcutaneous electrical nerve stimulation) devices for use with skin electrodes, and also to implantable epidural and "deep brain" stimulators. The invasive devices have found considerably less popularity than the TENS units.

The same general principles are felt to explain beneficial effects of acupuncture, a traditional Chinese art often combined with moxibustion. In current practice, it is often combined with electrical stimulation rather than manual manipulation of the needles. Though both techniques produce considerable interest among the lay public, no controlled trials demonstrating effectiveness of either technique are available. While acupuncture requires a trained specialist to implant and manipulate the needles, the TENS unit can be applied by the patient and, after the initial purchase price is covered, only minimal additional cost is necessary regardless of duration of usage.

Temperature-Related Modalities

A wide variety of modalities to provide superficial or deep heat have been used extensively, and are particularly popular in the United States. Local massage, heating pads, and hot showers are frequently combined with techniques that provide deep heat or energy transfer, including ultrasound, diathermy, and lasers.

By contrast, cold, in the form of ice packs or cold massage, has been advocated for acute injury, with the same rationale of controlling bleeding, edema, and blood flow that is used in acute athletic injuries. While it is practically impossible to demonstrate any short-term efficacy of such techniques in a controlled study, patient report and popularlity among clinicians keep these methods in wide use. Long-term effectiveness has never been seriously suggested.

Drugs and Nerve Blocks

Analgesics and Muscle Relaxants

A wide variety of opiate and semisynthetic narcotics for pain relief have been advocated for acute back episodes. Occasionally, injectable narcotics prove necessary for a short period of time. The so-called "muscle relaxants," which are really minor tranquilizers, apparently decrease muscle irritability temporarily, and are useful in acute muscle spasm. Unfortunately, both classes of drugs have substantial habituating potential, and their long-term use is not advocated. In practice, however, patients demand these medications in lieu of other pain-relieving mechanisms, and long-term habituation in the small percentage of patients who become chronic is endemic.

NSAIDs and Steroids

Over the past 10 years, use of nonsteroidal anti-inflammatory drugs (NSAIDs) for low back episodes, both acute and chronic, has become widespread. The use of aspirin, because of its gastric side effects, has probably declined slightly, though it remains extremely popular also. Short courses of oral or injectable steroids may also be used for severe acute episodes.

Antidepressants

These medications have recently been shown to have an effect on chronic pain in low doses (Ward, 1986). This mechanism is poorly understood, and requires further study. Their use will be discussed in greater detail later in this book.

Epidural Steroids

Filling the epidural space, either through the sacral hiatus or through the midlumbar posterior route, has been advocated for treating lumbar radicular syndrome, postoperative epidural fibrosis, or back and leg pain in which nerve root findings are equivocal. Evidence of effectiveness, other than patient self-report, is difficult to obtain. It is, however, a relatively widely used method.

Facet Blocks

Injection into the facet joints, under x-ray control with or without use of dye, is a commonly performed procedure for a well described clinical syndrome. However, results of injection have been unpredictable for pain relief and recurrence, with recent studies being considerably less hopeful concerning efficacy than initial ones (Mooney, Robertson, 1976; Jackson, Montesano, Jacobs, 1986). The procedure is also often used diagnostically to assess a patient's response to pain, and to assist in evaluating segmental instability.

Trigger Point Injections

"Trigger points" represent localized tender areas, often with pain radiating from them to a distant point, and sometimes associated with induration that appears to simulate "localized muscle spasm." Pathologic studies have failed to demonstrate significant abnormalities in the local tissue, but injection of local anesthetic and steroids into these areas is often temporarily effective in relieving pain.

SPINAL SURGERY

Only a small fraction of patients with low back pain require surgery, but as the problem becomes more chronic, the likelihood of surgical intervention grows larger.

Disc Surgery for Herniated Nucleus Pulposus (HNP)

This commonest of lumbar procedures is also the one performed most frequently on younger patients in the 3rd to 5th decades, and thus is most significant in its relation to disability. As has been shown by Weber (1978, 1983), disc surgery is likely to produce better short-term results, but even in myelogram-proven disc herniation with sciatica, long-term comparison of surgical versus nonsurgical treatment is indifferent. Furthermore, surgery performed after a long delay (more than 3 months) after onset of sciatica appears to be no better than nonsurgical treatment, even in relieving short-term disability. This has led to the concept of a "golden period" between 60 to 90 days post-sciatica onset, by which time disc surgery should be performed, if it is to be performed at all. Though surgery may be performed prior to 8 weeks if neurologic findings are relatively severe, a trial of conservative care until this point is reached is advocated in most cases.

The actual technique of disc surgery appears relatively unimportant. The most commonly performed surgical procedure continues to be the open discectomy, in which a small laminotomy exposes the nerve root and underlying disc protrusion or extruded fragment. Mechanical removal of disc contents rarely extirpates more than 25 to 40% of the disc material, and the dead space is resolved by partial collapse and scarring. Some degree of epidural fibrosis usually binds the nerve root anteriorly, and ultimately calcification of the peripheral anulus occurs. Postoperative changes may also leave asymmetric function of paravertebral musculature, intersegmental ligaments, and facet joints if partial facetectomy or inadvertent capsulotomy is performed. Disc collapse also narrows the neuroforamen, but a sufficient "fail-safe" usually exists, making lateral entrapment uncommon. Fat grafts placed over the laminotomy site, replacing ligamentum flavum between muscle and dura, are felt to reduce epidural scarring in most cases.

Microdiscectomy has been proposed to produce less damage to musculoskeletal tissues, and is advocated by some surgeons. However, results appear to be strongly related to the skill of the surgeon, and potential for creating unobserved injury or incompletely removing disc material appears to balance the potential advantages of the technique.

Percutaneous discectomy as an outpatient procedure through a posterolateral approach is currently entering clinical practice with attendant potential decrease in surgical costs and morbidity. However, this procedure can only be performed for the protruded disc, in which a change in the nuclear environment appears to cause the perineural inflammatory response. Extruded or sequestered fragments, necessitating removal to prevent further mechanical compression, cannot be reached through this technique.

Chemonucleolysis

Chemonucleolysis refers to the chemical alteration of the nucleus pulposus. This has been extensively studied using *chymopapain,* an enzyme from the papaya plant which appears to separate the water from the proteoglycan matrix of the nucleus, leading to rapid disc decompression. While there is evidence to show that some discs may rehydrate within months following chemonucleolysis, the efficacy of the procedure evolves from initial relief of sciatica. Recently, *collagenase,* another enzymatic nuclear degrading agent, has been utilized in clinical trials for similar purposes.

The advantage of chemonucleolysis is its performance through a percutaneous approach, with potential for lower-cost treatment and shorter hospitalization. However, a number of factors have complicated this hope, and have slowly decreased the popularity of chemonucleolysis. Because the results of the initial procedure are less effective than open discectomy in relieving sciatica, many patients go on to a second procedure, usually an open discectomy. Whether the problem is in the chymopapain, in a procedure that fails to visualize the nerve root, or in looser surgical indications because the procedure is "only an injection," is not clear at this time. Several studies have demonstrated, however, statistically significant higher cost of treatment for HNP when chemonucleolysis is the initial procedure. When combined with problems of a small but disastrous set of complications (anaphylaxis, CVA, transverse myelitis), a decrease in use of the enzyme has occurred.

Decompressive Laminectomy

Decompression of the spinal canal, generally by removing all or a significant part of the neural arch, is generally performed in an older age group. The procedure is specifically performed for those lesions in which the spinal canal is stenotic, or when "kinking" of the canal is present as in a higher grade spondylolisthesis. The procedure inevitably exposes a large area of dura posteriorly, predisposing to epidural fibrosis. Free fat grafts have been used in an effort to prevent fibrous adhesions to the muscle previously stripped from the periosteum.

In younger individuals, particularly those involved in relatively heavy occupations, there is concern about the potential for instability. Frequently in these individuals, posterolateral fusion is performed, with or without spinal instrumentation. In older individuals, on the other hand, fusion is rarely necessary, though there are some indications now that a small percentage of this group may become unstable even in the 8th or subsequent decades.

Posterior and Posterolateral Fusions

Posterior fusions are rarely performed any longer because of the tendency toward bony overgrowth over many years, ultimately encroaching on the spinal canal. If posterior stabilization is desired, the bilateral posterolateral mass fusion is generally utilized. In this procedure, the "gutter" between transverse process and neural arch is exposed and decorticated to provide a bed for corticocancellous grafts spanning the segments to be fused. Generally, these fusions involve one or two segments above the sacrum, with the grafts running inferiorly to the sacral alae (Fig. 6–10).

Interbody Fusion

Interbody fusion has, in the past, been performed only in unusual circumstances when posterolateral fusion was thought to be biomechanically unsound. However, there is currently increasing popularity for interbody fusion as a primary procedure for the "painful disc" demonstrated by discography, or for fusion from the posterior approach at the time of discectomy (Cloward, 1963; Crock, 1970; Flinn, Hogue, 1979; Holt, 1968; Collis, Gardner, 1962) (Fig. 6–11).

The role of lumbar fusion in the treatment of backache remains controversial. Although there are clear-cut indications such as obvious instability created by high-grade spondylolisthesis, or post-traumatic injury to the motion segment, these are relatively rare compared to the common complaint of severe disabling back pain. The problem is complex. We are aware that simple degeneration of the disc is no more disabling than wrinkles on the face, which is a similar process from a pathophysiologic point of view. The desiccation process occurs in association with aging. On the other hand, it is quite clear that some discs are extremely painful when disc injection occurs with contrast medium—discography. Sometimes the radiographic changes of the acutely painful disc, which reproduces the patient's own pain complaint, are relatively minor. Occasionally, even optimal, prolonged conservative care fails to resolve the pain complaints. On this basis, some surgeons have felt it appropriate to totally remove the disc and replace it by bone graft. Although this has been accomplished from a posterior approach (posterior lumbar interbody fusion: PLIF) an anterior approach creates less opportunity for spinal canal scarring and posterior extrusion of bone graft. This procedure is known as an anterior lumbar interbody fusion (ALIF). It is a technically demanding procedure but with appropriate selection, good results have been described (Fujimaki, Crock, Be-

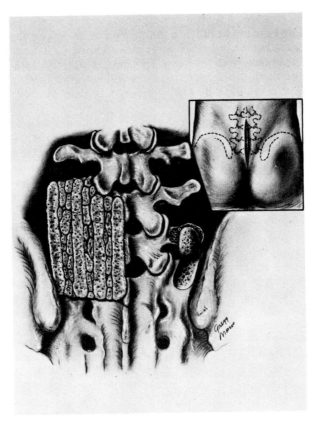

Fig. 6–10. Fusion of L4 to sacrum through a midline approach utilizing strips of graft from posterior ilium. The grafts are laid from sacrum to transverse process of L4. (From Ruge, D., and Wiltse, L.L.: Spinal Disorders: Diagnosis and Treatment. Philadelphia, Lea & Febiger, 1977.)

drook, 1982), though other authors have found the procedure less successful (Flinn, Hogue, 1974). An additional advantage of an anterior approach is minimal intrusion into the posterior trunk musculature. The posterior approach for spinal exposure creates the opportunity for muscular and posterior ramus denervation. In certain circumstances, frequently after multiple discectomies or significant trauma which creates degenerative arthritis of the facets and motion segments, a posterolateral fusion of the lower lumbar spine becomes necessary. In general, this fusion requires autogenous bone graft donated from the iliac crest and placed across the transverse processes and into the facet joints, and may also demand internal fixation to maintain stability (Fig. 6–12). Obviously, considerable dissection is necessary for both approaches, with morbidity after surgical procedure frequently lasting 4 to 6 months or longer. There is no question that care of chronic back pain by fusion forces the patient to pay a large price in terms of structural impairment, but it may be acceptable if ultimate disability is reduced in the appropriately selected patient.

THE PAIN CLINIC TREATMENT APPROACH

As we discussed in Chapter 4, Fordyce and colleagues developed a behavioral-operant treatment program for chronic pain (Fordyce, Fowler, Lehmann,

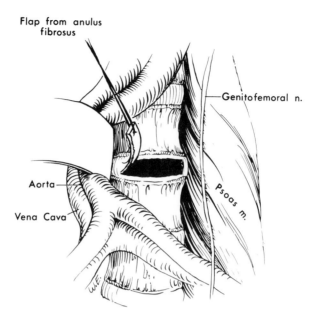

Fig. 6–11. Anterior interbody fusion. (From Ruge, D., and Wiltse, L.L.: Spinal Disorders: Diagnosis and Treatment. Philadelphia, Lea & Febiger, 1977.)

DeLateur, 1968). It involved a comprehensive 4- to 8-week inpatient approach designed to gradually increase the general activity level and decrease pain report of the patient. The program was based on the assumption that, although pain may initially result from some underlying organic disorder, learning and environmental reinforcement contingencies (such as secondary gain factors) can modify and further maintain various aspects of chronic pain behavior. Although such a program was not viewed as necessarily eliminating pain totally, it was found to make a difference in changing unbearable to bearable pain, and in changing an unproductive, sedentary existence to a relatively active lifestyle.

This multidisciplinary behavioral modification program served as the prototype for the subsequent emergence of a large number of "pain clinics" throughout the country. Unfortunately, however, most of these clinics developed into a "hodge-podge" of techniques aimed primarily at altering the patient's self-report of pain. Most employed primarily passive physical modalities such as spinal manipulation, acupuncture, or electrical stimulation, which often simply increased the patient's dependence on the medical care system. In addition, most used the same treatment strategy across a wide range of different chronic pain behaviors (low back pain, myofascial pain, etc.)

It is not surprising that there have been some major problems associated with these pain clinic approaches. We earlier discussed these problems in Chapter 1. Indeed, the effectiveness of such pain clinics in modifying back pain disability has recently been strongly questioned (Sturgess, Schaefer, Sikora, 1984). Although Fordyce's original behavioral concept was good, it became quite significantly diluted and modified by the rapid commercialization of the pain clinic concept.

When we review the functional restoration program in the next chapter, the

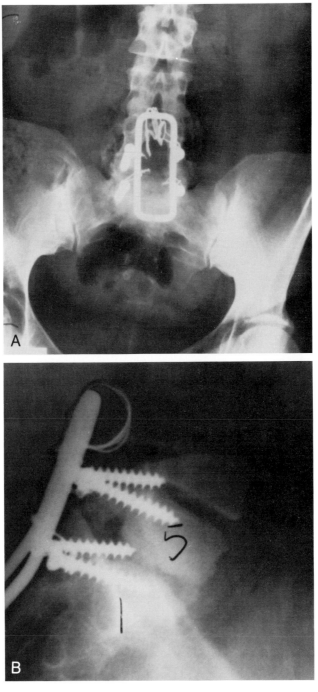

Fig. 6–12. AP (A) and lateral (B) roentgenograms of lumbar fusion supplemented by Luque ring fixation, L4 to the sacrum. Pedicular screws and laminar wires are both utilized for fixation.

reader will become aware of the important role that behavioral treatment components play. As with Fordyce and colleagues, learning and environmental reinforcement contingencies are viewed as significant. They are incorporated into a comprehensive approach aimed at increasing function and activity level. This approach differs from past approaches, though, because of the inclusion of objective measurement of function which is used in continuously guiding and evaluating the treatment process.

CHAPTER REFERENCES

Cloward R: Lesions of the intervertebral disks and their treatment by interbody fusion methods. Clin Orthop *27*:51–77, 1963.

Collis J, Gardner W: Lumbar discography: an analysis of 1,000 cases. J. Neurosurg *19*:452–461, 1962.

Crock H: A re-appraisal of intervertebral disc lesions. Med J Aust *1*:983–989, 1970.

Deyo R: Conservative Therapy for low back pain: distinguishing useful from useless therapy. JAMA *250*:1057–1062, 1983.

Deyo R, Diehl A, Rosenthal M: How many days of bedrest for acute low back pain? N Engl J Med *315*:1064–1070, 1986.

Flinn J, Hogue A: Anterior fusion of the lumbar spine: end-result study with long-term follow-up. J Bone Joint Surg *61*-A:1143–1150, 1979.

Fordyce W, Fowler R, Lehmann J, DeLateur B: Some implications of learning in problems of chronic pain. J Chron Dis *21*:179–190, 1968.

Fujimaki A, Crock H, Bedbrook G: The result of 150 anterior lumbar interbody fusion operations performed by two surgeons in Australia. Clin Orthop & Rel Res *165*:164–167, 1982.

Holt E: The question of lumbar discography. J Bone Joint Surg *50*A:720–726, 1968.

Jackson R, Montesano P, Jacobs R: Facet joint injections in mechanical low back pain patients: a prospective statistical study. Proceedings of Int'l Soc for Study of Lumbar Spine. Orthop Trans *10*:509, 1986.

McKenzie R: The Lumbar Spine: Mechanical Diagnosis and Therapy, Upper Hutt, New Zealand, Spinal Publications, 1981.

Melzack R, Wall P: Pain mechanisms: a new theory. Science, *150*:971–979, 1965.

Mooney V, Robertson J: The facet syndrome. Clin Orthop *115*:149–156, 1976.

Scavone J, Latshaw R, Rohrer G: Use of lumbar spine films: statistical evaluation at a university teaching hospital. JAMA *246*:1105–1108, 1981.

Sturgess E, Schaefer C, Sikora T: Pain center follow-up study of treated and untreated patients. Arch Phys Med Rehabil *65*:301–303, 1984.

Vanharanta H, Videman T, Mooney V: McKenzie exercises, back-trac and back school in lumbar syndrome. Proceedings of Int'l Soc for Study of Lumbar Spine. Orthop Trans *10*:533, 1986.

Waddell G, McColloch J, Kummel E, Venner R: Non-organic physical signs in low back pain. Spine *5*:117–125, 1979.

Ward N: 1986 Volvo Award in Clinical Sciences: tricyclic antidepressants for chronic low-back pain: mechanisms of action and predictors of response. Spine *11*:661–665, 1986.

Weber H: Lumbar disc herniation: a prospective study of prognostic factors including a controlled trial. Part I. J Oslo City Hosp *28*:33–64, 1978.

Weber H: Lumbar disc herniation: a prospective study of prognostic factors including a controlled trial. Part II. J Oslo City Hosp *28*:89–120, 1978.

Weber H: Lumbar disc herniation: A Controlled Prospective Study with 10 Years of Observation. Spine *8*:131–140, 1983.

Wiesel S, Tsourmas N, Feffer H, Citrin C, Patronas N: 1984 Volvo Award in Clinical Sciences. a study of computer assisted tomography: 1. The incidence of positive CAT scans in an asymptomatic group of patients. Spine *9*:549–551, 1984.

Williams P: Examination and conservative treatment for disc lesions of the lower spine. Clin Orthop *5*:28–40, 1955.

ADDITIONAL REFERENCES

Bell G, Rothman R, Booth R, Cuckler J, Garfin S, Herkowitz H, Simeone F, Dolinskas C, Han S: 1984 Volvo Award in clinical sciences: a study of computer assisted tomography: II. Comparison of metrizamide myelography and computer tomography in the diagnosis of herniated lumbar disk and spinal stenosis. Spine *9*:552–556, 1984.

Breig A, Troup J: Biomechanical considerations in the straight leg raising test: cadaveric and clinical studies of the effects of medial hip rotation. Spine *4*:242–250, 1979.

Brown M: Diagnosis of pain syndromes of the spine. Orthop Clin No Am *6*:233–248, 1975.

Crawshaw C, Frazer A, Merriam W, Mulholland R, Webb J: A comparison of surgery and chemo-nucleolysis in the treatment of sciatica: a prospective randomized trial. Spine *9*:195–198, 1984.

Cuckler J, Bernini P, Wiesel S, Booth R, Rothman R, Pickens G: The use of epidural steroids in the treatment of lumbar radicular pain. J Bone Joint Surg *67*-A:63–66, 1985.

Farfan H: Mechanical Disorders in the Low Back. Philadelphia, Lea & Febiger, 1973.

Florence DW: The chronic pain syndrome. Postgrad Med *70*:217–228, 1981.

Frymoyer J, Donaghy R: The ruptured intervertebral disc: follow-up report on the first case 50 years after recognition of the syndrome and its surgical significance. J Bone Joint Surg *67*A:1113–1116, 1985.

Godfrey C, Morgan P, Schatzker J: A randomized trial of manipulation for low-back pain in a medical setting. Spine *9*:301–304, 1984.

Jackson R, Boston D, Edge A: Lateral mass fusion: a prospective study of a consecutive series with long-term follow-up. Spine *10*:828–832, 1985.

Lawrence J: Disc degeneration. Its frequency and relationship to symptoms. Ann Rheum Dis *28*:121–137, 1969.

Magora A, Schwartz A: Relation between the low back pain syndrome and x-ray findings. I. Degenerative osteoarthritis. Scand J Rehabil Med *8*:115–125, 1976.

Mayer T: Rehabilitation of the patient with spinal pain. Orthop Clin No Am *14*:623–639, 1983.

Nachemson A: Lumbar Spine Instability: A critical update and symposium summary. Spine *10*:290–291, 1985.

Norten P, Brown T: The immobilizing efficiency of back braces: their effect on the posture and motion of the lumbosacral spine. J Bone Joint Surg *39*A:111–138, 1957.

Ottenbacher K, DeFabio R: Efficacy of spinal manipulation/mobilization therapy: a meta-analysis. Spine *10*:833–837, 1985.

Perry J: The use of external support in the treatment of low back pain. Artif Limbs *14*:49–57, 1970.

Thorstensson G, Stonnington H, Stillwell G: The placebo effect of transcutaneous electrical stimulation. Pain *5*:31–41, 1978.

Troup J: Straight leg raising (SLR) and the qualifying tests for increased root tension: their predictive value after back and sciatic pain. Spine *6*:526–529, 1981.

Wiesel S, Cuckler J, DeLuca F, Jones F, Zeide M, Rothman R: Acute low-back pain: an objective analysis of conservative therapy. Spine *5*:324–330, 1980.

Wiltse L: Chemonucleolysis in the treatment of lumbar disc disease. Orthop Clin No Am *14*:605–622, 1983.

Chapter 7

What Is Functional Restoration?

We can now begin our discussion of the functional restoration approach. This approach was developed in response to the obvious clinical need for a more effective method of treating chronic low back pain. Rehabilitation for spinal disorders has fallen into disrepute in recent years because of lack of standardization and questionable effectiveness. In contrast to other areas of musculoskeletal medicine, in which sports medicine rehabilitation generally implies restoring physical functional capacity to the highest level possible, low back care has taken another turn. The fine work of early psychologic investigators such as Fordyce and colleagues into psychosocial concomitants of long-term disability led to recognition of the relationships between illness behavior and operant conditioning. Also noted were relationships between stress and muscular tension and joint stiffness. Other psychophysiologic factors are also clearly identified (Fordyce, Roberts, Sternbach, 1985; Turk, Meichenbaum, Genest, 1983). This led to the present mosaic of 2000 American treatment facilities known as "pain clinics" which have mushroomed in the past 25 years. However, as noted in the last chapter, these clinics became quite "diluted" and nonspecific in their attempt to treat all kinds of different pain behaviors. The high cost and lack of quantifiable benefits attributed to these facilities also subsequently led to adverse attitudes toward *any* type of spinal rehabilitation among most American third-party payers.

As we have noted, important barriers to restoring function may be inherent in the "disability system." A generation of employers has grown up convinced that the high incidence of recurrent back problems in the previously back-injured population, and the frequently ambiguous circumstances of back injury, make these patients of dubious re-employment value. This thinking is magnified by insurance companies, attorneys, and state workers' compensation boards who, lacking objective criteria, are inevitably disagreeing over financial compensation to be granted to back "claimants." Unfortunately, but understandably, a hostile, adverse atmosphere is created.

The complex financial and social costs of disability have been discussed earlier in detail. Moreover, we have also considered the basics of conservative care, structural diagnostic testing, and surgical treatment for the large majority of back injuries. However, this leaves a relatively large group of 40 to 50% of patients with recurrent back pain after initial episodes. More importantly, it leaves a small group of chronic back pain patients who become the most seriously disabled, unproductive, and psychologically crippled, and who demand constant access to the medical care system.

It is into this strained atmosphere that a new approach to spinal rehabilitation, termed "functional restoration," has been introduced. The treatment basically consists of an amalgam of a "sports medicine" approach to restoring physical capacity and a cognitive "crisis intervention" technique for dealing with psychosocial issues in the patient suffering from chronic spinal disability. A key element of this approach is the objective quantification of this physical and psychologic functioning.

THE IMPORTANCE OF QUANTIFICATION OF FUNCTION

The basic diagnostic component in the functional restoration approach is quantification of physical and psychologic function. The derivation of this concept results, quite simply, from the recognition of the hidden nature of spinal impairments. Unlike the extremities, spinal anatomy does not lend itself to simple visual inspection or palpation. We, as clinicians, have been seduced by progressively more sophisticated imaging techniques into believing that: (1) a correctable structural lesion usually exists, and (2) an anatomic lesion is the most common basis for ongoing complaints. We have inadvertently lent credence to the grossly erroneous conclusion that "if surgery can't fix it, the lesion must be in the head." An error equally damaging to the doctor/patient relationship is the belief that "if the imaging tests are normal, there is probably nothing wrong."

Subsequent chapters will discuss the concept of the "Deconditioning Syndrome" in greater detail. In essence, this represents the loss of physical capacity attendant upon disuse that leads to many manifestations of chronic disability. As we shall see, the technology now exists to objectively measure this syndrome. When combined with barriers to functional recovery such as fear of injury, neuromuscular inhibition, psychologic distress, and inappropriate advice from family, physicians and attorneys, this deconditioning syndrome can become a potent organic determinant of continued psychophysiologic deficits. Extensive information concerning these issues is now available in the literature, specifically regarding measurement of range of motion (Mayer, Kishino, Keeley, Mayer, Mooney, 1985; Pearcy, 1986; Keeley, Mayer, Cox, Gatchel, Smith, Mooney, 1986); trunk strength in sagittal and axial planes (Davies, Gould, 1982; Mayer, Smith, Keeley, Mooney, 1986; Smith, Mayer, Gatchel, Becker, 1985; Thompson, Gould, Davies, Ross, Price, 1985); aerobic capacity (Mayer, in press); and functional task performance such as lifting and bending (Chaffin, Herrin, Keyserling, 1979; Kishino, Mayer, Gatchel, Parrish, Anderson, Gustin, Mooney, 1986; Mayer, Kishino, Keeley, Mayer, Mooney, 1985).

It should also be noted that recent evidence suggests that a large number of postoperative patients, even those with relatively minimal symptoms, continue with physical capacity deficits that make them susceptible to recurrent injury (Mayer, 1986). In general, it appears that the longer the time of disability and the more extensive the surgical procedure, the greater are the postoperative physical capacity deficits that need to be addressed as part of the recovery process. Since pain perception is an individual phenomenon with wide population variance, self-report is an extremely unreliable method for judging who may or may not be at risk (Gatchel, Smith, Barnes, Mayer, 1986). For these postoperative individuals, relatively simple outpatient reconditioning or work hardening programs may be instituted with subsequent use of home equipment or a fitness center to maintain higher levels of physical capacity. Routine re-employment physicals and education programs that stress the importance of maintaining high fitness levels in industry to prevent recurrence may well be established in the future.

MAJOR COMPONENTS OF FUNCTIONAL RESTORATION TREATMENT

The functional restoration treatment program for the chronic back patient involves an interdisciplinary team approach utilizing physical and occupational therapy, psychology, and nursing, and is guided by a supervising physician who is not necessarily a surgeon. The physician must have an understanding of neurologic and musculoskeletal disorders, and must clearly recognize the difference between previous passive interventions and the patient's *active* participation in functional restoration. He or she must be prepared to evaluate structural diagnostic tests to determine need for additional surgical treatment. He or she must also understand issues of disability evaluation and management, and be prepared to participate in medicolegal proceedings. Nursing generally functions as a "physician-extender," providing counseling on medical matters, patient education, medication control, communication with outside agencies, and examinations for minor intercurrent illnesses.

Physical therapists provide a vital service to this program. They are concerned with mobilizing and strengthening the injured part of the body. Their focus on the "weak link" or functional unit causing the problem involves them in guiding a sequential reconditioning program, and dealing with the minor overuse problems accompanying rebuilding a severely deconditioned anatomic area.

Occupational therapists also play an important role in this program. They have two main roles. The first is to provide training in task performance; that is, synchronizing the injured part with the whole body in tasks such as lifting, bending, twisting, squatting, and climbing. A variety of activities simulating tasks of a physical nature are employed. Improving positional tolerance for sitting and standing are also major training goals. Their second major role is to become involved in the socioeconomic consequences of disability, and the various societal outcomes that must be dealt with to promote the patient's recovery, such as employment and litigation.

Psychologists involved in this type of program also have a dual role. First, they have a general crisis intervention role in which they must coordinate with the occupational therapists to help the patients deal with the termination of disability, as well as the economic, vocational, and family goals associated with this change. Secondly, they must help other team members recognize the barriers to functional recovery in an individual patient and help the patient to deal with these barriers. We have found that a cognitive-behavioral treatment orientation is appropriate and effective for a functional restoration approach. This orientation emphasizes the importance of simultaneously dealing with thoughts and feelings, as well as overt behavior in correcting maladaptive behaviors and dysfunctions.

Under medical supervision, the psychologist may also provide valuable assistance in dealing with habituating drugs, as well as with appropriate medication for withdrawal, depression or anxiety neurosis. Counseling for specific individual problems identified through psychologic testing is a critical part of the program. Long-term psychotherapy, however, is inappropriate in such a program. Certainly, getting to the "root causes" of maladaptive behaviors is a laudable goal, but the cost and lack of objective measures of success for long-term psychotherapy makes these techniques inappropriate for functional restoration. If patients were working in gainful employment prior to injury, functional restoration seeks to return them to this previous level of functioning. Any treatment going beyond this goal must be considered adjunctive.

There are other important "players" involved in this treatment process. As we have emphasized earlier, low back disability is not just a disease but a manifestation of a complex system. The process also involves employers, attorneys, physicians, unions, insurance companies, and governmental agencies, all of whom may have fixed perceptions and deeply rooted resistance to change. These groups must be made aware of not only the problems of disability, but also multiple accompanying problems that range from the loss of productivity to the financial drain on society. Once aware of the problems, these groups will, in time, be able to accept the fact that functional restoration plays a crucial role in the ultimate solution.

All industrialized societies have a variety of social systems set aside to compensate individuals for injury, illness, or lost wages. From the relatively low reporting rates of back disability in emerging third-world countries which have limited compensation systems, we can deduce that compensation for lost time may also be a factor in a worker's decision to miss work after an injury. However, the literature is ambiguous regarding its role in *maintaining* disability. When we discuss the deconditioning syndrome in later chapters, it will become clearer to the reader that once the disability process has begun, a new set of mediators may take over to maintain it.

Unlike the pain clinics, whose goal is generally to alter patients' self-report of their pain complaints, functional restoration is similar to modern musculoskeletal extremity rehabilitation, whose primary goal is the return of the patients to the highest level of physical capacity and productivity. Extensive evaluation now documents the ability of such a program to significantly influence important societal issues such as return to work, settlement of litigation, additional medical cost, recurrent injury, functional capacity and pain reduction. (Mayer, Gatchel, Kishino, Keeley, Capra, Mayer, Barnett, Mooney, 1985; Mayer, 1986).

SPORTS MEDICINE PRINCIPLES AND FUNCTIONAL RESTORATION

Sports medicine principles have been used, not merely to treat the competitive athlete, but in a modified way to treat all individuals wishing to return to high levels of function after extremity injury. The following summary will focus on some of the basic principles of sports medicine rehabilitation that have been used in the extremities, primarily focusing on the knee. Many of these principles are applied to the back in functional restoration.

In simplified terms, the initial phases of injury are characterized by hemorrhage and edema. Within the first few days, cellular infiltration and enzymatic degradation occur, involving prostaglandins, bradykinins, and kallikreins. This inflammatory process involves clearing of necrotic substances. A proliferative phase follows, with its timing and duration related to the quality of the blood supply in the area; random deposition of collagen fibrils takes place initially.

In subsequent phases, the collagen fibrils align along lines of stress (Wolff's Law of Mesothelial Tissues). Quite understandably, a small amount of tissue injury with relatively good nutrition and low grade stresses, such as a wrist sprain or muscle contusion, will proceed through this process quickly. However, for the extremely high stresses, large musculoligamentous structures and poor blood supply (particularly involving the discs) probably make for considerably delayed healing in the lumbar spine area. At its end, however, the injured area is left with a scar, visible or hidden, which has matured to fill the injured area, but lacks the resilience, strength, and durability of the original tissue. Such an asymmetric scar, produced either by injury, degeneration, or surgical trauma, may produce severe disturbances of biomechanical performance in the critical lumbar spine articulations.

As we have noted, a particular characteristic of the injured individual is to splint and protect the injured area. This leads, in time, to delayed maturation of collagen (Gelberman, Manske, Akeson, Woo, Lundborg, Amiel, 1986; Akeson, Amiel, Woo, 1980); muscle atrophy (Mongomery, Steadman, 1985); adhesions and deficits in joint lubrication (Salter, Field, 1961); ligament atrophy (Akeson, Amiel, Woo, 1980); and bone loss (Ruben, 1985).

Subsequently, muscular endurance and tone, and cardiovascular aerobic capacity decline, leading to neuromuscular difficulties with decrease in proprioception, agility and coordination. This, then, leads to a vicious cycle with recurrent injury occurring more easily due to the decreased physical capacity, termed the "deconditioning syndrome." As inactivity leads to ever lower physical demands, including loss of responsibilities at work and in the home, and greater periods of time reclining, the physical capacity deficits continue in a downward spiral. "Psychologic deconditioning" then follows as a natural consequence of physiologic deconditioning.

The physiologic approach to the deconditioning syndrome involves exercise to address mobility, strength, endurance, and cardiovascular deficits. The exercises must then progress to involve simulation of customary physical activities to restore task-specific endurance, coordination and agility through restoring neuromuscular inputs (Gould, Davies, 1985). Obviously, these exercises must be focused at the specific functional units that have become deconditioned. Finally, psychologic deconditioning and a continued maintenance program, including returning to the sport or work and activities of daily living characteristic of productivity, must be entered into once again.

Strength may be restored after injury in a variety of modes. Initially, soon after injury when continued immobilization may be necessary, isometric exercise may be the only type that can be performed by the patient. This involves exercising against a fixed resistance without accompanying joint motion. These exercises may be done in a cast or splint, but the method has many drawbacks. First, it is the most fatiguing and least effective type of exercise (Hoshizaki, Massey, 1986). There is specificity of strength training to the length of the muscle fibers at the time of training, with rapid fall-off in training efficiency at different muscle fiber lengths. Additionally, there is limited translation of endurance and agility from isometric training to specific functional activiites, though it can be used during the early rest phases to maintain strength and produce relative resistance to muscle atrophy. There is also some suggestion of a benefit of electrical muscle stimulation in combination with isometric exercise, but some question of higher injury potential may be associated with overvigorous acceleration into a static pull (Haggmark, 1979).

Dynamic muscle training, which has been shown to be the most efficient method of muscle training, can also be employed. It involves three basic modes: isotonic, isokinetic, and psychophysical (free weights) (Eriksson, 1976). *Isotonic* exercises are those in which the same force is applied throughout the dynamic range, and is often inappropriately used for exercises in which a changing lever arm actually alters the weight applied. This type of exercise is most appropriate to the variable resistance devices, utilizing a cam to maximize and equalize muscular demands throughout the dynamic range of motion.

By contrast, *isokinetic* devices require a sophisticated dynamometer which limits the speed to a preset level. Thus, isokinetics maintains speed while allowing the production of torque around a central axis, thereby eliminating the effect of acceleration on energy production. These devices are generally accommodating to force application (providing injury protection), but also do not simulate the "real world" because of the compromises of the speed selection system. Unlike variable resistance devices, however, high-speed training is possible to develop some specific agility and coordination goals.

Finally, psychophysical strength training, utilizing free weights, is limited to those positions in which weights can be attached to the body or held in the hands. The method is so termed because the subject self-selects the amount of weight that is acceptable. While this is the closest to the "real world"strengthening, the maximum weight that can be handled is limited by the weakest portion of the dynamic range of motion and further compromised by limitations of the changing lever arm. However, if the exercise can be produced to simulate actual tasks or motions of the sport or work activity to which the patient is returning, this may be an effective training tool. Psychophysical and variable resistance lifting devices automatically provide concentric and eccentric contraction capability. This is more difficult and dangerous to provide in isokinetic devices, though computerized devices to produce these effects are being developed.

Secondary effects of a sports medicine program are also critically important. Training appears to have a specific beneficial effect on pain, and has been specifically demonstrated to prevent scarring and adhesions while improving cartilage nutrition (Gelberman et al., 1986). This may be done initially through passive, and later through active, means (Akeson, Amiel, Woo, 1980; Salter, Field, 1961; Noyes, 1977). Development of supernormal strength and endurance may be of benefit in protecting the damaged or unstable joint, particularly when complete return of normal architecture can no longer be anticipated.

This discussion was meant to be just a brief introduction of sports medicine principles, and how they are fundamental to a functional restoration approach. In the next part, these principles, and how they are integrated into the functional restoration approach, will be reviewed in greater detail.

CHAPTER REFERENCES

Akeson W, Amiel D, Woo S: Immobility effects on synovial joints. The pathomechanics of joint contracture. Biorheology *17*:95–100, 1980.
Chaffin D, Herrin G, Keyserling W: Pre-employment strength testing: an updated position. J Occup Med *20*:403–408, 1979.

Davies G, Gould J: Trunk testing using a prototype Cybex II isokinetic stabilization system. J Orthop Sports Phys Ther *3*:164–170, 1982.

Eriksson E: Sports injuries of knee ligaments. Their diagnosis, treatment, rehabilitation and prevention. Med Sci Sports *8*:133–144, 1976.

Florence D: The chronic pain syndrome. Postgrad Med *70*:217–228, 1981.

Fordyce W, Roberts A, Sternbach, R: The behavioral management of chronic pain: a response to critics. Pain *22*:112–125, 1985.

Gatchel R, Smith D, Barnes D, Mayer T: Relationships Among Common Self-Report Measures of Pain and Disability In Chronic Back Pain Patients. Proceedings of the International Society For The Study Of The Lumbar Spine, Dallas, Texas, May 1986.

Gelberman R, Manske P, Akeson W, Woo S, Lundborg G, Amiel D: Kappa Delta Award paper: flexor tendon repair. J Orthop Res *4*:119–128, 1986.

Gould J, Davis G: Orthopaedic and Sports Physical Therapy, St. Louis, C.V. Mosby, 1985.

Haggmark T: Comparison of isometric muscle training and electrical stimulation supplementing isometric muscle training in the recovery after major knee ligament surgery. Am J Sports Med *7*:169–171, 1979.

Hoshizaki T, Massey B: Relationships of muscular endurance among specific muscle groups for continuous and intermittent static contractions. Res Quart for Exercise and Sport *57*:229–235, 1986.

Keeley J, Mayer T, Cox R, Gatchel R, Smith J, Mooney V: Quantitification of lumbar function Part 5: reliability of range-of-motion measures in the sagittal plane and *in vivo* torso rotation measurement technique. Spine *11*:31–35, 1986.

Kishino N, Mayer T, Gatchel R, Parrish M, Anderson C, Gustin L, Mooney V: Quantification of lumbar 4: isometric and isokinetic lifting simulation in normal subjects and low back dysfunction patients. Spine *10*:921–927, 1985.

Mayer T: Lumbar Spine Assessment: In Assessment of Musculoskeletal Function (Ed. V. Mooney) Philadelphia, J.B. Lippincott Co, (in press).

Mayer T: Quantifying Postoperative Functional Capacity Deficits Utilizing Novel Technology. Proceedings of the International Society For The Study Of The Lumbar Spine, Dallas, Texas, May, 1986.

Mayer T: A Two-Year Follow-up Study of Functional Restoration In Industrial Back Pain Patients Utilizing Physical Capacity Quantification Technology. Proceedings of the International Society For The Study Of The Lumbar Spine, Dallas, Texas, May, 1986.

Mayer T, Gatchel R, Kishino N, Keeley J, Capra P, Mayer H, Barnett J, Mooney V: Objective assessment of spine function following industrial injury: a prospective study with comparison group and one-year follow-up. Volvo Award In Clinical Sciences, 1985. Spine *10*:482–493, 1985.

Mayer T. Kishino N, Keeley J, Mayer S, Mooney V: Using physical measurements to assess low back pain. J Musc Med *2*:44–59, 1985.

Mayer T, Smith S, Keeley J, Mooney V: Quantification of lumbar function Part 2: Sagittal plane trunk strength in chronic low back pain patients. Spine *10*:765–772, 1985.

Montgomery J, Steadman J: Rehabilitation of the injured knee. Clin Sports Med *4*:333–343, 1985.

Noyes F: Functional properties of knee ligaments and alterations induced by immobilization. Clin Orthop *123*:210–242, 1977.

Pearcy M: Measurement of back and spinal mobility. Clin Biomech *1*:44–51, 1986.

Ruben C: Osteoregulatory Mechanism . . . Kappa Delta Award in Transactions of Annual Meeting, American Academy of Orthopedic Surgeons, New Orleans, LA, 1985.

Salter R, Field P: The effects of continuous compression on living articular cartilage. An experimental study. J Bone Joint Surg *43*B:376–386, 1961.

Smith S, Mayer T, Gatchel R, Becker T: Quantification of lumbar function Part 1: isometric and multispeed isokinetic trunk strength measures in sagittal and axial planes in normal subject patients. Spine *10*:757–764, 1985.

Thompson N, Gould J, Davies G, Ross D, Price S: Descriptive measures of isokinetic trunk testing. J Orthop Sports Phys Ther *7*:43–49, 1985.

Turk D, Meichenbaum D, Genest M: Pain and Behavioral Medicine: A Cognitive-Behavioral Perspective. New York, Gilford Press, 1983.

Part II

Objective Quantification of Lumbar Function: The New Technology

Chapter 8

Quantitative Lumbar Spine Assessment to Address the Deconditioning Syndrome

The recognition of the deconditioning syndrome as an important factor in low back disability is quite recent and is one of the central concepts of this text. Physiologic and psychologic deconditioning have been discussed in Chapter 7, and have been well understood as the primary pathologic determinants of sports medicine rehabilitation for more than 25 years. Yet, prior to development of a variety of physical capacity measurements of the lumbopelvic functional unit, relatively little training has taken place to address this syndrome. In retrospect, quite obviously, this is due to the absence of visual feedback to structural components of the back, and the concomitant necessity of relying solely on patient self-report to guide treatment. Such habits are difficult to extinguish, and the transition to reliance on measurement technology to guide treatment in low back care is just beginning. Physicians, whose clinical judgments have been based only on what they can see directly, or what they are told, still continue to make subjective judgments of disability, support passive rather than active care, and continue to apply unqualified or misguided principles such as "If it hurts, let it rest indefinitely."

As we have discussed, the *deconditioning syndrome* refers to the loss of physical functional capacity, which is responsible for maintaining the organic component of disability in most chronic spine patients. There is increasing documentation of this relationship available in the literature, specifically regarding measurement of range of motion (Keeley, Mayer, Cox, Gatchel, Smith, Mooney, 1986; Mayer, Kishino, Keeley, Mayer, Mooney, 1985; Mayer, Tencer, Kristofferson, Mooney, 1984; Pearcy, 1986), trunk strength in sagittal and axial planes (Davies, Gould, 1982; Mayer, Smith, Keeley, Mooney, 1985; Mayer, Smith, Konraske, Gatchel, Carmichael, Mooney, 1985; Smith, Mayer, Gatchel, Becker, 1985; Thompson, Gould, Davies, Rose, Price, 1985), aerobic capacity (Mayer, 1987), and functional task performance such as lifting and bending (Chaffin, Herrin, Keyserling, 1979; Kishino, Mayer, Gatchel, Parrish, Anderson, Gustin, Mooney, 1985; Mayer, Kishino, 1985; Ayoub, Mital, Bakken, Asfour, Bethea, 1980). In this chapter, we will review the philosophy behind this objective measurement of physical functional capacity, and its recent development.

WHAT IS FUNCTIONAL CAPACITY EVALUATION?

Many terms encompass this form of physical evaluation. For the purposes of this text, it is the measurement of function quantitatively, by direct or indirect means, of a dynamic aspect of bodily activity necessary in daily living. It does not mean the measurement of *pain* which presently implies a subjective response to peripheral or central nervous system stimuli, producing a patient's verbalization of discomfort. Neither does it imply an anatomic description, such as whether a disc is protruding into the spinal canal or whether the spinal canal is stenotic. An x ray or magnetic resonance image would *not* be included as a test of functional capacity, while the physiologic measure of electromyographic change over time might be included under certain circumstances.

In essence, then, functional capacity evaluation involves the examination of the human body, including external physical examination, direct physiologic measurement such as pulse and blood pressure, as well as indirect measures for trunk strength and mobility. Blood tests for changes in certain metabolites under varying physical conditions might also be encompassed.

The testing of functional capacity can be anatomically subdivided into two groups of tests. Some tests examine certain isolated parts of the body or "functional units" such as the lumbar region. Others measure the ability of the functional unit to interact with, or be substituted for, alternative body functional units (we discussed the concept of functional units in Chapter 5). An example of the latter type of test would be a measurement of lifting capacity, which involves the interplay of a biomechanical chain (transferring forces from the hands through the upper extremity functional unit, to shoulder girdle, lumbar spine and lower extremity functional unit until the forces are transmitted to the ground at foot/floor contact). The spine, in lifting, serves as a segmented crane to allow movement from various heights and distances with a certain radius. After the load is placed into stable position, the "crane" can become a "forklift" carrying the object through the spine-driven locomotion system. The lumbopelvic functional unit is the critical component in both of these important human physical demands (Figs. 8–1 and 8–2).

The human mind can acquire and process only a limited number of dynamic

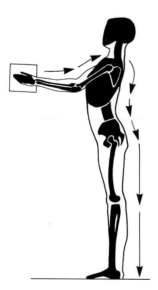
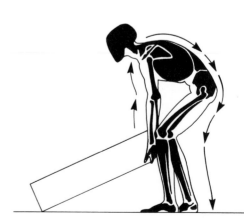

Fig. 8–1.   The "biomechanical chain" by which loads are transmitted from hands within a certain bodily radius to a stable foot/floor contact.

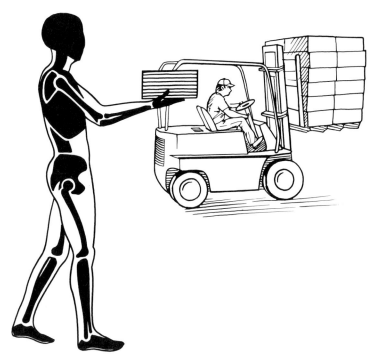

Fig. 8–2. The human as "forklift," maintaining objects in a stable position by using the human locomotion system.

variables at a time. For this reason, it is essential to select the functional parameters of greatest importance in defining the action of each functional unit. For instance, in describing the functional capacity of the hand, one must choose those parameters which most specifically describe its manipulative skill such as pinch or grasp. In the lumbopelvic functional unit, however, we must recognize that we have a weight-bearing structure with several purposes, including: (1) maintaining an upright posture; (2) protecting neurovascular elements traveling to lower extremities; (3) providing adequate space and stability for reproductive organs as well as abdominal and retroperitoneal contents; (4) providing the "spinal engine for locomotion" (Gracovetsky, Farfan, 1986); (5) supporting the upper extremities while bending, thus extending the reach of manual manipulation range.

Broadly speaking, the performance elements that lead to a reasonably complete functional assessment of the isolated lumbopelvic functional unit are: neurologic capacity, stability, flexibility, strength, and endurance. In addition, measures which quantify the lumbopelvic functional unit's ability to coordinate with other functional units to perform whole body tasks such as the capacity for lifting, bending, walking, and carrying, would also provide desirable information.

IMPORTANT COMPONENTS OF FUNCTIONAL CAPACITY EVALUATION

In making a determination of what to include in the evaluation of function, finding the most desirable measures is only one part of the process. One must then find a technique for providing accurate information and standardize the technique. For example, a simple, direct measure of cardiac output may be highly desirable, but the absence of a simple measure and the availablity of easy pulse and blood pressure measures have made a direct cardiac output measure less of a necessity. In some cases, however, it is worthwhile to take the trouble to obtain more sophisticated, direct measures to complement the simple ones.

In the lumbar spine, unlike most of the rest of the musculoskeletal system, right/left segmentation is incomplete and thus does not allow for intra-individual comparison from a normal side to an abnormal contralateral side. This leads to one of the first critical principles of functional capacity evaluation in the lumbopelvic region: a normal database is necessary for each functional capacity measure, since only inter-individual comparisons are possible. In this way, lumbar spine assessment is more akin to cardiovascular assessment than it is to extremity musculoskeletal assessment.

Beside the absence of a contralateral side, there is a second striking similarity between lumbosacral and cardiovascular assessment. This involves the often clinically unrecognized fact that, like the internal organs, there is little visual feedback to lumbar spine function. To appreciate this, the clinician must only observe the lack of accessibility to spinal motion segments whereas visual feedback is taken for granted in the extremities when palpating tender areas, taking simple joint goniometric measurements, or testing for stability. Similarly, simple extremity muscle assessment through circumferential measures, and comparison with the contralateral side, are not possible in the spine. This lack of visual feedback, without even the benefit of palpation feedback as in the cardiovascular system, has made functional capacity assessment of the lumbopelvic region one of the most difficult, and thus primitive, in medicine.

FACTORS IMPEDING EMERGENCE OF LUMBAR SPINE ASSESSMENT TECHNOLOGY

Two factors have thwarted the emergence of lumbar spine assessment technology. The first is the very mundane nature of low back pain. Since it is not life-threatening, back pain languished in medical disinterest as one of the minor, temporary ills to be tolerated by the working man. The least powerful elements of society were the ones forced to rely on a "strong back." Leisure time was less available or strenuously utilized by a middle class with a shorter lifespan than we know today. It is only as our average lifespans have soared into the 70s that quality-of-life issues have begun to supersede mortality issues. In addition, the high prevalence, financial and social cost, and loss of societal productivity through low back pain have also helped bring this problem to greater medical attention.

The second factor blocking emergence of low back functional assessment was, paradoxically, the discovery of the surgical disc lesion by Mixter and Barr (1934). Because of the unique proximity of nervous structures to musculoskeletal elements in the lumbar spine, a soft tissue injury to disc contents could produce severe disruption of extremity and bowel/bladder function. This discovery, like that of the symptoms associated with disruption of knee meniscus, led to a large number of successful surgical procedures to relieve nerve root compression over the ensuing 50 years. As might be expected, this success led to an overwhelming emphasis on surgical treatment of this disorder, as well as the imaging techniques necessary to document it. Less noted by the enthusiasts, however, was the fact that in correcting the nerve root compression, more damage was done to the lumbar spine than if no intervention had taken place at all; that is, bone and posterior ligament complexes are disrupted asymmetrically, facet joints may be invaded, scar is left perineurally and in the neuroforamen, and the disc structure is variably injured by incising and blindly removing large amounts of central disc material. In fact, overexuberant curetting may perforate the vertebral end-plate, resulting in permanent invasion of the disc space by vertebral neurovascular elements. Since back symptoms may also be improved postoperatively, or at least be of secondary importance to the relief of leg pain, these anatomic alterations may not be of substantial interest to the surgeon, who perceives them as unrelated to symptoms.

Thus, due mostly to the success of the disc operation in resolving leg pain and neurologic deficits, the surgical community sought, and continues to seek, ever more sophisticated means for imaging the spinal structures to demonstrate the structural (presumably pain-producing) lesion that can be surgically altered. The imaging techniques have evolved from simple x ray and oil-based myelography to CT scanning and water-soluble myelography. Now, MRI and three-dimensional CT scan reconstructions are becoming commonplace. Yet, while the cost effectiveness of these tests is rarely questioned, and despite misperceptions rampant in both the medical and lay communities, they are *only* capable of finding what is to be operated on, *not* "what is wrong." The inescapable conclusion is that tremendous cost and effort are exerted by the surgical community to find the small percentage of low back pain patients requiring surgical intervention, while the vast majority are left to a variety of therapies. These may include chiropractic, physical therapy modalities, or even psychotherapy, all of which are currently almost invariably applied without a structural anatomic or functional diagnosis. In most cases, the treatments are palliative at best. In some, it appears that a variety of socioeconomic factors have predisposed the medical community to ignore assessment of low back physical functional capacity, and its obvious utility in guiding therapeutics, at least until recently.

Anyone having spent long hours with partially or totally disabled chronic back pain sufferers (reportedly about 3% of the population of most industrialized countries) cannot help but observe the inactivity and disuse to which these individuals subject their spines, if not their bodies. More often than not, this is done with the advice and consent of treating physicians, therapists, and alternate professionals, most of whom subscribe to the principle "If it hurts, don't do it." Personal experience made this situation tellingly clear to the authors, and over several years led many members of a University of Texas Southwestern Medical Center research team in efforts to quantify physical functional capacity. In this way, they sought to develop a more rational approach to identifying physical deficits and rehabilitating these patients. The first step in this process was to develop a normative database of physical functional capacity for the various functional measures to use in objectively evaluating these deficits.

NORMATIVE DATABASE, EFFORT FACTOR, AND DATA DISPLAY

Measurement of physical capacity in the lumbar spine imposes test demands not usually encountered in the extremities. To reiterate, non-bilaterality implies that use of intra-individual controls, long utilized in the extremities, must be replaced by a reliance on a large *inter-individual normative database* in the spine. It also has become empirically evident that such databases must be made specific for gender and age. Furthermore, tests of muscular performance (i.e., trunk strength or lifting capacity) can have reduced population variability if normalized to body weight, and, in some instances, to the Davenport Index. Ultimately, databases may become large enough to relate anticipated physical capacities to the ergonomic demands of a specific job. A clinical example of a functional capacity evaluation utilizing physical measurement technology is shown in Figure 8–3.

In developing such a database, it became obvious that, because there are no intra-individual controls, an "effort factor" must be identified for each test. Terminology may be confusing, though, and the reader must understand that limitations of effort are only infrequently the result of conscious attempts by a patient to defraud the examiner and misrepresent his or her true abilities. They usually result, at least on initial testing, from pain, fear of injury and neuromuscular inhibition. Patients usually have been conditioned by personal experience, as well as advice from friends and physicians, that "If it hurts, don't do it." This results in a vicious cycle of overprotectiveness, leading to additional disuse, and resultant susceptibility to recurrent injury with minimal additional trauma, until a steady state is reached at low activity tolerance. The effort factor, together with a variety of psychologic tests and patient self-report measures, identifies the cognitive and psychosocial barriers to function. The clinician's recognition of suboptimal effort helps direct subsequent interventions to a greater emphasis on education and counseling. It also identifies the degree to which the testing has been invalidated, and shows the clinician that a higher degree of physical performance than was demonstrated may be expected from this individual on subsequent testing.

The range-of-motion effort factor has been clearly delineated in other publications (Keeley, Mayer, Cox, Gatchel, Smith, Mooney, 1986; Mayer, Kishino, Keeley, Mayer, Mooney, 1985). Endurance tests can usually be calibrated for effort by use of a target heart rate (with notable exceptions, such as intercurrent cardiovascular disease or use of rate-limiting medications). Reaching the target heart rate in bicycle ergometry, upper body ergometry, or psychophysical lifting tests indicates that the patient has high motivation in achieving his or her ultimate work performance level. From this point on, the patient is usually able to continue reaching the target heart rate as reconditioning leads to achievement of progressively higher work rates.

Dynamic strength testing (sagittal and axial trunk strength and isokinetic lifting) permits identification of another effort factor. This factor is related to the empirical observation that only a maximum voluntary contraction (MVC) is truly reproducible through multiple trials. It has already been established in several studies that reproducibility of isometric lifting tasks (multiple functional units in a single dimension) leads to measurement precision of better than 10%. However, conscious suboptimal performance attempting to duplicate similar tasks results in variances above 20% (Carlsoo, 1986). Though isometric testing may provide for comparison of peak forces, a dynamic test gives a curve of force versus distance, which allows for improved characterization of function through comparison of curve shape and work integral (or area beneath the

This patient underwent a Quantitative Impairment Evaluation which is a battery of tests of spinal physical functional capacity. This information may be used to determine medical impairment of function. % Normal ratings are based on a limited clinical sample: a large standardized normative database is being assembled and constantly updated.

Test Date	1/12/87		2/6/87	
I SELF-REPORT SCORES				
1. Back Depression Inventory	18		5	
2. Pain Drawing				
a. Intensity Score	9/10		7/10	
b. Trunk	10/72		3/72	
c. Extremities	9/136		10/136	
3. Dallas Analog Score	104/150		78/150	
4. Oswestry Rating	42%		18%	
II. PHYSICAL CAPACITY				
1. PHYSICAL STATUS	RIGHT/LEFT		RIGHT/LEFT	
a. Neurological Deficit	Negative/Negative		Negative/Negative	
b. FABER	Negative/Positive		Negative/Positive	
c. Spasm	Negative/Negative		Negative/Negative	
2. DEFORMITIES/POSTURE	RIGHT/LEFT		RIGHT/LEFT	
a. Surgical Scar	Yes		Yes	
3. RANGE-OF-MOTION	DEGREES	% NORMAL	DEGREES	% NORMAL
a Sagittal				
1. Gross Motion F/E	70(MoD)/25(MoD)	58/56	120(NL)/30(MoD)	100/67
2. True Lumbar (T12-S1 only) F/E	40(MoD)/15(MoD)	62/50	55(MiD)/20(MoD)	85/67
3. Hip Motion F/E	30(MoD)/10(MoD)	55/67	65(NL)/10(MoD)	118/67
4. Straight Leg Raise R/L	75(NL)/70(Ad)	100/93	80(NL)/80(NL)	107/107
5. True Spine/Hip Flex Ratio	133% Borderline: Possible true lumbar flexion deficit		85% Abnormal: True spine flexion deficit	
4. TRUNK STRENGTH (CYBEX)				
a. Isokinetic Sagittal Peak	TORQUE(ft-lb)	% NORMAL	TORQUE(ft-lb)	% NORMAL
1. 60°/second F/E	151(MiD)/148(MoD)	77/58	183(Ad)/253(Ad)	91/96
2. 120°/second F/E	196(NL)/146(MoD)	100/61	172(MiD)/212(MiD)	85/87
3. 150°/second F/E	223(NL)/141(MoD)	116/65	170(MiD)/218(Ad)	86/98
4. F/E Ratios (60°/120°/150°)	102%/134%/158%	(Abn)/(Abn)/(Abn)	72%/81%/78%	(NL)/(Abn)/(NL)
5. High Speed Dropoff (120°/60°)	129%/99%	(NL)/(NL)	94%/84%	(Abn)/(Abn)
b. Isokinetic Axial	TORQUE(ft-lb)	% NORMAL	TORQUE(ft-lb)	% NORMAL
1. 60°/second R/L	78(SeD)/61(SeD)	45/29	115(MoD)/106(SeD)	64/49
2. 120°/second R/L	69(SeD)/39(SeD)	40/20	104(MoD)/95(SeD)	58/47
3. 180°/second R/L	53(SeD)/34(SeD)	37/22	101(MoD)/90(MoD)	68/56
4. R/L Ratios (60°/120°/180°)	129%/177%/158%	(Abn)/(Abn)/(Abn)	109%/110%/112%	(Abn)/(Abn)/(Abn)
5. High Speed Dropoff (180°/60°)	68%/43%	(NL)/(NL)	87%/78%	(Abn)/(Abn)

	BICYCLE ERGOMETRY	UPPER BODY ERGOMETRY	BICYCLE ERGOMETRY	UPPER BODY ERGOMETRY
5. CARDIOVASCULAR ENDURANCE				
a. Target Heart Rate (BPM)	162	162	162	162
b. Work Rate (KGM)	700(MoD)	600(MoD)	900(NL)	900(NL)
c. Endurance Time	8	6	12	12
d. Heart Rate Achieved	140	144	162	162
e. Effort Factor	Fair	Fair	Excellent	Excellent

	FLOOR-WAIST	WAIST-OVERHEAD	FLOOR-WAIST	WAIST-OVERHEAD
6. LIFTING CAPACITY				
a. Frequent Lifting Capacity				
1. Weight Lifted (lbs.)	23	23	73	73
2. Force/Body Weight	13(SeD)	13(SeD)	40(MiD)	29(MiD)
3. Endurance Time	60	60	140	120
4. Heart Rate Achieved	120	120	160	160
5. Effort Factor	Poor	Fair	Good	Good

b. Dynamic Isokinetic Lift (Cybex)	MAX. FORCE (lbs.)	% NORMAL	MAX. FORCE (lbs.)	% NORMAL
1. Lumbar (0–4 ft.)				
a. 18″/second	37	17(SeD)	270	123(NL+)
b. 30″/second	39	19(SeD)	240	114(NL)
c. 36″/second	38	19(SeD)	230	114(NL)

7. GLOBAL EFFORT RATING			7. GLOBAL EFFORT RATING	
a. Physical Therapy	Fair		a. Physical Therapy	Excellent
b. Occupational Therapy	Poor		b. Occupational Therapy	Excellent

8. CUMULATIVE TEST SCORE				
Performance This Test EXCELLENT	Performance Last Test FAIR		Performance Initial Test FAIR	

SUMMARY

Fig. 8–3. Quantitative evaluation of physical functional capacity. A lumbar quantitative functional evaluation (QFE) report from the Productive Rehabilitation Institute of Dallas for Ergonomics (PRIDE) demonstrates patient results in quantified self-report, range of motion, trunk strength, and aerobic and lifting capacities. Normal databases are utilized to calculate a "% normal" based on the mean scores of the specific test group. Symbols categorize the degree of physical deficit into simplified groupings. NL = normal; Ad = adequate; Abn = abnormal; MiD = mildly deficient; MoD = moderately deficient; SeD = severely deficient.

curve). In time, it should be possible to provide a normal database of "acceptable variability" between trials with regard to peak forces, curve shape or work performance, leading to a fully quantified "strength effort factor."

Finally, a variety of quantified psychosocial tests and self-report measures are combined (Capra, Mayer, Gatchel, 1985) to give a comprehensive view of other potential barriers to functional recovery. Armed with this information, including repeated self-report testing of patient pain/disability/depression at scheduled intervals, the psychologic counselor can become a potent force in advising the physical treatment team, and in supporting the patient through the functional restoration program. In turn, effort factors, if not improving with education and training, alert the counselor to those individuals most in need of their intervention.

PHYSICAL CAPACITY MEASUREMENT TECHNOLOGY

In developing a normative database, the measurement technology used in collecting it becomes an important issue. In subsequent chapters we will discuss the specific techniques used to measure physical capacity in the lumbopelvic functional unit. This will be added to data on psychosocioeconomic function to provide a true assessment based on a combination of measures. The word assessment implies an *interpretation* has been made to guide the treatment approach, based on a series of *valid and relevant* observations that comprise the assessment. At this point in time, just at the dawning of recognition of the importance of measurements of spine function, there is considerable controversy regarding a number of competing technologies emerging to dominate the vast area of spine rehabilitation. The devices often have overlapping functions, variable accuracy of measurement, and no standardization whatsoever. Comparison between one database and another is currently impossible.

Though many claims are made in the highly competitive marketplace, the reader must carefully assess the rapidly changing technology to answer several questions (Table 8–1):

1. Is the test truly objective, with observations unaffected by patient effort, or, at least, with a mechanism for identifying or controlling for patient effort?
2. Has the test demonstrated its accuracy and reproducibility for measuring the specific function it purports to measure?
3. Is the functional characteristic measured *relevant* to the back disability process, or does it reflect extraneous information?
4. Has a sufficiently large normal database been provided to make meaningful statements concerning the deviation from "normal?"

Table 8–1. Critical Factors in Evaluating Physical Capacity Measurement Technology

Validity/Accuracy
Reproducibility/Reliability
Relevance
Effort factor
Normative database

5. Has the normal database been sufficiently refined to reflect specific phys- ical, ergonomic demands of a job, daily living activity, or sport?

6. Has the test been shown to have predictive value in a prospective study for injury or recurrence?

The answers to these questions will determine the usefulness of physical capacity measures to the clinician for purposes of defining capabilities and disability and guiding the rehabilitation approach. Such information is also useful to psychologically reassure the fearful or concerned patient, and to demonstrate progress to both the patient and the clinician through a rehabil- itation program. The techniques and devices discussed in subsequent chapters represent one of the first attempts to codify such methodologies, but it will certainly not be the last. In our rapidly changing technologic world, new devices are being introduced even as this book goes to press, and the astute clinician must be careful to utilize the principles enumerated above to discern the "wheat from the chaff."

CHAPTER REFERENCES

Ayoub M, Mital A, Bakken G, Asfour S, Bethea N: Development of strength and capacity norms for manual materials handling activities. The state-of-the-art. Human Factors *22*:271–283, 1980.

Capra P, Mayer T, Gatchel R: Adding psychological scales to your back pain assessment. J Musc Med *2*:41–52, 1985.

Carlsoo S: With what degree of precision can voluntary static muscle force be repeated? Scand J Rehab Med *18*:1–3, 1986.

Chaffin D, Herrin G, Keyserling W: Pre-employment strength testing: an updated position. J Occup Med *20*:403–408, 1979.

Davies G, Gould J: Trunk testing using a prototype Cybex II isokinetic stabilization system. J Orthop Sports Phys Ther *3*:164–170, 1982.

Fordyce W, Roberts A, Sternbach, R: The behavioral management of chronic pain: a response to critics. Pain *22*:112–125, 1985.

Gracovetsky S, Farfan H: The optimum spine. Spine *11*:543–573, 1986.

Keeley J, Mayer T, Cox R, Gatchel R, Smith J, Mooney V: Quantification of function 5: reliability range of motion measures in the sagittal plane and *in vivo* torso rotation measurement tech- nique. Spine *11*:31–35, 1986.

Kishino N, Mayer T, Gatchel R, Parrish M, Anderson C, Gustin L, Mooney V: Quantification of lumbar 4: isometric and isokinetic lifting simulation in normal subjects and low back dys- function patients. Spine *10*:921–927, 1985.

Mayer T, Kishino N, Keeley J, Mayer S. Mooney V: Using physical measurements to assess low back pain. J Musc Med *2*:44–59, 1985.

Mayer T, Smith S, Keeley J, Mooney V: Quantification Of Lumbar Function Part 2: Sagittal plane trunk strength in chronic low back pain patients. Spine *10*:765–772, 1985.

Mayer T, Smith S, Kondraske G, Gatchel R, Carmichael T, Mooney V: Quantification of function Part 3: preliminary data on isokinetic torso rotation testing with myoelectric spectral analysis in normal and low back pain subjects. Spine *10*:912–920, 1985.

Mayer T, Tencer A, Kristofferson S, Mooney V: Use of noninvasive techniques for quantification of spinal range-of-motion in normal subjects and chronic low-back dysfunction patients. Spine *9*:588–595, 1984.

Mixter W, Barr J: Rupture of the intervertebral disc with involvement of the spinal canal. N Engl J Med *211*:210, 1934.

Pearcy M: Measurement of back and spinal mobility. Clin Biomech *1*:44–51, 1986.

Smith S, Mayer T, Gatchel R, Becker T: Quantification of lumbar function Part 1: isometric and multispeed isokinetic trunk strength measures in sagittal and axial planes in normal subject patients. Spine *10*:757–764, 1985.

Thompson N, Gould J, Davies G, Ross D, Price S: Descriptive measures of isokinetic trunk testing. J Orthop Sports Phys Ther *7*:43–49, 1985.

Chapter 9

Objective Measurement of Spinal Joint Function

The measurement of spine joint mobility and stability will be considered in this chapter. Such tests of range of motion are of vital importance to extremity function. The adverse impact on the ability to perform tasks in the extremities caused by contracture or ankylosis has long been recognized. In judging the desirability of surgical fusion for pain, the price to be paid in terms of mobility loss at the involved segment and its impact on adjacent joints is always carefully assessed. The goal of a large portion of the therapist's efforts is the restoration, through active or passive means, of joint flexibility. The absence of joint mobility is considered, by the American Medical Association guidelines, to be the only physical examination criterion required for assessment of impairment, and the simple goniometer as the only necessary instrument (AMA, 1983).

Yet, until recently, the assessment of spinal mobility, as displayed in publications produced both by the American Medical Association and the American Academy of Orthopedic Surgeons, has remained crude and inaccurate. Their method uses a simple plastic goniometer, which is commonly and effectively used for extremity measures, to assess multi-joint function of up to 24 spinal segments plus the hips. However, a more complex technique than the method currently described in AMA and AAOS literature is required (Fig. 9–1). Simple angular tests have actually provided a disservice because they not only have produced inaccurate measurements leading to erroneous conclusions for many years, but also have prejudiced the current generation of clinicians. Obtaining physicians' interest in new techniques for spine measurement, or demonstrating its relevance to a skeptical audience, is an extremely difficult task. In this chapter, after reviewing some of the traditional evaluation techniques, we will present the newer techniques for such measurement.

RANGE-OF-MOTION MEASURES

Goniometric Measurements

The simple goniometric measurements that have been utilized under current guidelines assume that a patient is standing vertically erect in a "neutral" or "zero" position, and then bending from this position in coronal and sagittal planes with knees locked. One arm of the goniometer is maintained in the vertical position while the upper arm is visually "aimed" along the spine, either at C7 or at the thoracolumbar junction, depending on which segments are to be measured. Unfortunately, this method suffers from many difficulties, including: (1) in the erect position, the angulation of T12-L1 is not truly vertical;

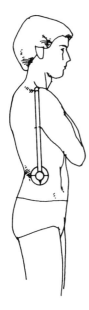

Fig. 9–1. A and B, Spine flexion and extension as measured by AMA and AAOS techniques. (A reproduced with permission from Guides to the Evaluation of Permanent Impairment, 2nd Edition, Chicago, Illinois, American Medical Association, 1984, p. 53. B reproduced with permission from Joint Motion—Method of Measuring and Recording. Park Ridge, Illinois, American Academy of Orthopaedic Surgeons, 1965, p. 53. The information found in this publication is presently being revised and updated by the American Academy of Orthopaedic Surgeons.)

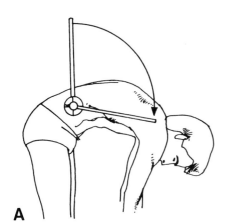

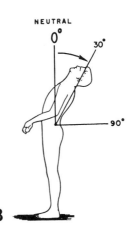

A   **B**

(2) hip range of motion is not considered and therefore not separated from true lumbar spine motion; (3) there is no way for the examiner to sight the angle of the upper arm accurately or reproducibly; (4) attempts are not usually made to mark the T12-L1 interspace, producing additional variability in positioning of the upper arms; (5) there is no "effort factor" to assess patient motivation in performing the test. These difficulties make the simple goniometric technique, though it is the most widely performed, of low validity in terms of accuracy and repeatability. For this reason, recommendations for its abandonment have been widespread (Moll, Wright, 1976).

"Fingertip to Floor" Method

Two other motion quantification techniques measure only sagittal flexion. The first is the "fingertip to floor" method. The patient bends in an identical manner as in the 2-piece goniometric method, but the distance between the fingertips and the floor is measured. This method has all of the inherent inaccuracies of the goniometric measures, with the added difficulty that variability in arm length makes it impossible to develop population standards for this distance. This test remains popular because of its simplicity. However, because it is hopelessly inaccurate, it misleads the examiner into believing he or she has a valid measure of spinal movement. This is clearly not the case. This method, too, deserves an "early retirement."

Tape Measure Method

The tape measure method of Schöber (Schöber, 1937) has been modified by several authors. In the most recent form described by MacRae and Wright (McRae, Wright, 1969), a mark is made (presumed without verification to be at the lumbosacral junction), at a midline point along the line connecting the "dimples of Venus." Additional marks are made 5 cm below and 10 cm above, with the patient in the erect position. With forward flexion, the distraction between the most superior and inferior points is measured, with the increase in the original 15 cm length being calculated. In this method, relatively minimal equipment is necessary, and the tests can be performed quickly. It has the advantage of eliminating the hip motion component, but it sacrifices the ability to measure extension or coronal bend. The absence of any hip motion measure, when it is usually the largest component to forward flexion, eliminates considerable information.

Test accuracy is controversial with this method, and no effort factor can be identified (MacRae, Wright, 1969; Reynolds, 1975). Furthermore, test relevance is questionable because of the arbitrary choice of measurement length and anatomic reference point. The "dimples of Venus" may be so large that a decision to standardize the horizontal line at either upper or lower borders of the dimples may result in addition or deletion of the mobility of an entire segment. Alternatively, the dimples may be completely absent to visual inspection in 20 to 35% of subject populations. The modified Schöber technique, usually based on identifying the lumbosacral junction, depends greatly on the clinical skills of the examiner, and may also produce at least a 1-segment error, particularly in a postoperative patient with lower lumbar hypomobility. In a small subject, if the horizontal line is drawn at the upper border of the "dimples of Venus," the technique might actually include 4 or 5 lumbar segments. Conversely, in a tall individual, in whom a low transverse line is chosen, it is possible to include only 1 or 2 segments. If this individual has a stable L4-S1 fusion, the technique may show no motion whatsoever, even if 50 degrees or more flexion is present from T12 to L4.

The Spondylometer

A device developed primarily for flexion is the *spondylometer,* which is a type of protractor with a multi-angled arm for measuring thoracolumbar spine mobility between C7 and the sacrum. Here too, the readings are misleading, since the angle measured on the protractor does not necessarily duplicate the actual flexion developed through the thoracolumbar spine. Variability is large, hip motion is excluded, and effort cannot be assessed. The device is also relatively large and somewhat cumbersome to use.

Flexicurves

Flexicurves are draftsmen's devices that can also be made to conform to a patient's spine. The curve shape then must be transferred to paper and tangents constructed to obtain an estimate of the angular position of the back at end-range (Anderson, Sweetman, 1975; Burton, 1986). Like the spondylometer, the device is cumbersome and measurements are time-consuming. Continuous movement cannot be monitored. However, advantages of the device are that actual angular displacement of the spine can be dependably measured, and the hip mobility can be separated from the spine mobility.

Inclinometers

Use of inclinometers involving the pendulum principle was first described by Asmussen, and further developed by Loebl and Troup (Asmussen, Heeboll-Nielsen, 1959; Loebl, 1973). Hand-held, fluid-filled inclinometers (Fig. 9–2A), available from several sources (MedDesign, Liverpool, U.K.; M.I.E. Goniometer, Leeds, U.K.), have long been used under the sponsorship of the British Back Pain Association. The technique for separating hip from true lumbar spine motion components (Mayer, Tencer, Kristofferson, Mooney, 1984) allows identification of sagittal plane factors such as: (1) motion of T12-S1 (or any multisegmental spine) component; (2) motion of hip component; (3) spine/hip ratio showing whether spine motion pattern is normal or whether physiologic contracture is present; (4) hip/straight leg raising ratio, providing an "effort factor." More sophisticated, computerized motion devices are now also commercially available (Fig. 9–2B and C).

The inclinometer is the only one of these methods universally applicable to sagittal, coronal, and even axial plane movements (Keeley, Mayer, Cox, Gatchel, Smith, Mooney, 1986). The other flexion methods developed earlier must be supplemented by special techniques such as the *plumb line pointer* used by Moll for spinal extension. The line is held at the thoracolumbar junction at the side of the trunk, while the distance in centimeters traversed by the pointer is measured as the patient extends. Several obvious criticisms arise, not the least of which are test variability, lack of precise placement, and absence of an effort factor. Furthermore, an angular motion is expressed as a translation distance, a disadvantage also associated with the Schöber distraction method. Moreover, this technique fails to separate hip from true spine motion. The spondylometer may also be used to assess extension, but not lateral bend or torsion.

Three-Dimensional Digitizer

Three-dimensional digitizers have been used in research settings for some time, but a commercial device has now been produced known as the *Metrocom* (FARO Medical Technologies Inc., Montreal, CN). While the device has other measurement capabilities, the primary feature is the 3-D digitizer incorporating an electromechanical linkage with a precise angular displacement transducer at each joint in the system. With its IBM-PC software, the free-standing device is extremely accurate, permitting tolerances of 1.5 mm over its full range of 200 cm. Reproducibility of limb-length measurements and curve tracing, as would be done in scoliosis screening, also appears accurate and reproducible in a laboratory setting. However, because the digitizer depends on *absolute*

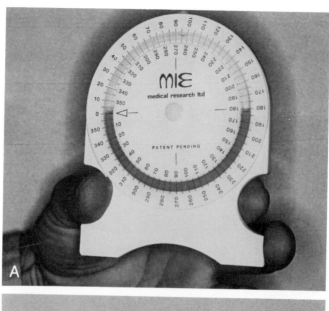

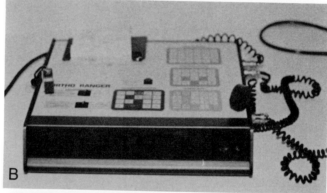

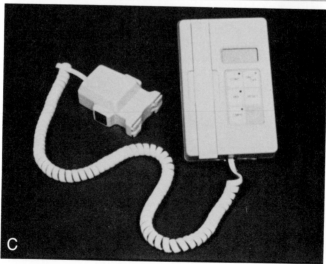

Fig. 9–2. A, Fluid-filled inclinometer. B, OrthoRanger motion measurement device (Orthotronics, Daytona Beach, FL). C, New hand-held computerized range-of-motion measuring device (EDI-320) (Cybex Inc., Ronkonkoma, NY).

orientation in space relative to its fixed base, any shift of body position in the process of changing from one position to another will produce significant error in clinical practice. This will be compounded by any difficulty the examiner may have in localizing anatomic landmarks, such as the spinous processes, in the course of running the digitizer tip down the spine. If these problems can be overcome, however, another potentially accurate and relevant spine mobility measure may become clinically available. Also on the positive side is the ability to assess limb lengths and x-ray angles. Drawbacks are high cost, equipment bulk, and the current absence of an effort factor or normative database. Actual laboratory and clinical experience with this device may alter some of these findings.

RADIOLOGIC EVALUATION

Radiologic evaluation has also been used to assess spinal range of motion. The obvious concern about x-ray exposure has been only partially addressed by development of special screens requiring less radiation. The simple flexion and extension x ray is subject to too much error due to subject positioning of the beam and slight variations of lateral bend or torsion. However, x rays have been used to confirm findings of non-invasive techniques (Mayer, Tencer, Kristofferson, Mooney, 1984).

Stereoradiography

More recently, biplanar or stereo radiographs have been used (Seligman, Gertzbein, Tile, Kapasouri, 1984). These techniques involve simultaneous x-ray exposure of the lumbar spine in a fixed position. In the biplanar, two x-ray sources are usually oriented orthogonally to give the best three-dimensional discrimination. In stereoradiogaphy, the x-ray sources are usually used while sequentially changing the film in a single x-ray plate. Angular asymmetry leads the observer to some appreciation of a three-dimensional effect. All radiographic mobility measuring methods depend on the identification of specific anatomic points on the vertebrae for orientation in each of the positions or postures assumed for each exposure. Problems are introduced by micro-motion between exposures, and x-ray landmarks are visually difficult to reproducibly identify. While radiation exposure, cost, and the need for cumbersome equipment with stabilizing frames necessary for x-ray techniques make them inapplicable for routine clinical use, considerable promise is held out for identifying segmental instability and confirming intersegmental mobility norms through its use. At this point, it seems that no noninvasive technique will discriminate intersegmental mobility at a single level.

Vector Stereography

Vector stereography requires an electromechanical device which, currently, only has limited availability. It offers three-dimensional measurements through movement of a pointer through space whose position is constantly computed from a fixed base. Three orthogonally mounted potentiometers gauge the distance moved, while a computer calculates the position in space. Variations due to the movement of the subject can be limited by attaching the entire device to the patient's back, though this introduces other disadvantages. A stablilizing frame is thus usually required as the device is sensitive to small translations of the body (Grew, Harris, 1979). The main advantage of this complex research device is the potential for measurement of dynamic movement and recording postures utilized during actual work and sports activities.

OPTICAL METHODS

A variety of optical methods for assessing range of motion also show some promise. Simple photography using skin markers has been used, often supplemented by film or videotape. In advances that parallel the development of gait analysis laboratories, complex computer-controlled video systems focusing on light emitting diodes (LEDs) or reflective markers have been used to assess spinal range of motion (Thurston, Harris, 1983). Dynamic measurements during daily living activities such as walking and carrying are promising; however, the limiting factor of accuracy continues to be due to the spatial relation of a skin contour mark to the underlying spinal segment, particularly without a firm skeletal attachment. Significant expense and inconvenience, as well as specialized equipment needs including emitters on outriggers, will make this system unavailable for general use and will tend to slow development for some time to come.

Finally, other technologies such as ultrasound or Moire fringe photography have been suggested as having potential for noninvasive measurement of spinal mobility. Their entry onto the clinical scene, however, is not expected for an extended period.

PRIDE RANGE-OF-MOTION ASSESSMENT TECHNIQUE

The technique utilized at PRIDE involves a hand-held computerized device, the EDI-320 (Cybex, Ronkonkoma, NY), which allows the separation of hip from lumbar spine mobility, and provides assessment of an "effort factor" to confirm test validity. It also allows comparison to a normal database (Fig. 9–3). The device somewhat modifies the measurement technique previously described using two inclinometers (Mayer, 1984; Keeley, Mayer, Cox, Gatchel, Smith, Mooney, 1986). Normal ranges of true spinal and hip mobility are reproduced in Table 9–1.

The EDI-320 computerized inclinometer allows a full 360-degree measurement. As such, it is contrasted to the OrthoRanger (Orthotronics, Daytona Beach, FL) whose pendulum sensor contains a "dead space" in its measurement arc. However, the latter more expensive device has dual sensor inputs, permitting simultaneous calculations of motion from two separate points. An additional feature is the presence of a printer built into the portable console, providing reports directly for clinical records.

The full-arc capability of the EDI-320 permits a "posture measurement" as a prelude to spine range-of-motion measurements. A "standardization measurement" is initially taken against a flat, vertical wall or carpenter's level to provide truly absolute, rather than relative, measurements. With the patient in the erect position, skin marks are placed over the proposed contact points of the sensor on the sacrum and thoracolumbar junction. Initial measurements taken at this point reflect actual postural inclination. During the course of testing in sagittal and coronal planes, a return to the subject's original position is required for accuracy after each measurement. Postural comparisons can also be made among subjects by measuring spinal inclination at a specific, easily

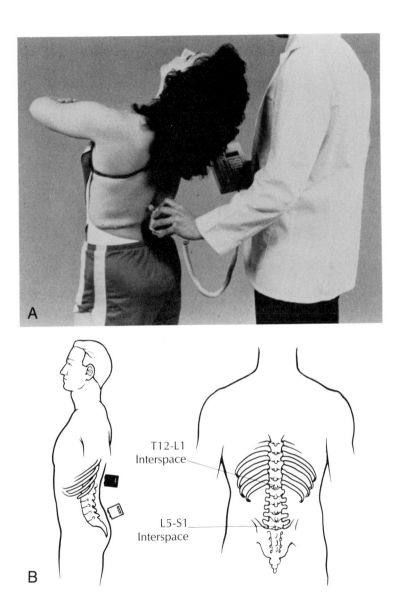

Fig. 9–3. A, The technique for utilizing the hand-held computer range-of-motion device for spine/hip mobility measurements. First, one must obtain starting reference points as compared to a vertical plane on "continuous" mode. B, Palpate the T12-L1 interspace. Place the device over the interspace and place a skin mark opposite the upper limb of the device. Similarly, place the device over the sacrum, marking opposite the upper limb.

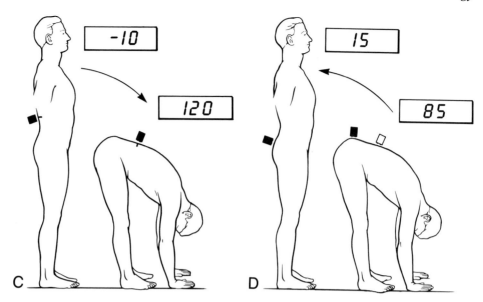

Fig. 9–3 (cont.) C, Press device to compound mode. Place the device on sacrum and press the activator. Return the device back on T12-L1; press the activator. Keeping the device on T12-L1, ask the patient to flex fully forward with knees straight and at terminal position; again trigger the activator. D, Immediately place the device opposite the original mark on the sacrum; trigger activator and ask patient to resume the erect position. Record hip and true spinal flexion readings.

identifiable anatomic landmark, such as the thoracolumbar junction or cervicothoracic junction. Since a large number of subjects can all be compared to the "standardized vertical measurement," frequent postural checks of a large group can be simply performed. The identical "continuous read-out" mode of operation, utilized for postural measurements, can also be utilized for assessing angulation of body parts on work postures, or assessing relative angles on x rays.

The identification of an effort factor to confirm test validity involves the comparison of straight leg raising to hip flexion and extension components of the test. Since hip flexion is ultimately limited by the tightest hamstring, supine straight leg raising should be closely coupled to the hip flexion component of spine mobility testing if the subject produces full effort. If the straight leg raising component is, on either side, considerably less than the hip flexion component, the patient has "consciously" restricted supine leg raising on that side. Conversely, if hip flexion is less than supine straight leg raising, which is most commonly the case, maximal bending has not been performed by the subject. When differences are large (> 30 degrees), there is no doubt that a psychophysiologic barrier to function has been identified. However, in some cases a small amount of this difference may be accounted for by the fact that the hamstring's extensibility may vary in the supine and standing positions due to the hamstring's contraction. Alternatively, the apparent straight leg raising may be artifically increased by hip extension hypermobility, in which the examiner fails to detect that the straight leg raising end-point is occurring only after the pelvis has flexed maximally to the extent of contralateral side hip extension. This is particularly likely to occur when a strong clinician examines a small and hypermobile subject.

Great discrepancies between pelvic mobility and supine leg raising should

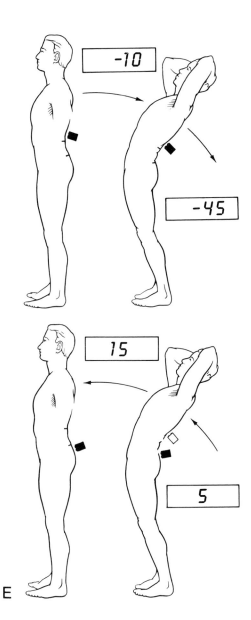

Fig. 9–3 (cont.) E, After making certain that the patient has returned to the starting reference points, repeat the sequence, with patient bending into extension, to obtain hip and true spinal extension readings.

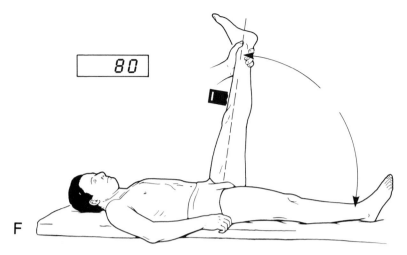

Fig. 9–3 (cont.)   F, Supine straight leg raising using the inclinometer in its continuous or reference mode requires performing the straight leg raise after triggering the activator with leg extended and reading maximum inclination with contralateral leg maintained straight.

alert the clinician to the possibility of suboptimal motivation. If this is identified, a further check on the consistency of the examination is provided by comparison of relative lumbar and pelvic measurement, the so-called "spine/hip ratio" (Fig. 9–4). In the normal subject, lumbar motion predominates, representing 60 to 70% of the gross motion component. As the midline ligaments and lumbodorsal fascia are gradually tightened, hip flexion gradually assumes a greater proportion of the total mobility until a cross-over point is reached. At this point, the spine is "hanging on its ligaments," and the lumbar spine musculature is in its "silent period." Terminal bending with knees straight is therefore almost entirely a hip flexion phenomenon. Ultimately, flexion (lumbar or gross) depends on the degree of hamstring tightness. It has been our experience that this relationship, termed the spine/hip ratio, is reproducible, although it may change with added upper body load.

In our patient population, however, initial true lumbar spine flexion represents a smaller proportion of the total mobility component. Yet, after a relatively brief intensive stretching program, the true lumbar mobility in patients can be dramatically increased, except when bony fusion or fibrous ankylosis has occurred. In a patient with true spine stiffness due to prolonged immobility causing facet capsular stiffness and ligament/fascia contractures, the pattern demonstrated in Figure 9–4 will be dramatically altered, with "reversal" of the spine/hip ratio. If this is noted in a patient, regardless of suboptimal effort demonstrated on the hip/straight leg raising (SLR) ratio, spinal dysfunction may be accurately diagnosed. Conversely, individuals with flexion limited by pain perception or poor motivation, but no organic soft tissue alteration, will likely demonstrate a normal spine/hip ratio in the presence of a decrease in the hip/SLR ratio (effort factor). Treatment strategies should be geared more to intensive stretching for the "stiff" group, and emotional support, education, and counseling for the "suboptimal effort" group.

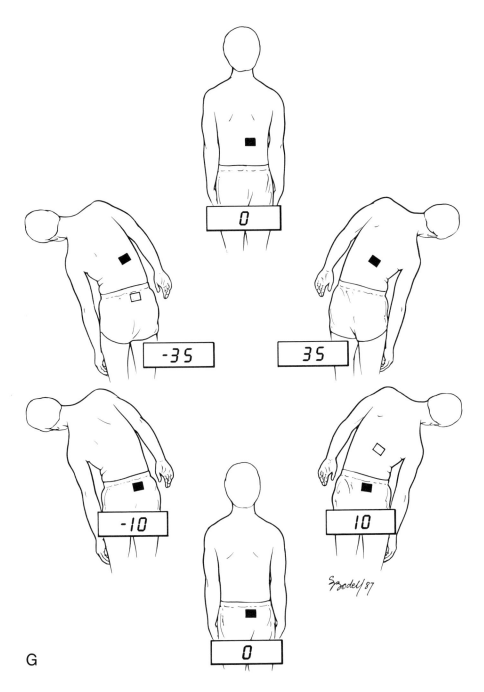

Fig. 9–3 (cont.)   G, Place device at T12-L1 level in coronal plane and repeat identical sequence to obtain true lumbar and hip right/left lateral bend mobility.

Table 9–1. Norms for True Lumbar Spine (T12–S1) and Hip Mobility Components of Compound Lumbar Spine Movements (from Keeley et al., 1985)

Motion	Mean for Normal Subjects	
	Males	Females
Gross flexion	118.6	123.2
Gross extension	40.4	41.4
Hip flexion	53.6	58.9
Hip extension	13.7	14.1
True lumbar spine Flexion (T12–S1)	65.0	64.4
True lumbar spine Extension (T12–S1)	26.6	27.3
Straight leg raise	73.6	82.9

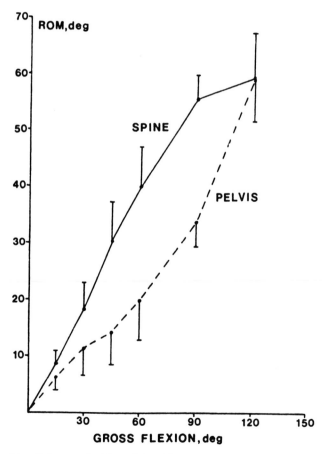

Fig. 9–4. Spine/hip ratio in normal subjects. (From Mayer, T, Tencer, A., Kristofferson, S., and Mooney, V.: Use of noninvasive techniques for quantification of spinal range-of-motion in normal subjects and chronic low-back dysfunction patients. Spine, 9:588, 1984.)

THE PROBLEM OF MEASURING SPINAL STABILITY

Joint stability may be extremely important in weight-bearing joints, in which ligament disruption may produce significant loss of function. The knee and ankle are specific, important examples. In the spine, we have a paradox in this area that typifies the difficulties of spinal assessment. While the lumbar spine does not have the ribs or a contralateral side as stabilizing structures, the three-joint complex usually provides an extremely stable intersegmental link even in pathologic cases. Even with experimental cadaveric serial ablation of stabilizing connective tissue structures, production of true segmental instability is quite difficult. Because of the small deep, inaccessible joints, no simple physical examination method for detecting segmental instability has yet emerged. Radiographic techniques for demonstration of dynamic instability are controverisal, subject to inter-observer variability, and are often not repeatable. Testing for stability is commonly done in candidates for spinal fusion, usually post-disc surgery. Performing *routine* fusion after disc surgery for presumed mechanical instability has resulted in no improvement in outcome and has been discontinued in almost all clinical settings. However, as a result of their surgery, these patients frequently develop chronic deconditioning syndromes, often brought about by prolonged immobilization and disuse. Lack of flexibility, particularly at the operated level, tends to produce abnormal stresses, encouraging hypomobility at adjacent levels (Pearcy, Portek, Shepherd, 1985; Pearcy, Shepherd, 1985; Tibrewal, Pearcy, Portek, Spivey, 1985). Disruption of stabilizing structures, such as facet capsules or midline ligaments, may occur with the original surgery, commonly leading to scar tissue that is stiffer and weaker than the original, and may produce asymmetric stresses on a contralateral, unoperated side. In this case, stability testing preceded by forced spinal manipulation or loaded bending may be expected to produce excessive strain at the "weak link" operated level. To interpret motion as segmental instability, however, even if detected, may well be unwarranted. Load transferred from hypomobile adjacent segments may alter strains in the operated level much as an oiled chain distributes loads better than a rusted one with incomplete motion of all links. Thus, until a repeatable and valid dynamic test for spinal stability becomes available, this will remain one of the most nebulous, but most interesting, areas of spinal assessment.

CHAPTER REFERENCES

American Academy of Orthopaedic Surgeons. Joint Motion—Method of Measuring and Recording. Park Ridge, Illinois, 1965.

American Medical Association Guides to the Evaluation of Permanent Impairment. Chicago, AMA, 1984.

Anderson J, Sweetman B: A combined flexi-rule/hydrogoniometer for measurement of lumbar spine and its sagittal movement. Rheumatol Rehab *14*:173–179, 1975.

Asmussen E, Heeboll-Nielsen K: Posture, mobility and strength of the back in boys, 7–16 years of age. Acta Orthop Scand *28*:174, 1959.

Burton A: Regional lumbar sagittal mobility: measurement of flexicurves. Clin Biomech *1*:20–26, 1986.

Grew N, Harris J: A method of measuring human body shape and movement—the "Vector Stereograph." Engineering Med *8*:115–118, 1979.

Keeley J, Mayer T, Cox R, Gatchel R, Smith J, Mooney V: Quantification of Lumbar Function Part 5: Reliability of range of motion measures in the sagittal plane and in *in vivo* torso rotation measurement technique. Spine *11*:31–35, 1986.

Loebl W: Measurement of spinal posture and range in spinal movements. Ann Phys Med *9*:103, 1967.

MacRae I, Wright V: Measurement of back movement. Ann Rheum Dis *28*:584, 1969.

Mayer T: Using physical measurement to assess low back pain. J Musculoskel Med *6*:44–59, 1985.

Mayer T, Tencer A, Kristofferson S, Mooney V: Use of noninvasive techniques for quantification of spinal range of motion in normal subjects and chronic low-back dysfunction patients. Spine *9*:588–595, 1984.

Moll J, Wright V: Measurement of Spinal Movement, In: The Lumbar Spine in The Back Pain Patient, Ed. J Jayson. New York, Grune & Stratton, 1976, pp. 93–112.

Pearcy M, Portek I, Shepherd J: The effect of low back pain on lumbar spinal movements measured by three-dimensional x-ray analysis. Spine *10*:150–153, 1985.

Pearcy M, Shepherd J: Is there instability in spondylolisthesis? Spine *10*:175–177, 1985.

Reynolds P: Measurement of spinal mobility: a comparison of three methods. Rheum and Rehab *14*:180–185, 1975.

Schöber P: Lendenwirbelsaule und kreuzschmerzen. Munch Med Wschr *84*:336, 1937.

Seligman J, Gertzbein S, Tile M, Kapasouri A: Computer analysis of spinal segment motion in degenerative disk disease with and without axial loading. Spine *9*:566–573, 1984.

Thurston A, Harris G: Normal kinematics of the lumbar spine and pelvis. Spine *8*:199–205, 1983.

Tibrewal S, Pearcy J, Portek I, Spivey J: A prospective study of lumbar spinal movements before and after discectomy using bi-planar radiography. Spine *10*:455–460, 1985.

Chapter 10

Objective Trunk Strength, Endurance, and Aerobic Capacity Measurements

Like range of motion, the strength of para-articular musculature has long been recognized as a critical factor in describing dynamic functional capacity of extremity joints. The loss of muscle strength, as occurs with prolonged cast immobilization or excessive rest/inactivity, particularly in weight-bearing joints, leads to loss of joint function and endurance. As a typical example, loss of thigh muscle strength after knee injuries and/or surgical procedures leads to a tendency of the knee to "buckle" in the flexed position. In addition, we note loss of stair climbing, long distance walking and running ability, and considerable risk to ligamentous structures when subjecting them to excessive strain, as in "cutting." Extremity deficits are easily noted because they are susceptible to simple visual observation of atrophy through muscle circumference measures and comparison with the contralateral side. For this reason, sports medicine programs have focused considerable therapist effort on restoring strength/endurance in the para-articular musculature as a natural part of any rehabilitation process.

In the spine, due to lack of visual feedback and a comparison side, these connections have not generally been made. While certain "wasting" neuromuscular conditions (polio, muscular dystrophy, spinal cord injury) have been recognized as causing lumbar dysfunction and increased incidence of low back pain, clinicians usually accept the relationship only when spine deformity results from gross, asymmetric loss of muscle bulk. More subtle forms of loss of trunk strength are generally not observed and therefore not taken into consideration as a cause of symptoms. While considerably more research has been done relating trunk muscle strength to low back pain (Mayer, Greenberg, 1942; Flint, 1955; Nachemson, Lindh, 1969) than relating pain to range of motion, most clinicians tend to recognize motion deficits much more rapidly as a reflection of lumbar spine dysfunction. Again, we may speculate that the lack of visual feedback and the consequent need for mechanical devices to supplement the senses for strength assessment are the reasons.

TRUNK STRENGTH TESTING

While strength measurement devices have at least a 40-year history, it is only recently that the number of publications in this area has risen dramatically (Andersson, Ortengren, Herberts, 1977; Alston, Carlson, Feldman, Grimm, Gerontinos, 1966; Cady, Bischoff, O'Connel, Thomas, Allan, 1979; Davies, Gould, 1982; Flint, 1955; Hasue, Fuguwara, Kikuchi, 1980; Langrana, Lee, Alexander, Mayott, 1984; Mayer, Greenberg, 1942; McNeill, Warwick, Andersson, Schultz, 1980; Oneidi, Petersen, Staffeldt, 1975; Smidt, Herring, Admundsen, Rogers, Russell, Lehmann, 1983; Suzuki, Endo, 1983; Thorstensson, Nilsson, 1982; Thorstensson, Arvidson, 1982). The generally utilized approach has been for individual investigators to use a strain gauge or modify a standard Cybex dynamometer (Lumex Corp., Ronkonkoma, NY) for use in trunk testing units in various positions. These include sagittal measurement devices in standing, sitting, side-lying and prone/supine positioning, thus offering a variety of starting positions, physiologically-induced motion restriction, and gravity effects (Davies, Gould, 1982; Hasue, Fuguwara, Kikuchi, 1980; Langrana, Lee, Alexander, Mayott, 1984; Smidt, Herring, Admundsen, Rogers, Russell, Lehmann, 1983; Suzuki, Endo, 1983; Thorstensson, Nilsson, 1982; Thorstensson, Arvidson, 1982). While most of these publications concerned muscle strength testing in normal individuals, the link between trunk muscle strength deficits and deconditioned chronic back pain patients has most recently been shown (Mayer, Gatchel, Kishino, Keeley, Capra, Mayer, Barnett, Mooney, 1985; Mayer, Smith, Keeley, Mooney, 1985). Thus, two critical points appear to be established: (1) trunk muscle strength is one important factor in functional capacity assessment of the lumbar spine; and (2) because of lack of visual feedback, mechanical devices to directly measure trunk strength are essential. Because strength and endurance measures require subject motivation, and the clinician lacks a validity check, an "effort factor" to assure optimal subject compliance is also necessary.

At this point we must distinguish among some terminologies in muscle function measurements. *Trunk strength* measures, as used in this chapter, will refer to those that measure the isolated functional capacity of the lumbopelvic functional unit; that is, the anatomic segment between scapulae and thighs which transmits axial forces involved in lifting and ambulation. This distinguishes trunk strength measurement from *lifting capacity* measurement, which is a whole-body technique that will be discussed separately in Chapter 11. *Strength* is a term used loosely to connote a variety of muscular functions. These include the capacity to produce *force* or *torque* (around an axis), both statically and dynamically. It also includes the ability to produce *work* (force times distance traveled) and *power* (work divided by time). *Curve shape* refers to the graphic display of the force (or torque) versus distance, or force versus time, that can be produced by most of the measurement devices. *Endurance* generally refers to the muscle's ability to perform repeated contractions or work during a specified time interval. It is generally considered the measure of muscle fatigue resistance. Additionally, the traditional tri-planar anatomic descriptions are used, with *sagittal* referring to the flexion-extension plane, *axial* to the rotary or torsional plane, and *coronal* to the lateral bending plane.

While most experimental work has been done on one-of-a-kind laboratory models, a sitting device has been duplicated for use in a few centers by one of the orignal investigators in the field (Langrana, Lee, 1984). This machine was probably the first available for multicenter testing, and utilizes a sturdy frame with the patient in the sitting position with a Cybex dynamometer linked to an Apple computer for summation of key measurements and graphic display.

As in all units employing Cybex dynamomometers, both isokinetic and iso-metric tests are available. With the patient in the sitting position, the trunk is already flexed 90 degrees through a combination of hip and true spine flexion, so that only limited additional flexion is possible. Extension can take place for at least 60 degrees, still falling short of the posturally neutral (equivalent of erect standing) position, while non-physiologic gravity effects must be taken into account. This device has the longest history of any of the commercially sold devices, though it has not been widely disseminated. It is useful purely for sagittal (flexion/extension) measurements.

SPECIFIC COMMERCIALLY AVAILABLE UNITS

Several commerical companies, having recognized the need for computerized trunk strength measurement devices, have jumped into the market place. Un-doubtedly, many others will follow. We will review the most widely used current devices in this section.

Cybex Sagittal Strength Device

The first group to be reviewed is Cybex (Lumex Corp., Ronkonkoma, NY), which has been involved in dynamic isolated joint testing since 1969. Recog-nizing that the extremely high torques and stabilization requirements for lumbar spine measurement merited a totally separate back testing system, they devel-oped a series of prototype devices. Two commercial trunk strength machines have resulted, measuring isolated sagittal and axial plane motions. Both ma-chines perform isometric and isokinetic dynamic tests, sacrificing uncon-strained physiologic motions for control of variables in order to produce valid measurements. Both devices attempt to constrain pelvic and lower extremity motion in order to isolate the spinal muscular "functional unit." In the sagittal device, this is done with a standing machine with stablization occurring across the chest between sternum and scapulae, at the pelvis across the pubis and iliac crest, and above and below the slightly flexed knees. Motion occurs through an axis set at the lumbosacral level beginning in a "posturally neutral" position, inclined backwards about 10 degrees from the erect position, and allowing motion of up to 120 degrees flexion. Isometric measurements may be taken at any point along the range of motion, and multispeed isokinetic pro-tocols are available. Gravity correction may also be selected. A computer with individual diskettes for each subject resets the original position for repeated tests, and records machine output in terms of several parameters, including peak torque, acceleration time, work, power consumption, and curve variability (as an effort measure). The computer permits data summation from multiple patients and normals to obtain appropriate databases (Fig. 10–1). Endurance and recovery protocols also permit mechanical documentation of fatigue re-sistance.

The Cybex device has been employed extensively in our facility, and we are familiar with its use and capabilities. For specific strength testing, reciprocal flexion and extension are performed over an 80-degree arc, as long as the patient is capable of combined hip/spine flexion to this degree. In practice, as discussed in Chapter 9, most unfused patients will produce spine flexion of 45 to 60 degrees before pelvic tilt through the hips becomes a major factor in flexion.

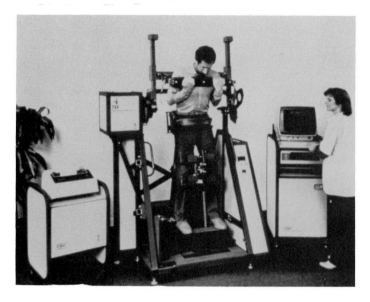

Fig. 10–1. Cybex sagittal plane measurement device. (Lumex, Ronkonkoma, NY).

In extension, patients will generally extend first and then "crane up" the rigid spine using hip extensors.

A series of computer print-outs will display some typical curve outputs produced by the device. These illustrate the printed data output of an individual test for a given subject and generally display three specific lines:

1. The Average Points Curve (APC): The average score at each point (in 10ths of seconds) summated over the total number of repetitions performed;
2. The Maximum Points Curve (MPC): The maximum value (each 0.1 second) for the duration of the test summated over the total number of repetitions performed;
3. The Best Work Repetition Curve (BWRC): The actual repetition which produces the best work, or integrated computation of the area beneath the curve. This is the only curve which is an actual (or real) curve.

In Figure 10–2, a typical curve for a normal subject at 60 degrees/second is shown. A is the flexion curve (read from left to right) and B is the extension curve (read from right to left). Note the essentially "square wave" type of curve, particularly at its endpoint, showing that once a maximum torque has been reached, the muscular function required to maintain the force throughout the dynamic range is present. Note the initial "sine wave" at the outset of the curve, most pronounced in flexion, which represents the only partially damped "explosiveness" or acceleration/impulse produced by the body catching up to the isokinetic device. The sine wave appearance represents the rebound that occurs with rapid deceleration once the fixed speed has been reached. This ability to "attack" the device can be quantified as a method to measure effort and explosiveness, although it is not available at this time.

Next, look at the delay, minimal in this patient, between onset of measurement and acceleration to peak torque. The delay interval of zero torque is the time required to catch up to the device, while the slope of the increasing torque

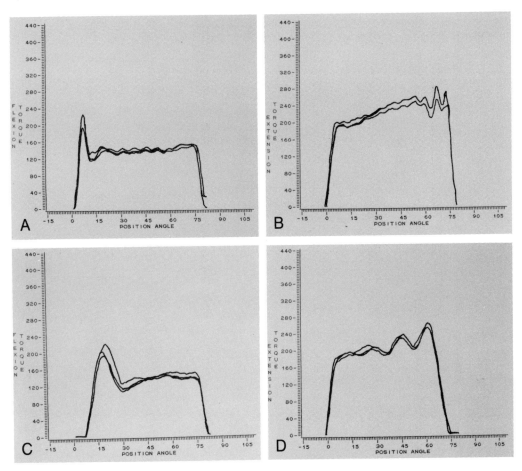

Fig. 10–2.   This figure represents a series of computer curves demonstrating the three curves (APC, MPC and BWPC) in flexion and extension. A through D show a normal at 60 and 150 degrees per second, and E through H show a patient at the initiation and midpoint of rehabilitation (at 150 degrees/second). A, Flexion curve at 60 degrees/second in a normal subject (read left to right). Note large impulse and "square wave" pattern. B, Extension curve at 60 degrees/second in a normal subject (read right to left). Note torque considerably higher than flexion curve with minimal "lag" prior to torque development. C, Flexion curve at 150 degrees/second. Note slower development of torque and wider "impulse" oscillations, still maintaining minimum curve variability and "square wave" form. D, Extension curve at 150 degrees/ second. Note "high-speed dropoff" with some lag in torque development compared to extension at 60 degrees/second.

also represents the patient's motivation or inhibition in producing high muscular effort initially. Finally, the area beneath the curve represents average, maximal, and single repetition actual work production during a trial.

Figure 10–2 C and D represent curves for the same patient at the much higher speed of 150 degrees/second. Note the much more pronounced sine wave impulse, particularly noted in flexion. However, the curves continue essentially in a "square wave" pattern, with extensor strength greater than flexor strength. Similarly, both peak torque and work rate performance shows only small decrements from values noted at the lower speed, though work drop-off is more pronounced. It is important to note that the "peak torque" calculation screens

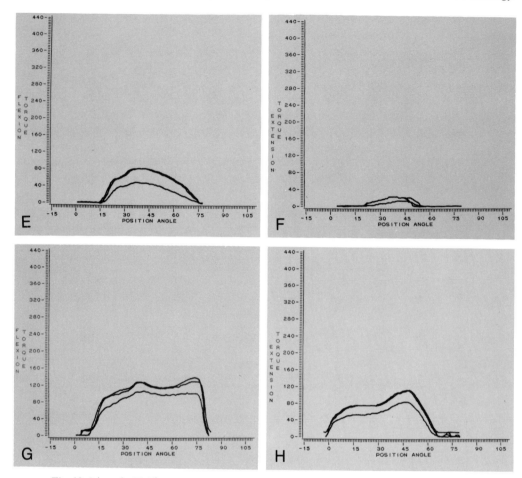

Fig. 10–2 (cont.) E, Flexion curve on initial testing in patient at 150 degrees/second. Note extreme lag in torque development and curve variability with low torque and end-curve dropoff. F, Extension curve in patient at 150 degrees/second (initial test). Note extremely low torque produced only in limited range with extreme lag in torque production. Also note reversal of extensor/flexor ratio. G, Flexion curve in patient at 150 degrees/second (midpoint of rehabilitation): Relatively low torque production with torque lag. Note gradual torque acceleration without significant "impulse." H, Extension curve in patient at 150 degrees/second (midpoint of rehabilitation). Note lag time with relatively low torque and persistent reversal of extensor/flexor ratio.

out the first portion of the curve, thus eliminating the impulse from peak torque calculations. This software characteristic allows the peak torque to more accurately reflect strength rather than the "acceleration variable," or impulse, which is more subject to patient training. Ultimately, calculations of "impulse work" should be able to define this variable, which shows potential for assessing explosiveness and/or motivation.

In Figure 10–2 E and F, we see flexor and extensor curves at 150 degrees/ second for a deconditioned back-injured patient prior to entering a spine rehabilitation program. This patient previously had undergone 3 weeks of simple home stretching exercises and some "desensitization" to the testing device, though considerable fear of injury persisted. On initial testing, the patient was unable to produce any torque whatsoever at this high speed, but on the second test prior to entering a real functional restoration program, these torques were produced. Particularly noteworthy are the extremely low peak torques and work rates leading to very low torque/body weight ratios. The variability between the maximum and average point curves is important as a measure of inconsistent effort, although the primary effort factor relies on repeat testing at 60 degrees/second at the end of a trial. The long delay between onset of contraction and "catching up" with the device, and the slow rise time with some fall-off in torque toward the end of the contraction, as well as lack of the sine wave representing the impulse against the device, are also apparent.

Finally, Figure 10-2 G and H demonstrate testing in the same patient some 3 weeks later at the same speed of 150 degrees/second. Rehabilitation has progressed, with some increase in strength, but probably more significantly, a decrease in neuromuscular inhibition. Both flexor and extensor torque have improved, now with a small impulse demonstrated showing the patient's willingness to "attack" the device. The initial delay and rise time have also improved, as has the variability between average and maximum point curves. Flexion has shown the most significant change, with a square wave pattern now present, though peak torque and work are still suboptimal. However, the extensor curve shows significant dropoff at the end of the curve, demonstrating the patient's inability to sustain the initial force production throughout this high speed movement. This incomplete rehabilitation of extensor function, which is quantified through a discrepancy between normal and patient peak torque/work ratios, could be expected to correct to normal values with continued training.

In addition, protocols for documenting endurance and recovery are available in the software. The *Endurance Protocol* compares work performed during the first 20% contractions with the last 20% in a preselected number of repetitions. The *Recovery Protocol* measures recovery potential and evaluates total work performed in two identical fatiguing trials separated by a predetermined recovery period (Fig. 10–3).

In essence, these protocols measure additional dimensions of the lumbo-pelvic functional unit's basic elements of performance. Endurance measures demonstrate the decay of the subject's ability to sustain force output through repetitive dynamic contractions over a predetermined arc at predetermined speed. The test is set over a short enough interval that the muscle performs its tasks anaerobically without inducing a significant oxygen debt, thus avoiding confusion with deficits in cardiovascular capacity. With this information, statements can be made concerning comparison of a patient's endurance profile to a normative database. Specific databases can be developed, such as for athletes in specific sports or workers performing a certain amount of work involving the back over the course of an 8-hour day, to provide an added dimension in analyzing a patient's potential for whole-day activity in a brief testing sequence.

The recovery protocol assesses another phase of the muscle function dimension. After a short burst of anaerobic activity, a normal individual should return to a nearly equivalent level of capacity after a short rest period. With deficits in muscular regulatory mechanisms, blood flow, or cardiovascular aerobic capacity, the ability to recover will be affected. The software program offers several comparisons including: (1) ratio of work output over the first 20% of pre- and post-recovery curves; (2) comparison of end-trial 20% repetitions work performance pre- and post-recovery; and (3) comparison of first/end-trial work

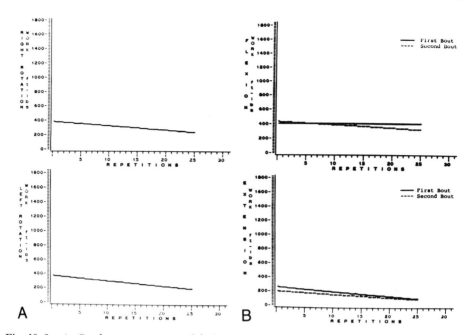

Fig. 10–3. A, Graphic representation of decline in work output per repetition over the course of a fatiguing set of repetitions. Represented separately for left rotation and right rotation. B, Graphic representation of Endurance Protocol and Recovery Protocol. The comparison between the two pairs of lines represents recovery potential (second set versus first set). These protocols are represented separately for flexion and extension.

ratios pre- and post-recovery. A great many applications of this measurement capability can be anticipated in the future.

Cybex Torsional Strength Device

The second device is similar to the first in all functional concepts, but measures *torsional* strength instead. It takes advantage of the pelvic stabilization supplied by the sitting, hip-abducted position, with an axially mounted dynamometer. Its output is displayed through the same computer system as the sagittal device, with identical computer features (Fig. 10–4).

The rotation device has similar outputs to those noted for the trunk extension/flexion device (Fig. 10–5A and B). A normal subject at low speed will show general symmetry between force outputs, rapid rise time, and a characteristic peak torque/work ratio and variability that is quite consistent. Though there is "high speed dropoff" for torsion, this activity appears capable of higher speeds in normal individuals than sagittal motion, and the dropoff does not occur until higher velocities are reached. In this case, a high speed test at 180 degrees/second is shown for the same normal subject (Fig. 10–5C and D).

The remaining figures of this group (Fig. 10–5E and F) demonstrate characteristics of a patient in torsion. While not all patients show asymmetric torsional strength, a certain subgroup appeared to display significant differences in torque and work output from side to side. In particular, the capability for high speed production is decreased and total torque/body weight and work/

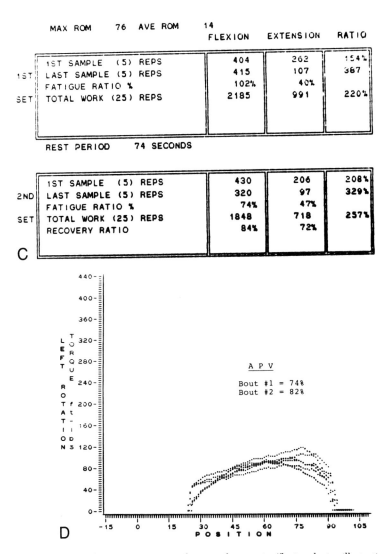

MAX ROM 76 AVE ROM 14	FLEXION	EXTENSION	RATIO
1ST SAMPLE (5) REPS	404	262	154%
1ST LAST SAMPLE (5) REPS	415	107	387
FATIGUE RATIO %	102%	40%	
SET TOTAL WORK (25) REPS	2185	991	220%

REST PERIOD   74 SECONDS

	FLEXION	EXTENSION	RATIO
1ST SAMPLE (5) REPS	430	206	208%
2ND LAST SAMPLE (5) REPS	320	97	329%
FATIGUE RATIO %	74%	47%	
SET TOTAL WORK (25) REPS	1848	718	257%
RECOVERY RATIO	84%	72%	

C

A P V

Bout #1 = 74%
Bout #2 = 82%

D

Fig. 10–3 (cont.)   C, Typical computer printout from trunk extension/flexion device illustrating numeric calculations of Endurance and Recovery Protocols based on work/repetitions and cumulative work. D, Graphic representation of *Average Points Variance* (APV) measuring point-to-point variation between curves on two separate sets of repetitions at the same velocity. The APV is sensitive to suboptimal effort.

body weight ratios are dramatically lowered in both male and female back-injured patients.

Characteristic databases have also been indentified for a small group of normals and patients (Mayer, Smith, Kondraske, Gatchel, Carmichael, Mooney, 1985). In this testing, a total of 67 normal subjects and 33 patients were evaluated. The results of the peak torque/body weight test for left rotation are shown (Fig. 10–6). Right rotation was almost identical to left rotation, with no asymmetry being identified in mean values (work calculations were not available at that time).

Interestingly, EMG testing was also performed during a series of isometric contractions going both right and left in various positions. The finding was

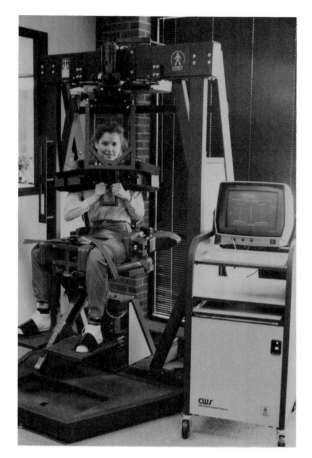

Fig. 10–4.   Cybex torso rotation measurement device (Lumex, Ronkonkoma, NY).

that the highest RMS voltages (corresponding to the highest force outputs) were produced by the obliques, with by far the highest voltages produced by the ipsilateral oblique to the side to which the patient was attempting to rotate. The contralateral oblique produced about half this amount of voltage, while a much smaller voltage was produced by the contralateral erector spinae muscle measured at the level of L3, 3 cm lateral to the midline. A negligible EMG RMS voltage was produced by the ipsilateral oblique (Fig. 10–7).

Isotechnologies Device

Another device already commerically available is the B-100 (recently replaced by the B-200) (Isotechnologies, Hillsboro, NC) which measures the torques and position changes occurring about multiple centers. This relatively compact device can measure torques in all three axes simultaneously, or a single axis can be isolated for sagittal or coronal measures. The subject stands on a platform with pelvis stabilized and with a shoulder harness arrangement holding the upper trunk. The axis lies posteriorly near the lumbosacral junction. The measurement system is termed "isodynamic," a technology unique to these machines. Essentially an electronically monitored hydraulic system, the device permits no motion until a preselected minimal torque is produced, after which the acceleration and velocity are controlled only by the degree to which the

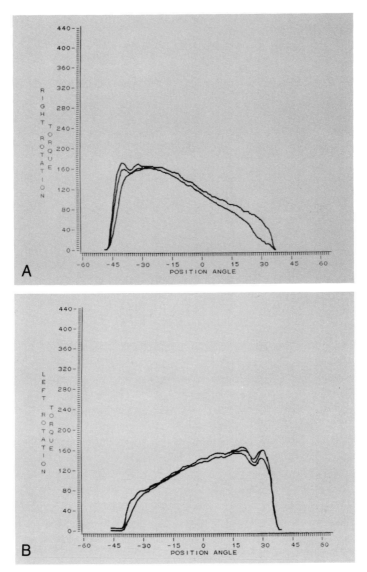

Fig. 10–5. A and B, Right and left rotation curves, respectively, in a normal subject at 60 degrees per second.

torque exceeds the preset minimum, as in any hydraulic device. As torque varies, acceleration and velocity also vary without control. Its computerization is relatively simple, being monitored by IBM PC or Apple computers, with substantial manufacturing cost savings resulting. Data from current users are being gathered at a central data compilation site under a common protocol to provide population specific profiles. At present, the computer is capable of comparing trials with graphs, tables and user-selected analysis routines. Future development calls for dynamic computer control of velocity and resistance which may resolve some of the controversy about "isodynamics." At this time, however, there is no scientific basis for the term "isodynamic," and the B-200 is *not* capable of performing isokinetic measurement.

In summary, this device is presently available and has major advantages in

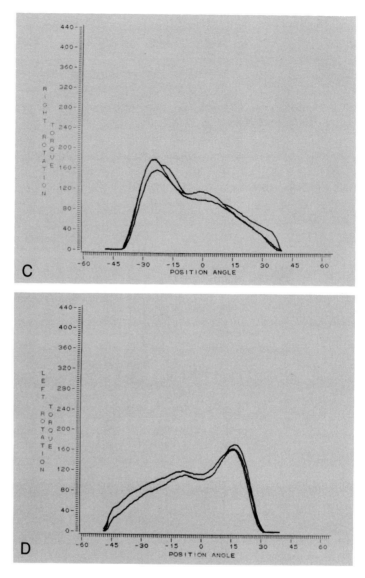

Fig. 10–5 (cont.)   C and D, Right and left rotation curves respectively in a normal subject at 180 degrees per second. Note, delay and diminution in torque production at a higher speed.

flexibility and versatility. However, it must sacrifice measurement accuracy in two major areas: (1) anatomic stabilization and location of the axis of rotation; (2) control of primary variables of either velocity or resistance. Until a repeatable, variable-stabilizing dynamic measurement technique (either isokinetic or isoinertial) is built into the machine, questions will remain about validity and relevance for quantification of functional capacity purposes, and users will be discouraged from the arduous task of collecting normative data in a consistent manner. As a training tool, however, its utility seems significant.

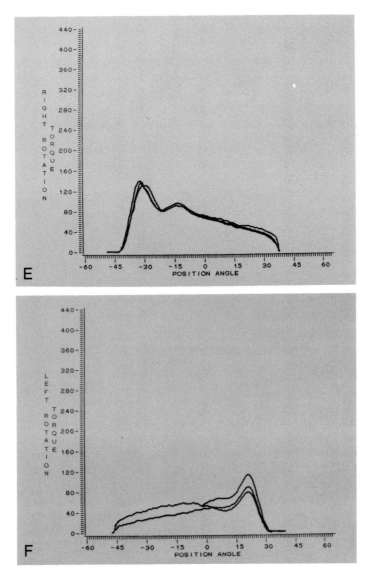

Fig. 10–5 (cont.) E and F, Asymmetric right and left rotation curves, respectively, in a patient at midpoint of rehabilitation at 180 degrees/second. Note greater delay, diminution, and variability in torque production in left rotation as compared to the right.

Kin-Com Device

The Kin-Com device (Chatteck Corp., Chattanooga, TN) has an attachment to its extremity dynamometer, making it amenable for use as a back testing device. The regular Kin-Com machine allows for isometric and multispeed isokinetic measurement, but also has a motor-driven forced-resistance capability that allows measurement of eccentric (muscle lengthening while contracting), as well as concentric (muscle shortening while contracting) strength. The pelvis is stabilized in the sitting position by two rigid locking arms pressed against the pelvis, with dynamic range-of-motion quite limited as is charac-

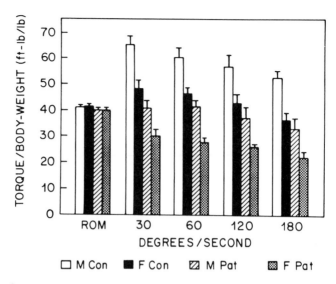

Fig. 10–6. Male patients (M Pat) and female patients (F Pat) versus normal controls (M Con, F Con) on left rotation measures demonstrating range-of-motion in degrees and torque production normalized to body weight.

teristic of most sitting devices. The machine is capable of measuring either flexion or extension at one time only (Fig. 10–8A and B), with the interscapular bar being pushed by the subject in extension. Risk of injury in the eccentric mode is decreased by a computer-controlled "lockout feature" that instantaneously halts the motion of the dynamometer arm when the subject breaks contact with the arm, causing the resistance to drop below a predetermined minimum.

Many investigators have found eccentric contractions to be characteristic of many bodily activities, and have established that specificity of training carries over to the concentric/eccentric dichotomy. Bending the back while lowering a weight is a typical example. Because of training specificity, concentric training may leave a significant gap in eccentric capability, just as isometric training fails to strengthen the muscle throughout its dynamic range or at different speeds. While most training is done with free weights or variable resistance weight machines that generally provide eccentric, as well as concentric, capability, eccentric measurement capability may be desirable, and only partially offset by potential risk of injury from equipment malfunction.

Since the sagittal extension measurement attachment can be added to a device already available to the user, low cost is a prominent advantage, particularly for a low-volume facility doing both spine and extremity testing. Isometric, as well as isotonic, measurement and training capability is available on the same device. The specifically designed computer produces high resolution graphics and numeric calculations of velocity, torque, angular displacement and power consumption. Other analysis modes can be selected, and a unique voice synthesizer provides auditory feedback to operator and subject. In addition, the company has a fine reputation for quality, with a national sales and service organization typical only of the largest manufacturers in this area.

The hydraulically-driven computerized dynamometer has previously been

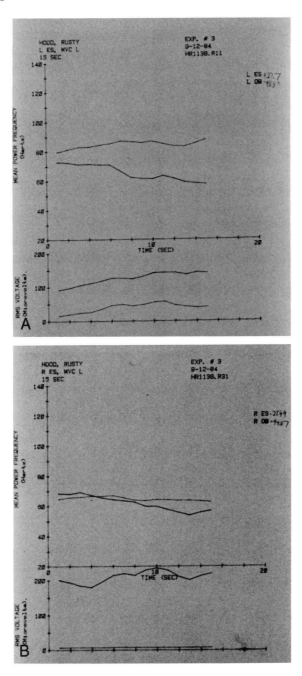

Fig. 10–7.   Patient undergoing maximal voluntary rotation isometric contraction to the left in the neutral position. Upper graph shows fatigue as documented by change in slope of mean power spectrum. Lower graph shows force production as documented by RMS voltage utilizing surface electrodes. A, Results of fatigue analysis and EMG force production monitoring on *ipsilateral* abdominal oblique and erector spinae musculature. Note moderate force production in abdominal obliques with low (but present) force production in left erector spinae. Fatigue in the 15-second trial is only demonstrated in the abdominal obliques. B, Fatigue and force production in *contralateral* abdominal oblique and erector spinae. Note extremely high force production in right abdominal oblique (possibly due to more superficial location of external oblique muscle). By contrast, there is extremely low force production by the contralateral erector spinae (or multifidus). Fatigue is demonstrated only in the abdominal obliques.

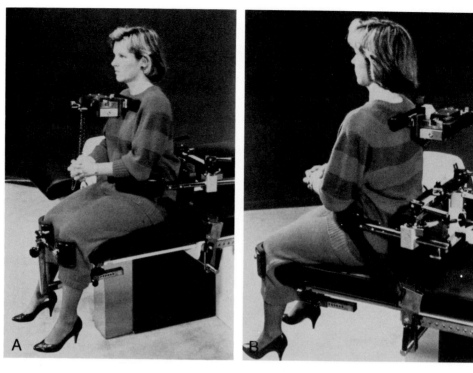

Fig. 10–8.   Kin-Com sitting sagittal strength testing device (Chatteck Corp., Chattanooga, TN).

evaluated for accuracy against alternate devices, with the finding that lever arm speed never varied more than 1.5% from target speed, and force measurements were within 4% of independently measured levels (Farrell, Richards, 1986). A feature allows a variable preload to be set requiring a subject to exceed this level before motion can be initiated. The effect is to produce a motion motivating factor, as well as simultaneously eliminating the initial "acceleration" impulse present on most isokinetic devices. Truly isokinetic movement is achieved after overcoming the preload. Work is currently progressing on a research device in an academic setting to develop a normative database. The device provides sagittal plane measurement only, and is currently improving the sophistication of its software.

Biodex System Back Attachment

The Biodex Back Attachment (Biodex, Inc., Shirley, NY) is, like the Kin-Com, an attachment to an already existing extremity system (Fig. 10–9). Unlike the Kin-Com, however, the attachment is a stand-alone reclining chair hinged in the lumbar spinal region in which the subject is seated and stabilized. The mobile dynamometer with its free-standing base is disconnected from the extremity attachment and connected in line with the axis of rotation of the chair. The dynamometer operates in isokinetic and isometric modes, but is also directly coupled to the computer which drives the device actively in both directions. Accuracy of the dynamometer is reported as +/− 2%, but whether this is altered by speed, torque, or both is not specified. The calibration mechanism is not identified.

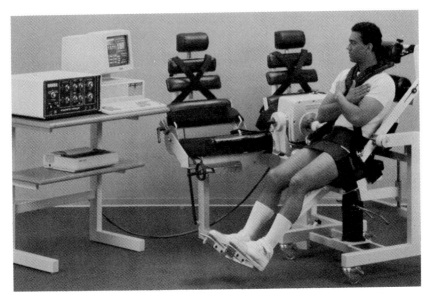

Fig. 10–9.   Biodex isokinetic dynamometer connects to semi-reclining back attachment for trunk flexion/extension measurements.

The patient is positioned in a partially reclining, full body extended position. The lower extremities are stabilized with slight knee flexion with a lumbosacral pad that attempts to maintain posterior pelvic tilt through full sagittal flexion/extension mobility. The chest harness has a soft anterior restraint allowing some uncontrolled upper torso motion to occur. Like the other sitting devices, and unlike the standing devices, extension is assisted by gravity while flexion is resisted. The lumbar support is designed less for stabilization than for comfort and accommodation to motion. The chair permits considerable motion from flexion to hyperextension with electronic stops provided by the dynamometer, as well as back-up mechanical stops on the back attachment. Dynamometer speed ranges from 0 to 450 degrees/second, though the manufacturer suggests a maximum of 120 degrees/second. A project to obtain normative data is currently in process in a large midwestern medical clinic.

Like the Kin-Com, the Biodex System has the advantage of an attachment added to a free-standing extremity system which provides space savings. Though not as frugal as the Kin-Com, it also provides cost savings. In facilities doing both back and extremity measurements, these may be significiant advantages for this device, but careful consideration of the problems of sitting versus standing techniques is important for the prospective purchaser. The clinical data station allows control of the active/passive motion of the dynamometer, as well as impressive computer software measurement capability built into the entire multi-joint system.

Lido Sagittal Tester

The Lido Isokinetic Sagittal Tester (Loredan, Inc., Davis, CA) is a new contender in the strength testing manufacturer's derby (Fig. 10–10A and B). Introduced commercially for distribution only in 1987, it resembles the Cybex sagittal testing unit, but with the added feature of testing either in a standing

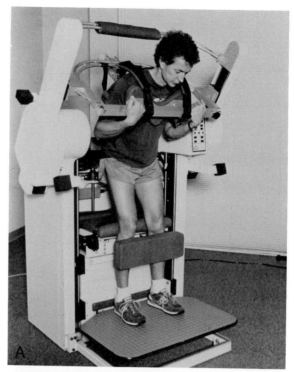

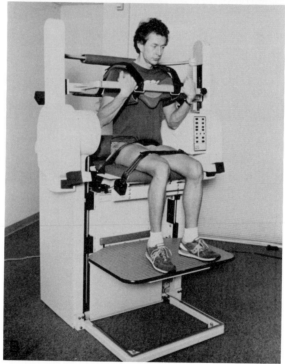

Fig. 10–10.   A and B, Lido sagittal sitting/standing isokinetic strength testing device. (Loredan, Inc., Davis, CA)

or sitting mode utilizing a sliding seat in the appropriate sagittal axis. There is some slight sacrifice in stabilization characteristics, but this appears to be offset by a unique sliding upper torso harness which permits the subject to bend farther in this device than is permitted with a static arm. The sliding harness in the mobile upper torso arm prevents the "binding" produced in other devices by changing length of the trunk as flexion increases. The device is large, stable and attractive, and like the Cybex TEF unit, functions only in the sagittal plane with an axis mounted appropriately along the actual lumbopelvic axis of rotation rather than posteriorly as in some other units. The device permits isometric and isokinetic measurements at multiple speeds, with an IBM PC computer for monitoring and calculations.

The software available is already quite sophisticated, producing good graphics, calculating peak torques, acceleration, work and power. There is also an endurance protocol termed the fatigue index and a calculated effort factor based on curve slope. The device calculates the slope variance between any two curves at 0.1-second intervals and sums the result algebraically. The number that appears will have meaning only after more testing, but the manufacturer reports that initial indications by a few subjects "faking" tests show that the slope number is increased by a factor of at least 8 to 10.

Clinical research is currently taking place at 6 physical therapy facilities around the U.S.A. Testing on the hydraulic actuator with measurements taken by a pair of pressure transducers on each side of the actuator indicates high accuracy with reproducibility in the 2% range. "Internal calibration" by the computer through resetting of the torque baseline with no time-related measurement decay or scale drift is reported by the manufacturer. However, the concept of self-calibration is somewhat misleading, as the calibration test with weights is relatively lengthy to perform. A separate extremity device, but no other trunk measurement device, is currently produced by this company.

There are also other devices that are either not generally commercially available, currently under construction, or capable only of isometric measurement. They will not be considered at this time.

CONSIDERATIONS IN AN EXPANDING FIELD

Our research group has had extensive experience with the Cybex prototypes. Unfortunately, the recent availability of all commerical devices makes it impossible for any single group to have gained extensive familiarity with all of the machines. Cybex has had long and exclusive domain over isokinetic extremity measurement. There has been general acceptance in the industry of their concepts of joint stabilization, accommodation to resistance for injury prevention, and the need to control physiologic variables for *valid, repeatable,* and *relevant* measures in dynamic testing. While speed/acceleration control (isokinetic measures) is only one technique for controlling variables, no one, to our knowledge, has come up with a means of providing constant resistance, with accurate measures of velocity/acceleration. Even if such a technique were available, it would be less desirable than measuring force since we are used to expressing strength in terms of resistance rather than speed. Other methodologies (isotonic, isodynamic) may have an important place in training, but do not appear to have the potential to become equivalent in validity for measurement purposes. Thus, most manufacturers have chosen to do one of three things:

(1) employ isokinetic technology (Cybex, Kin-Com, Biodex, Lido); (2) employ no dynamic testing, but substitute multi-position isometric testing, or (3) do not control variables, allowing for physiologic movement (Isotechnologies). Only time and research by unbiased investigators comparing different devices will identify the optimal machine(s), while market factors will undoubtedly take their own toll irrespective of quality issues.

Because the Cybex prototypes have been available so long, there has been ample opportunity to develop relatively large normative databases, as well as experience in testing the deconditioned chronic pain patient (Thompson, Gould, Davies, Ross, Price, 1985; Smith, Mayer, Gatchel, Becker, 1985; Mayer, Smith, Keeley, Mooney, 1985; Mayer, Smith, Kondraske, Gatchel, Carmichael, Mooney, 1985). Initial disadvantages of the Cybex back system have been its high cost and large space requirements relative to the other available trunk strength devices. However, other manufacturers appear to be narrowing cost differentials as service and marketing rise. When a cost versus applicability comparison is made with structural diagnostic devices, such as CT scanners and MRI (magnetic resonance imagers), the 5 to 10% fractional cost of the isokinetic machines compares favorably.

A most disturbing feature of this burgeoning field is that the relatively sophisticated clinician will have a difficult time distinguishing the accuracy of the marketing claims of the many manufacturers who will inevitably be entering this field. Unlike x-ray technology, there are no generally accepted standards for strength testing likely to guide new manufacturers. At worst, diversity will produce a "Tower of Babel" phenomenon until research leads to optimal stabilization, variability control, machine design with accepted databases and protocols, and techniques for documenting degree of effort. Fortunately, the American Academy of Orthopedic Surgeons has recognized this problem, and has a committee on Occupational Health providing courses featuring opportunities for discussion by the manufacturers of these devices.

IMAGING OF SPINE MUSCULATURE

Another measure of spine musculature should also be discussed. Morphologic information on trunk musculature can now be obtained by computer tomography (Bulcke, Termote, Palmers, Crolla, 1979; Termote, Baert, Crolla, Palmers, Bulcke, 1980). At the present time, the criteria for muscle atrophy in CT scanning is: (*a*) decreased muscle volume or (*b*) fatty infiltration (increased fat/muscle fiber ratio or actual fatty replacement of fibers). Due to the latter phenomenon, the density of muscles through x-ray attenuation can be regarded as a measure of atrophy (Laasonen, 1984). Some reports indicate that in the multiply-operated chronic low back pain patient, the paraspinal and psoas muscles are often atrophic (Laasonen, 1984), and similar findings have been reported in ankylosing spondylitis (Gordon, Sage, Bertouch, Brooks, 1984). In a more recent study, CT scan measurements of a sample of patients having a single cut CT scan at the level of the inferior pedicle of L3, performed 3 months postoperatively, were compared to a normal population (Mayer, Terry, Smith, Gatchel, Mooney, 1987). While the difference in muscle bulk in both males and females was not statistically significant, the difference in muscle x-ray attenuation was. The postoperative patients could be distinguished from a non-operated population on the basis of muscle fiber density, most significantly in the erector spinae, but also in the psoas to a lesser extent. In addition, there was positive correlation in the tested postoperative population, between muscular density and sagittal trunk strength as measured on the Cybex TEF unit. While the data are only preliminary, they suggest the ultimate use of imaging devices such as CT scan or MRI to characterize refractory muscular deficits.

AEROBIC CAPACITY TESTING

Many volumes have been written concerning cardiovascular measures. These are, in some ways, linked to measures of endurance, as both extrinsic cardiovascular capacity and intrinsic muscle enzyme responses to fatiguing demands are involved in the complex process of endurance. Bicycle ergometry has been utilized to obtain physiologic information on patient work performance and oxygen consumption, which predicts cardiovascular capacity with considerable reliability.

Schmidt (1985) has shown that chronic back pain patients have lower levels of aerobic capacity than normal subjects. Standardized nomograms are available to provide oxygen consumption data based on heart rate and bicycle ergometry work rate that can be obtained using a number of exercise bicycles, such as the Fitron or Monarch. Normalization to age, gender and body weight through use of standard tables then permits an estimate of MVO_2 and a fitness level. Early extremity fatigue or an inadequate heart rate response invalidates the test. Errors may occur in a deconditioned or poorly motivated population through failure to comply fully with the protocol, poor maintenance of a stable work rate, or failure to achieve a stable final heart rate at a high enough level. Effort may be difficult to assess.

A simple standardized alternative bicycle ergometry protocol can also quantify a patient's response to an increasing work load. In the test, the rested patient is exercised at a set initial work rate utilizing a timer and pulse monitor. Before beginning the test, a target heart rate representing 85% of age-related maximum is selected. The test is not performed initially in patients with recent myocardial disorders, but is performed in a modified fashion in patients with a longer cardiac history or on rate-limiting medication, with heart rate limited to 120. Their training is delayed, however, until a cardiac stress test can be performed by a consulting internist, and a recommendation made as to an appropriate training heart rate.

In the protocol, testing begins at a predetermined work rate and progresses at regular intervals until the target heart rate is reached. At this point, the result is expressed as final work rate, time of test, and ratio of final heart rate achieved to the target heart rate (as a measure of effort). This "basic test" is designed to permit almost all patients to produce some work on the device. Naturally, if lower extremity strength or functional capability, rather than cardiovascular capacity, is the limiting factor to the ability to produce work on the bicycle, this will be reflected in the patient stopping the test before the target heart rate is achieved. Though this can occur with other lower extremity pathologies, there are a few patients with so much neurologic or muscular damage from back/extremity injury that they are permanently limited in aerobic measurement and training by their lower extremity deficits. In most cases, however, lower extremity weakness and fatigue are usually related to disuse and manifested only in the early stages of rehabilitation. When retested, patients are generally capable of hitting their target heart rate.

A similar device is the upper body ergometer (UBE). This is basically a bicycle for the arms, for which an identical test has been devised with a similarly established normal database. Upper body ergometry tends to be less a test of cardiovascular capacity than of upper extremity functional unit strength/endurance performance. This is apparently because the capacity to deliver blood to the upper extremities is limited by the size of the vessels, preventing even high stress activities in the upper extremities from placing a substantial load on the cardiopulmonary system. As a result, high-performance wheelchair athletes may show relatively low MVO_2. Therefore, while the bicycle ergometry test is primarily a measure of cardiopulmonary capacity, but may be limited by lower extremity fatigability, the UBE is primarily a test of upper extremity strength/endurance.

Cardiovascular deconditioning is generally rapidly reversible with training. For this reason, the basic test can become interminable and cumbersome. Therefore, a high performance level (HPL) test is used for testing most normal industrial subjects and patients who have achieved a certain training level. In the HPL, the subject begins training at a much higher work rate than in the basic test and continues ascending at 2-minute intervals. Target heart rate is generally achieved in about half the time required for the "basic test."

The Versa-climber (Heart Rate Inc., Costa Mesa, CA) will be discussed further in the next chapter. While its primary use is for functional task performance measurement, it has a unique upper and lower extremity simultaneous use capability supplementing the isolated testing on a bicycle or upper body ergometer. In terms of cardiovascular training, it certainly appears to be a valuable tool, but its usefulness in aerobic capacity testing is yet to be demonstrated.

SUMMARY OF METHODS

In summary, isolated trunk strength with skeletal stabilization, trunk muscle endurance, and aerobic capacity are important elements in the deconditioning syndrome of the lumbopelvic functional unit. Measurement of this physical capacity involves new and exciting technology, but data are quite expensive and time-consuming to obtain. However, since experience with rehabilitation programs shows that all three pieces of information are relevant to back injury, and progress in rehabilitation correlates with increases in general functional capacity, the use of such devices to provide this information is justified at this time. Presently, we have only begun to tap the information that can be obtained from the present devices. We must begin to sort out the most important measures and standardize them before we are swamped by an onslaught of meaningless numbers. It is hoped that, in time, general agreement on devices and protocols can be obtained, but this is not likely to occur in the next few years.

CHAPTER REFERENCES

Andersson B, Ortengren R, Herberts T: Quantitative electromyography studies of back muscle activity related to posture and loading. Orthop Clin N Am *8*:85–96, 1977.
Alston W, Carlson K, Feldman D, Grimm Z, Gerontinos E: A quantitative study of muscle fatigue in the chronic low back syndrome. J Am Geriatr Soc *14*:419–423, 1966.
Bulcke J, Termote J, Palmers Y, Crolla D: Computer tomography of the human skeletal muscular system. Neuroradiol *17*:127–136, 1979.

Cady L, Bischoff D, O'Connel E, Thomas P, Allan J: Strength and fitness and subsequent back injuries in firefighters. J Occup Med *21*:269–272, 1979.

Davies G, Gould J: Trunk testing using a prototype Cybex II Isokinetic Stabilization System. J Orthop Sports Phys Ther *3*:164–170, 1982.

Farrell M, Richards J: Analysis of the reliability and validity of the Kinetic Communicator exercise device. Med & Sci in Sports and Exer *18*:44–49, 1986.

Flint M: Effect of increasing back and abdominal muscle strength on low back pain. Res Quart *29*:160–171, 1955.

Gordon T, Sage M, Bertouch J, Brooks P: Computed tomography of paraspinal musculature in ankylosing spondylitis. J Rheum *11*:794–797, 1984.

Hasue M, Fuguwara M, Kikuchi S: A new method of quantitative measurement of abdominal and back muscle strength. Spine *5*:143–148, 1980.

Laasonen E: Atrophy of sacrospinal muscle groups in patients with chronic, diffusely radiating lumbar back pain. Neuroradiol *26*:9–13, 1984.

Langrana N, Lee C: Isokinetic evaluation of trunk muscles. Spine *9*:171–175, 1984.

Langrana N, Lee C, Alexander H, Mayott C: Quantitative assessment of back strength using isokinetic testing. Spine *9*:287–290, 1984.

Mayer L, Greenberg B: Measurements of the strength of trunk muscles. J Bone Joint Surg *24*:842–856, 1942.

Mayer T, Gatchel R, Kishino N, Keeley J, Capra P, Mayer H, Barnett J, Mooney V: Objective assessment of spine function following industrial injury: a prospective study with comparison group and one-year follow-up, Volvo Award paper. Spine *10*:482–493, 1985.

Mayer T, Smith S, Keeley J, Mooney V: Quantification of lumbar function Part 2: Sagittal plane trunk strength in chronic low-back patients. Spine *10*:765–772, 1985.

Mayer T, Smith S, Kondraske G, Gatchel R, Carmichael T, Mooney V: Quantification of lumbar function Part 3: Preliminary data on isokinetic torso rotation testing with myoelectric spectral analysis in normal and low-back pain subjects. Spine *10*:912–920, 1985.

Mayer T, Terry A, Smith S, Gatchel R, Mooney V: Quantitative Postoperative Deficits of Physical Capacity Following Spine Surgery. *In* Orthopedic Transactions for Proceedings of annual meeting of American Academy of Orthopedic Surgeons, San Francisco, CA, January 24–28, 1987.

McNeill, Warwick D, Andersson C, Schultz A: Trunk strength in attempted flexion, extension, and lateral bending in healthy subjects and patients with low back disorders. Spine *5*:529–538, 1980.

Nachemson A, Lindh M: Measurements of abdominal and back muscle strength with and without low back pain. Scand J Rehab Med *1*:60–69, 1969.

Oneidi O, Petersen R, Staffeldt E: Back pain and isometric back muscle strength of workers in a Danish factory. Scand J Rehab Med *7*:125–128, 1975.

Schmidt A: Cognitive factors in the performance level of chronic low back pain patients. J Psychosom Res *29*:183–189, 1985.

Smidt G, Herring T, Admundsen L, Rogers M, Russell A, Lehmann T: Assessment of abdominal and back extensor function: a quantitative approach and results for chronic low back patients. Spine *8*:211–219, 1983.

Smith S, Mayer T, Gatchel R, Becker T: Quantification of lumbar function Part 1: Isometric and multispeed isokinetic trunk strength measures in sagittal and axial planes in normal subjects. Spine *10*:757–764, 1985.

Suzuki N, Endo S: A quantitative study of trunk muscle strength and fatigability in the low-back pain syndrome. Spine *8*:69–74, 1983.

Termote J, Baert A, Crolla D, Palmers Y, Bulcke J: Computed tomography of the normal and pathologic muscular system. Radiol *137*:439–444, 1980.

Thompson N, Gould J, Davies G, Ross P, Price S: Descriptive measures of isokinetic trunk testing. J Orthop Sports Phys Ther *7*:43–49, 1985.

Thorstensson A, Nilsson J: Trunk muscle strength during constant and velocity movement. Scand J Rhab Med *14*:61–68, 1982.

Thorstensson A, Arvidson A: Trunk muscle strength and low-back pain. Scand J Rehab Med *14*:69–75, 1982.

Chapter 11

Objective Measurement of Functional Task Performance

While there are compelling reasons to study the spinal "functional unit" in isolation to gain information about the presumably injured body part, we all recognize that the lumbar spine is of greatest interest when it is operating in coordination with other functional units. Thus, we are interested in such activities as lifting, bending, standing, sitting, walking, carrying, climbing, and crawling, which involve interaction of multiple functional units extending from hands to feet. Except for lift testing, to be discussed next, this important area of study has been almost totally devoid of good research. While positional tolerance has long been noted as a characteristic complaint of low back dysfunction patients, evaluation of this process has usually been based simply on subjective self-report of patient to physician. More recently, prolonged observation of patients on obstacle courses has been used (Mayer, 1985). Such techniques, however, may be time-consuming and require special environments. Research and development in this area is only in its infancy, but will hopefully lead to some new reliable and effective methods.

LIFT TESTING

Much attention has been focused on lift measures as the quintessential total body functional capacity measure for several reasons. Lifting has traditionally been identified in industry with the highest correlation between reported activity and low back injury. It is a full body task involving transfer of forces along the biomechanical chain from hands down to feet. This has led to mathematical models of lifting, and simple educational concepts of modifying lift techniques (Chaffin, Andersson, 1984; Pope, Frymoyer, Andersson, 1984). The substitution of one functional unit for another promised easily attainable decreases in industrial injury rates. This promise has led to a combination of pre-employment lift capacity tests (erroneously referred to as "strength tests"), and a large compendium of knowledge on ergonomic analysis of job design and injury modes (Chaffin, Andersson, 1984; Pope, Frymoyer, Andersson, 1984). Effectiveness of these prevention methods remains controversial (Spengler, Bigos, Martin, Zeh, Fisher, Nachemson, 1986; Bigos, Spengler, Martin, Zeh, Fisher, Nachemson, Wang, 1986; Bigos, Spengler, Martin, Zeh, Fisher, Nachemson, 1986).

Essentially, analysis of lift capacity has encompassed several different techniques, moving along lines somewhat parallel to those more recently taken by trunk strength testing manufacturers. These include the psychophysical or isoinertial tests (Snook, Campanelli, Hart, 1978; Snook, Irvine, 1967; Kroemer, 1983; Ayoub, Mital, Bakken, Asfour, Bethea, 1980; Asfour, Ayoub, Mital, 1984), isometric lift tests (Chaffin, Herrin, Keyserling, 1978; Keyserling, Herrin, Chaffin, 1980; Harber, Sooho, 1984) and constrained isokinetic lifting (Kishino, Mayer, Gatchel, Parrish, Anderson, Gustin, Mooney, 1985; Mital, Channaveeraiah, Fard, Khaledi, 1986). Mathematical modeling, biomechanical analysis, and investigation of myoelectric signals have also been utilized by several investigators to calculate loads on the spine in various static postures encountered in industry.

The primary focus in employee screening for specific materials handling tasks has involved lift capacity testing. The first approach tried was *isoinertial,* in which the velocity is not controlled (or measured), but the mass is held constant. In effect, this is a typical *isotonic* lift, and the term *psychophysical* has been used to connote the fact that lifting capacity has frequently been set by the subject's self-report of his or her maximum capability, a point of discomfort, or feedback perception of impending injury.

Isometric testing is the most well-established technique. It has been used extensively as a means of employee selection by a number of groups in industry, either by itself or in conjunction with job redesign. Isometric strength testing has been recognized in the NIOSH (National Institute of Occupational Safety and Health) Work Practices Guide for Manual Lifting as a way to identify workers who would be at higher risk of over-exertion injury. A commercially available system for isometric evaluation has now been produced. The Isometric Strength Testing Unit (ISTU) (Dynadex Corp., Ann Arbor, MI) was developed in conjunction with the Center for Ergonomics at the University of Michigan, the dominant academic group in promoting understanding of ergonomic therapy and potential industrial applications. This updated ISTU is an adjustable device which measures static lift capacity of an individual using isometric principles (Arnold, Rauschenberger, Soubel, et al., 1982; Chaffin, 1974; Chaffin, Herrin, Keyserling, 1978; Jackson, Osburn, Laughery, 1984; Jackson, 1968; Kamon, Kiser, Pytel, 1982; Keyserling, Herrin, Chaffin, 1980; Marras, King, Joynt, 1984; Pytel, Kamon, 1981; Reilly, Zedeck, Tenopyr, 1979; Schultz, Andersson, Haderspeck, et al., 1982; White, Gordon, 1982). It has a platform with an attached strain gauge, a force monitor with timing, averaging and error detecting capability, and a strip chart recorder (Fig. 11–1). The computer software utilizes a biomechanical mathematical model based on postural assumptions, disc pressure measurements and body-segment links that attempts to make a statement of an individual's risk of injury when a given isometric lifting force is exerted.

A large industrial database has also been developed for isometric "leg lift," "torso lift," and "arm lift" (the new Dynadex device also allows a wider variety of postures to be utilized). The strength testing system is actually secondary, in the Center for Ergonomics model, to the job analysis. Ergonomic analysis is performed and typical postures are reviewed, after which a test individualized for this specific job is identified. This test, while usually consisting of an isometric lifting test and possibly a cardiovascular endurance test, may vary greatly based on the most prevalent tasks identified in the work evaluation. "Minimum standards" are generally set, based on testing incumbence within a given industry and related to defining groups of substandard individuals with higher historic injury records. Little use, however, has been made of this meth-

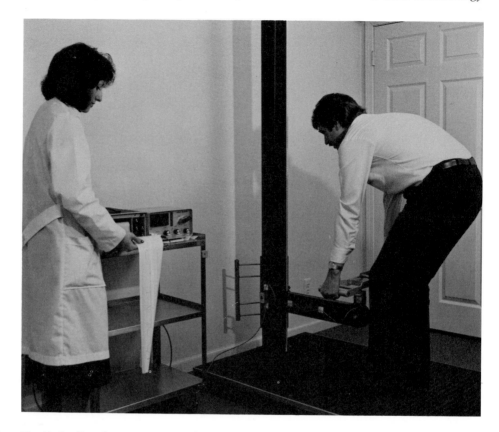

Fig. 11–1.   Dynadex isometric strength testing unit (ISTU) (Dynadex, Ann Arbor, MI).

odology in treating or rehabilitating patients. The primary focus has instead been on industry and worker selection.

The major limitation of the device, of course, is its lack of dynamic measurement capability. Moreover, the biomechanical model, like all mathematical models, often involves assumptions that prove to be inaccurate in the light of later developments, often leaving the degree of error induced difficult to identify. Finally, isometric contractions are much more likely to produce muscle strains with truly maximal exertions than dynamic contractions.

The commercially available Liftask (Cybex, Ronkonkoma, NY) (Fig. 11–2A) is an outgrowth of the same technology leading to the previously mentioned trunk strength measurement devices. It continues to use the isometric and multispeed isokinetic control of variables for valid measurement. For meaningful data, it requires a normal database, and computerized display of force, work, power consumption, curve shape variability, and endurance measures inherent in the other machines. However, it sacrifices the joint stabilization associated with isolated testing of a single joint or functional unit. Instead, it substitutes a lifting handle on a cable attached to the dynamometer permitting a wide selection of body positions and lifting styles during a test protocol. The device is relatively compact and also holds the potential for portability to test subjects at distant job sites.

A new dynamometer known as the Electronic Resistance System (ERS) has

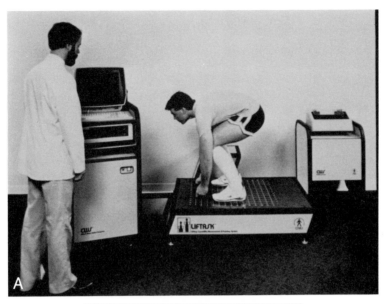

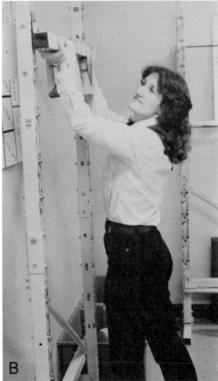

Fig. 11–2. A, Cybex Liftask isokinetic device with computerization (Lumex, Ronkonkoma, NY). B, Individual performing "lifting under load" isoinertial task on WEST 2 equipment (WEST, Huntington Beach, CA).

been developed (Digital Kinetics, Danville, CA) for use with a variety of mechanical systems. The resistance unit is currently sold as part of a gymnasium setup, but can be modified in any one of a number of ways. The system is actually a true electromagnetic break attached either to an IBM-PC or inexpensive Tandy computer for feedback and calculations. The break is purported to have superb stability on repeated cycling (0.1% drift in 5 million cycles, minimal power consumption) accuracy, varying from 2 to 5% for force resistance and from 1 to 3% for velocity (depending on computer choice) in the isokinetic mode. Both isokinetic and isotonic testing may be selected, with force/velocity repeatability in the 1 to 2% range. Velocity spectrum is only slightly limited relative to the Liftask, but force maximums topping out at 120 pounds significantly limit its clinical utility. Peak force, velocity and work readings are available on the computer screen or printout. No effort calculation is established in the software as yet, and the device is too new for development of a normative database. With selection of an appropriate mechanical system to which the ERS can be linked, significant acceptance of this inexpensive device may be anticipated in the future.

LIFT TESTING FOR FUNCTIONAL RESTORATION

Progressive Isoinertial Lifting Evaluation (PILE)

Standardized and widely accepted techniques for isoinertial lift testing have been slow to develop. Our technique, developed at the University of Texas Southwestern Medical Center at Dallas, will be described here (Mayer , Barnes, Kishino, Nichols, Gatchel, Mayer, Mooney, 1988, in press; Mayer, Barnes, Nichols, Kishino, Coval, Piel, Hoshino, Gatchel, 1988, in press). The principles of the testing are quite simple, involving both psychophysical and progressive isoinertial components. A sequence of incremental weight lifting, identical for groups of individuals separated by gender and normalized to body weight, is inherent to the protocol. A normal database must be developed, normalized to body weight, and ultimately be gender/age/work demand specific. Because lifting capacity incorporates aerobic activity, a cardiovascular end-point must be established that also functions as an "effort factor," while also establishing whether aerobic capacity or muscle fatigue in any of the functional units is the limiting factor of task performance.

The Progressive Isoinertial Lifting Evaluation (PILE) test protocol involves the lifting of weights in a plastic box from floor to waist (0 to 30 inches) and waist to shoulder height (30 to 54 inches). Women begin with a 5-pound load, while men begin with a 10-pound load (though weight lifted is not identified to the subject). Weight is incremented upward at a rate equal to the initial weight every 20 seconds, with a rate of 4 lifting movements in each 20-second interval. A "lifting movement" involves a single transfer from one level to the next, i.e., from floor to waist, or waist to shoulder. Lifting progresses in sequence: floor to waist to floor unless the patient reaches an end-point on one level of lifting. Tests from floor to waist and waist to shoulder are done separately, since norms differ for varying heights of lift. The test is terminated when the first of the following end-points is achieved: (1) Psychophysical End-point: voluntary test termination by the subject for complaints of fatigue or excessive pain; (2) Aerobic End-point: achievement of a specific aerobic capacity goal, usually 85% of age-determined "maximum heart rate:" (unless cardiac precautions are in force); or (3) Safety End-point: a predetermined "safe limit" of 45–55% of body weight. Results are expressed as: (1) maximum weight lifted at the lumbar and cervical levels (floor to waist and waist to overhead); (2) the endurance time to discontinuation at each level; and (3) the final end target heart rates. Since distance and repetitions are also known, calculations of work and power consumption can easily be made and normalized to body weight.

Low back pain patients or inadequately conditioned workers will usually discontinue testing because of stated fatigue (Psychophysical End-point). Larger, but well-conditioned, men and women will usually reach their target heart rates (Aerobic End-point), while smaller individuals may reach the Safety End-point of lifting first. The different weights based on gender and body weight are intended to smooth these discrepancies. It is felt that this type of standardization has adequate safeguards for an easily administered and reliable method of truly physiologic lift testing. With the endurance factor incorporated in the test, it gives a repeatable and objective measure of the subject's *frequent* lifting capacity, that can easily be translated to job requirements in the workplace, or training protocols for work simulation and hardening.

The WEST 2 (Work Evaluation Systems Technology, Huntington Beach, CA) is a commercially available device for testing isoinertial lifting over pre-set ranges. The device consists of a frame with a "lifting bar" holding weights in the center up to approximately 90 pounds (Fig. 11–2B). Testing can be performed under pre-selected ranges, not only involving lifting, but sufficient control of the bar to "hook" the bar ends over the projecting bolts. No effort factor is defined, nor has a normative database been made available. However, "standards" for lifting are determined, differentiated by gender and age (but not by weight), for the amount of weight lifted at set rates of 1 and 4 lifts/minute. Training rates are set as percentages of assessed patient maximums. Progression is dependent on patient self-report of symptomatology.

Dynamic/Isometric Testing

When choosing a commercial lift simulator, one is again limited by the recent advent of these devices and the limited number of manufacturers, as well as a lack of standardized and well-accepted methods for lifting assessment. Under the circumstances, it appears that the Cybex Liftask offers clear superiority in its incorporation of isometric as well as isokinetic measurement capacity. Its inability to allow "physiologic" movements is inherent in the need to control as many variables as possible for reproducible measures, and thus the psychophysical protocol described above must be utilized for direct documentation of "real lifting."

Isometric testing can be performed by locking the cable on the support bars at the appropriate height specified in the NIOSH protocols for the "leg lift," "torso lift," and "arm lift." Measures thus obtained can be compared with the large normal databases now available (Chaffin, Herrin, Keyserling, 1978; Kishino, Mayer, Gatchel, Parrish, Anderson, Gustin, Mooney, 1986).

Effort assessment for isometric testing is based on the reproducibility of the performance on multiple tests for the same individual. The variance for maximum effort has been shown to be less than 10%, while that for individuals attempting to display suboptimal effort is above 20% (Carlsoo, 1986; Caldwell, Grossman, 1973). It would appear that the standard "torso lift" and "leg lift" procedures would be broadly used in developing a general normative database. However, specific changes may be proposed following ergonomic job analysis, and different lifts based on set foot position and varying heights for isometric testing may be required. These tests can be performed on the ISTU or Liftask by resetting the lift height. A disadvantage of the Cybex dynamometer for this purpose is that a "jerky" lift impulse limits the averaging capability of the dynamometer when the force settles to a stable level. This probem is eliminated by the ISTU strain gauge.

Following this, isokinetic testing for dynamic lifting capacity can be performed on the same machine. At the University of Texas Southwestern Medical Center at Dallas, we have chosen not to restrict foot position or lifting technique, since we feel this imposes artificial restraints not justified by the current state of knowledge of "proper lifting style." Furthermore, externally imposed lift instructions are not likely to be used by the worker on the job. While weight-lifters do appear to have accepted training techniques and styles of lifting, they often require considerable education not generally available to the industrial population. It is still controversial whether these styles, even if learned by workers, would decrease rates of lifting injury. Certainly, the superb training and fitness of the athlete are key factors in injury resistance.

There are two possible styles of lifting evaluation, the *ergonomic* and the *anthropometric.* At present, computer software facilitates the latter technique because there is no electronic or mechanical way of stopping a test at a pre-determined height. However, even when such capability is available, each protocol will have its own advantages as follows:

1. *Ergonomic Protocol:* In this method, one attempts to simulate specific heights of lift one might actually encounter in industry. Loads typically need to be lifted on to certain height shelves, and for certain purposes tests, specific to a given job, can be designed according to this method. A convenient height for testing lumbopelvic functional unit capacity is generally in the range of 0 to 36 inches, while shoulder girdle and upper extremity functional units are tested from 36 to 72 inches. However, anthropometric considerations affect this test, so that a shorter individual will be at a relative disadvantage in producing work over this range compared to a taller person. The taller individual can "get his back into it" all the way to 36 inches, while the shorter subject may be completing the lift in an erect position using the "arm curl" musculature that is incapable of generating as much force. Similarly, the shorter individual is forced to transfer to an overhead "arm extension" position in the upper ranges of lifting. On the other hand, if appropriate height and weight normalization is used, this can be an effective test to stabilize the "impulse" variable isokinetically while simulating actual workplace conditions in all other ways. Moreover, because the distance is constant, work and work/body weight values can be compared from one individual to the next. By contrast, average force will be a far less consistent measure unless sufficient subjects are available to normalize directly to height as well as to weight.

2. *Anthropometric Protocol:* In this method, patients' anatomic landmarks are selected to set the lift termination point. In effect, the lumbopelvic and lower extremity functional units are active in lifting from floor to knuckle height in an erect posture, while the arm curl functions from

knuckle to shoulder height. Above this level, shoulder flexion and arm extension are operative. By utilizing this measure, height normalization is not required, which is a great advantage in decreasing the demands of normative database collection. The price paid, however, is that work and work/body weight values cannot be used because of the variable distance of lift between subjects. However, an important characteristic of isokinetic testing can be used to advantage here. Because isokinetic distance of lift is proportional to time of lift at any given speed (by definition), D/t is always a constant. Because power equals force × distance/time, power is actually proportional to an "average force" integrated over the distance of lift. Thus, at any given speed, both power and average force can be used in this protocol to compare subjects irrespective of lift distance. For this reason, the anthropometic protocol can be used at present even though no electronic or mechanical stops have been built into the system. In addition, because the power and average force calculations are based on different computer-manipulated curves (best work repetion curve vs. average points curve), they have different characteristics and can both be used for comparison as independent variables.

The computer calculates factors similar to the isolated sagittal and axial trunk testing devices including peak-torque, work, angle of peak, and acceleration time (effectively, a measure of lift "explosiveness"). Endurance and recovery protocols may be available, though they are probably of less importance than measuring this factor specifically in the injured functional unit, as would be tested with the isolated sagittal and axial trunk strength testing devices.

Lifting to set heights produces an *ergonomic protocol* in which test heights can be set actually simulating the shelf heights in a workplace. In comparing one individual to another for normalized physical capacity, however, heights of different individuals impose anatomic restraints which may provide an artificial advantage to one individual or another based on height. This means that ergonomic protocols, if standardized, must be normalized for height in addition to other factors such as weight, gender, and age. An advantage of ergonomic protocols is that peak forces, average forces, work and power can all be compared since the lifting distance is always the same. By contrast, anthropometric protocols are tests based on body position; i.e., floor to knuckle, knuckle to shoulder, etc. Because these tasks use anatomic landmarks, normalization for height is unnecessary. Fortunately, because distance is unstandardized between individuals of different heights, comparison of work performance is not possible. However, a feature of isokinetic devices is that at any given speed, distance is proportional to time (D/t = velocity, or a constant). Thus, power as calculated by the computer is comparable between individuals in an anthropometric protocol.

As in the isolated trunk strength measurement devices, computerization now permits analysis of curves with a printout superimposing an average points curve (APC), maximum points curve (MPC) and best work repetition curve (BWRC) (Fig. 11–3A). Poor patient effort can be documented by the variability between the APC/MPC displays, which may be a consistent display as seen with neuromuscular inhibition, or a variable display as seen in a "malingerer" who is trying to "defraud the machine" (Fig. 11–3B).

The Electronic Resistance System (Digital Kinetics, Danville, CA) is a device

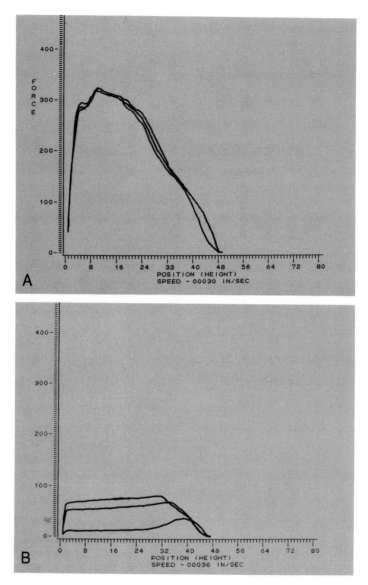

Fig. 11–3. A, Liftask curves through a standard range of motion on a normal subject with good effort. B, Liftask curve on a subject who is "malingering," thereby producing very variable forces on multiple repetitions.

just becoming commercially available for measurement of isokinetic and isotonic lifting. In addition, the Biodex System (Biodex, Inc., Shirley, NY) is currently introducing a Lift Simulation Attachment to permit isokinetic and isometric lift measurements. This attachment will allow utilization of the Biodex dynamometer and data collection capability. Further details on these devices are unavailable at this time.

POSITIONAL TOLERANCE TESTING

The testing of positional tolerance is truly in its infancy. While it is clear that patients with low back pain have difficulty performing a variety of tasks besides lifting, quantitative testing of these abilities remains primarily in a research setting. While lifting, and for that matter strength and range of motion, can be measured in short, time-limited tests, the measure of positional tolerance ultimately demands a length of observation that may be inconsistent with practical, clinical assessment. Philosophically, however, a test can provide a relevant functional measure if it is able to simulate a task, even incompletely, thereby correlating deficiencies in the test with deficiencies in performing physical demands of actual work. The tasks of standing, carrying, or crawling are limited primarily by endurance, though time constraints force therapists to evaluate the task with short tests failing to reach an endurance threshold.

Thus, the challenge in developing positional tolerance tests becomes two-fold: (a) designing a relevant, time-efficient measure which provides true simulation of the activity in question; and (b) comparing this information with known work demands. In addition, as before, an effort factor must be available and a normative database must be assembled. If these conditions can be satisfied, determination of the patient's capability to perform a specific job is feasible. Furthermore, training protocols can be established for improving the capability to do all of these tasks, while intensively emphasizing those which are particularly necessary for the patient's job.

Figure 11–4A illustrates one question from the Department of Labor's Duty Status Report, form CA-17, describing the subject's regular work and physical requirements. This information is to be provided to an evaluating physician by the patient's supervisor. Figure 11–4B illustrates a question in part B, to be filled out by the attending physician, in which the patient's physical limitations are indicated, for comparison to job demands of the patient's regular work position. If lower physical capabilities are identified than required in the regular job, "light duty" can be provided at the option of the employing agency. If total incapacity is documented, or if restricted duty is unavailable, the patient may be eligible for compensation. This is, by no means, intended as providing an exhaustive job analysis, and relies on information provided by a patient or supervisor which may be neither entirely accurate nor objective. At this point, a complete analysis provided by an industrial engineer trained in ergonomic procedures is not generally feasible within the medical milieu, and the number of industries which have already obtained such analyses within their facilities remains small and scattered. Therefore, the ultimate ability to obtain meaningful analyses of jobs, at least in major industries, is a goal of both the ergonomist and spine rehabilitation specialist, but such information is unlikely to be generally available in the near future.

Most tasks lend themselves to an initial categorization: Can the patient do the task or not? If confronted with the need to climb a ladder, crawl through a tunnel, or push an object requiring specific force output, a subject will declare if he or she is either able to perform the task or not. However, the issues of what a "normal subject" can perform, or the effort the patient is placing into the testing, are more difficult to quantitate. With regard to "normative data," we have taken the position that the same principles can be followed that were utilized in developing normal databases for mobility, strength, and lifting capacity. Appropriate numbers of "normal subjects" are tested, with a broad spectrum of age, body weight and gender characteristics available to provide the most specific data. In functional task performance, we ideally add testing

A

8. Specify the Usual Work Requirements of the Employee. Check Whether Employee Performs These Tasks or is Exposed Continuously or Intermittently, and Give Number of Hours.

Activity	Continuous	Intermittent		Activity/Exposure	Continuous	Intermittent	
a. Lifting/Carrying: Sedentary 0–10 lbs.			Hrs Per Day	p. Fine Manipulation			Hrs Per Day
b. Lifting/Carrying: Light 10–20 lbs.			Hrs Per Day	q. Reaching above Shoulder			Hrs Per Day
c. Lifting/Carrying: Moderate 20–50 lbs.			Hrs Per Day	r. Heat			degrees F
d. Lifting/Carrying: Heavy 50–100 lbs.			Hrs Per Day	s. Cold			degrees F
e. Sitting			Hrs Per Day	t. Excess Humidity			Hrs Per Day
f. Standing			Hrs Per Day	u. Chemicals, Solvents, etc. (Identify)			Hrs Per Day
g. Walking			Hrs Per Day	v. Fumes (Identify)			Hrs Per Day
h. Climbing Stairs			Hrs Per Day	w. Dust (Identify)			Hrs Per Day
i. Climbing Ladders			Hrs Per Day	x. Noise			dBA Hrs Per Day
j. Kneeling			Hrs Per Day	y. Other (Describe)			Hrs Per Day
k. Bending			Hrs Per Day	9. Does the Job Require Driving a Vehicle?			
l. Stooping			Hrs Per Day	☐ Yes (Specify____) ☐ No			
m. Twisting			Hrs Per Day	Operating Machinery? ☐ Yes (Specify____) ☐ No			
n. Pulling/Pushing			Hrs Per Day	10. The Employee Works			Hours Per Day
o. Simple Grasping			Hrs Per Day				Days Per Week

B

14. Is Employee Able to Perform His/Her Regular Work (Described on the Front of This Form)?

☐ Yes, If so, ☐ Full-Time or ☐ Part-Time____ Hours Per Day
(Fill In)

☐ No, If not, complete Item 15 below.

15. Complete the Following If the Answer To Item 14 is "No".

Activity/Exposure	Continuous	Intermittent		Activity/Exposure	Continuous	Intermittent	
a. Lifting/Carrying: Sedentary 0–10 lbs.			Hrs Per Day	p. Fine Manipulation			Hrs Per Day
b. Lifting/Carrying: Light 10–20 lbs			Hrs Per Day	q. Reaching Above Shoulder			Hrs Per Day
c. Lifting/Carrying: Moderate 20–50 lbs.			Hrs Per Day	r. Heat			degrees F
d. Lifting/Carrying: Heavy 50–100 lbs.			Hrs Per Day	s. Cold			degrees F
e. Sitting			Hrs Per Day	t. Excess Humidity			Hrs Per Day
f. Standing			Hrs Per Day	u. Chemicals, Solvents, etc. (Identify)			Hrs Per Day
g. Walking			Hrs Per Day	v. Fumes (Identify)			Hrs Per Day
h. Climbing Stairs			Hrs Per Day	w. Dust (Identify)			Hrs Per Day
i. Climbing Ladders			Hrs Per Day	x. Noise			dBA Hrs Per Day
j. Kneeling			Hrs Per Day	Y. Are Interpersonal Relations Affected Because of A Neuropsychiatric Condition? (e.g., Ability to Give or Take Supervision, Meet Deadlines, etc.)			
k. Bending			Hrs Per Day				
l. Stooping			Hrs Per Day	☐ Yes (Describe) ☐ No			
m. Twisting			Hrs Per Day				
n. Pulling/Pushing			Hrs Per Day				
o. Simple Grasping			Hrs Per Day				

Fig. 11–4. A, Department of Labor Duty Status Report, form CA–17: Question 8 to be filled out by supervisor describing physical requirements of regular work. B, Department of Labor Duty Status Report, form CA–17: Question 14 to be filled out by attending physician documenting the physician's perception of present work tolerance.

of new norms associated with a specific job, such as truck driver or nurse. Development of these databases may not be universally practicable, but should at least be done for particularly high risk ergonomic activities, or for those in which a particularly high demand for a specific activity, such as climbing, is inherent in the job. Patients returning to these positions should be at a particularly high state of fitness for carrying out necessary job-related tasks. When the workplace requires extreme emphasis on a specific task, such as balance for high-rise construction, special testing protocols may be required.

Effort testing may ultimately be quantified along the lines described in previous chapters. Patients whose performance is erratic and inconsistent may be supplying suboptimal effort for a variety of reasons (pain, neuromuscular inhibition, generalized deconditioning, fear of reinjury or conscious malingering). Most of the functional tasks measured require combinations of mobility, strength, endurance, and agility. Performance deficits are thus likely to be proportionately inhibited (albeit in non-linear fashion) by deficits in more than one of these general functions. Since most of these physical attributes obey the principle that, in general, maximum effort is reproducible and submaximal effort is not, measures of performance variability will probably evolve as commercial technology to document positional tolerance emerges. In this regard, it is interesting to note that patients whose performance is limited by legitimate pain generally manage to demonstrate minimal variability in effort measurements, particularly after periods of training. Thus, there is even the hope that some day pain itself may be "quantified" by the degree to which performance is impaired on physical measurement by evaluating the consistency with which the measurements are reproduced. Effort in tasks limited by aerobic capacity can be assessed alternatively. Heart rate monitoring of these tasks permits observation of a reproducible end-point. Use of this technique, already described for isoinertial lifting, may be appropriate for some positional tolerance tests.

TASK PERFORMANCE SIMULATION DEVICES

One particularly promising method is the computer-assisted functional measurement technology developed under grants from the National Institute of Disability Research and Rehabilitation (NIDRR) at the University of Texas Southwestern Medical Center at Dallas. This system, which tests a large number of musculoskeletal and neurologic parameters, offers promise for quantifying some specific physical characteristics which may have implications for specific tasks. Thus, certain jobs (e.g., a steel worker) require balance as a job demand criterion. This function can be measured by the Function Measurement Laboratory (FML) devices, and compared to a large normative database to quantify this capability. Other measurement capabilities of potential importance in this area are body stability, reaction time, and upper/lower extremity movement speed (Fig. 11–5A).

One of the multiple measures of human performance available at the FML is measurement of postural stability. A forced platform is used to detect the amount of fore-aft and lateral sway, taking into account ability to maintain stable stance over time in multiple testing modes, including eyes open/closed and single or both-leg stance (Kondraske, 1986). In cases where a subject cannot maintain stability for the required 15-second interval, their score (based on average center of pressure displacment on the platform) is normalized by dividing by the actual stance time. Upper and lower extremity test boards are used to implement reaction, speed and coordination tests (Fig. 11–5B and C) (Kondraske, Potvin, Tourtellotte, Syndulko, 1984). The boards consist of various touch-sensitive regions and visual stimuli (lights) used with special algorithms to obtain measures of specific dimensions of performance. Lateral reaching and finger-tapping coordination has been found to be a most useful test for both upper and lower extremities. Both speed and accuracy are stressed in this coordination test. For upper extremity reaction tests, simple and multichoice tests (from 1 to 8 choices) can be executed. In lower extremity reaction time, single and 2-choice modes are included. Speeds of finger, hand, and foot-

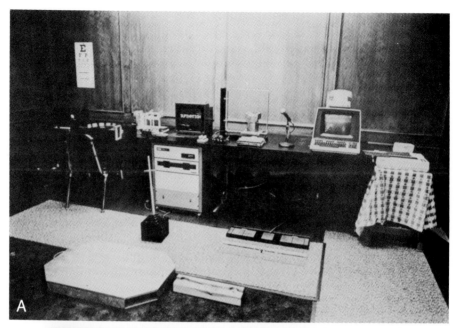

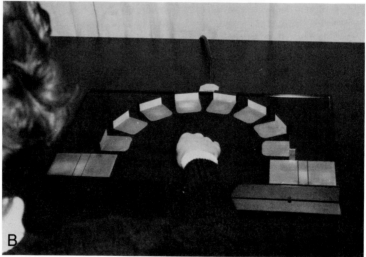

Fig. 11–5. A, The Function Measurement Laboratory at the Department of Physical Therapy, University of Texas Southwestern Medical Center at Dallas. B, Upper extremity reaction, speed and coordination test board.

tapping are also measured with these boards, counting the number of taps accomplished in a fixed time period.

Upper Extremity Devices

Another functional task assessment technique has been developed by Matheson and Ogden (1983) and is utilized in a variety of rehabilitation/work hardening programs with seminar presentations. Measurement tends to focus primarily on lifting characteristics, using equipment such as the WEST device

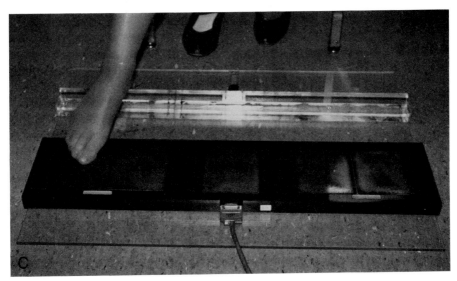

Fig. 11–5 (cont.) C, Lower extremity reaction, speed and coordination test board.

discussed previously for "lifting under load," but other techniques look at functional performance measurements. An example of this technology is the "Tool Sort," which measures the patient's ability to recognize and manipulate a variety of tools.

Upper extremity function, specifically as it relates to hand manipulation of tools, can also be assessed using the BTE computer-assisted measurement system (Baltimore Therapeutic Equipment, Inc., Baltimore, MD). The computer is connected to a transducer, allowing measurement of torque produced by a variety of tools which can be attached to the transducer. Hand and arm strength, as related to tool use, can be assessed. It can be quantified in comparison to the contralateral side, as well as, potentially, to a normative database. It is used primarily as an occupational therapy assessment tool for functional retraining following hand injuries or surgical procedures. However, this function can also be affected by problems in the cervical or shoulder girdle functional units, particularly in whole-body activities such as lifting. Therefore, in assessing whether the dysfunction noted in the whole-body activity is due primarily to axial or extremity difficulties, the therapist may utilize this tool.

The computer itself is compact and lends itself to easy storage, with a cart holding more than 20 "tools" allowing manipulations of individual fingertips or gross motion, such as rotating wheels or crossbars. There is also a somewhat cumbersome set of pulleys/ropes available to which weights (sandbags) can be attached for assessing lifting at a variey of positions. This "add-on" seems inferior to other assessment devices more specifically designed to measure lifting functions. Accuracy and an effort factor are difficult to assess from the manufacturer's information, but the relatively unique upper extremity assessment capability probably warrants the significant cost.

Another device for upper extremity evaluation is the upper body ergometer (UBE) (Cybex, Ronkonkoma, NY). This is basically a vertically mounted exercise bicycle with a unique bi-directional system and adjustable arm length that permits upper extremity work evaluation and exercise in a variety of postures. Endurance/work can be assessed grossly utilizing a progressive incremental work protocol, though relative inaccuracy of the hydraulic actuator must be considered. There is also another manufacturer with an upper extemity strength/fatigue assessment tool—the WEST 4 (Work Evaluation Systems Technology, Huntington Beach, CA). This technology, while used primarily for hand and upper extremity function measures, can be an important adjunct to assessing the patient's level of reconditioning and appropriateness for return to work.

Multiple-Task Obstacle Course

The approach taken at PRIDE and the University of Texas Southwestern Medical Center at Dallas has been to measure actual physical task performance on an "obstacle course," simulating the job demands of the workplace identified in Figure 11–4. A normal database is developed by testing the number of repetitions produced on each component during a fixed period of time. Results are expressed as percent normal for each individual activity (reaching, bending, crawling, etc.), as well as a cumulative time for the entire obstacle course. Effort ratings, at this time, are based on heart rate assessment by therapists observing the test. The present obstacle course quantifies a variety of tasks related to spine function. These are documented in Table 11–1 (Mayer, 1985).

A typical pair of obstacles is seen in Figure 11–6. In 11–6A, a patient is seen passing through the crawling tunnel. Its walls are padded to protect the individual's head and knees, and there is a sufficient diameter to permit large individuals to pass through unimpeded. An "electric eye" sensor detects the initial entry, and counts the number of passes (repetitions) through the tunnel in a predetermined period of time.

Figure 11–6B shows a subject using the squat push-pull device. The "drawer," really a bar mounted in a slide at 12 inches height, is mounted beneath a table

Table 11–1. Obstacle Course Tasks

Tasks	Technique
1. Walking push-pull	Waist-high slide with dynamometer providing higher work for greater movement velocity
2. Sitting reach	Stool with 45 degree angle slide mounted for motion from shoulder height to overhead using similar dynamometer
3. Squatting push-pull	Simulated "drawer" at 12″ height with dynamometer
4. Twisting	Rotate bar at table height with similar dynamometer forcing trunk torsion
5. Bending (without lifting)	Maneuver air pump behind thigh-high wall forcing task with bent posture
6. Crawling	Crawl through 6 ft tunnel
7. Balancing	Walking on 4″ × 6″ beam
8. Climbing	Climb a vertical or angled ladder or climbing simulator

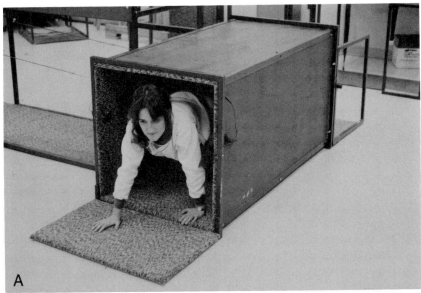

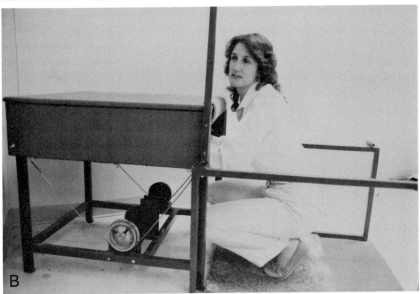

Fig. 11–6. A, Subject exiting from the tunnel portion of the Obstacle Course to test crawling and kneeling capacity. B, Subject being tested at the obstacle requiring push/pull forces to be exerted in the squatting position.

top which allows the movement to be done only when arms are at the level of the bar. For efficiency in a test, the subject will usually choose to squat; but in a training mode with prolonged movements in this position, the subject may choose the kneeling posture. Like several of the other obstacles, a dynamometer serves to produce push/pull resistance in both directions, with work performed in a fixed interval increasing with greater speed. Thus, the number of repetitions in a fixed period of time is a measure of work performance rather than merely speed of movement.

The Versa-Climber

The Versa-Climber (Heart Rate, Inc., Costa Mesa, CA) is an interesting device permitting vertical climbing simulation utilizing synchronous alternating upper/lower extremity training, or isolating upper from lower training (Fig. 11–7). It is a hydraulic device, with a direct relationship between velocity and force output: as work velocity increases, so does the force required. It includes a metronome to set climbing rate, a display which counts velocity, reps and distance traveled, and a heart rate monitor allowing the subject to self-select (or pre-select) a training protocol based on improving aerobic fitness. In effect, it is a cardiovascular training tool and hydraulic resistance strength/endurance training device, while also being useful for assessment of functional task performance. As such, it is one of the first devices to be available, other than lifting devices already discussed, to assess capability for performing specific tasks.

The device permits a pre-set 75-degree climb angle. In the conventional mode, the feet are placed into stirrups and hands grip a bar, and as hand and foot are depressed on one side, they rise on the other. Pulling down simulates climbing, but pushing upward can simulate descending. In addition, stationary footplates and hand grips permit the arm and leg portions of the device, respectively, to be used independently.

As in other task performance tests, standardized protocols can be developed

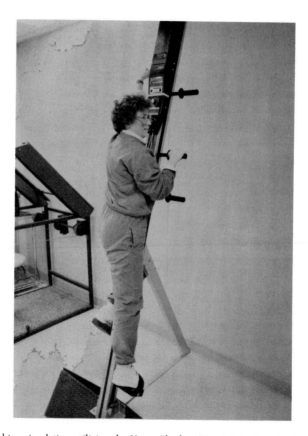

Fig. 11–7.   Climbing simulation utilizing the Versa-Climber (Heart Rate Inc., Costa Mess, CA).

in which repetitions in a fixed time interval can be assessed, with the knowledge that ascending speed also increases force necessary. Therefore, increased repetitions are indicative of increased work rates. The heart rate monitor can be used as an "effort factor" or a "training monitor" during strength/endurance/aerobic training.

Tolerance to Specific Daily Postures

Quantifying tolerance to specific daily postures, particularly sitting and standing, is in some ways simpler and in other ways more difficult. These postures are so frequently used that a time-limited test really can give only inadequate information concerning these tolerances. The challenge has additional practical implications for every occupational therapist confronted by the chronic low back pain patient skilled in sedentary work who reports, "I can only sit for 15 minutes." Sitting intolerance can be plausibly accentuated by the addition of vibratory factors, particularly in the range of 4.5 to 6 Hertz, such as is commonly encountered in driving trucks or heavy equipment (Pope, Frymoyer, Anderson, 1984; Chaffin, Anderson, 1984). As a practical matter, a time-limited system for evaluating this type of tolerance has not yet been devised. Therefore, we rely on more prolonged observation in the treatment program itself for measuring and building sitting and standing tolerance. In addition to their other roles, then, the physical and occupational therapists observe patients in a regimented program requiring specific periods of sitting and standing. While patients may initially be constantly changing position due to pain while participating in functional restoration, tolerance usually develops through the treatment program so that sitting and standing positions can each be documented many hours a day. For those individuals who do have a serious sitting/standing tolerance problem, treatment is routinely prescribed to lessen this problem. For those patients subjected to a one-time test, however, a functional measurement is not presently available.

Other Quantifiable Tasks

Though not included in the PRIDE obstacle course, other tasks can be quantified by the imaginative occupational therapist. For example, carrying can be observed over a measured course requiring the subject to hold specific weights, such as cinder blocks. Stairs or a platform simulating a loading dock may be added to the course. Areas for simulating house framing, heavy-equipment operation or plumbing tasks can also be assembled. Until more commercial devices appear on the market, this field will require continued creativity.

SUBJECTIVE FACTORS IN TASK PERFORMANCE

It is now proper to focus on the issues that task performance tests *cannot* measure. These issues are summed up in the following questions: *a)* does the subject have pain during the test? and *b) will* the patient do a specific job? These questions revolve partly around the previously described physical capacity measures, and partly around psychosocioeconomic factors which can be only partially quantified, or in some cases, not measured at all. Amount of pain magnification, level of motivation, and secondary gain are examples of these psychosocioeconomic factors. In most cases, the clinician is able to make a definitive statement in response to the following question: "*Could* the patient do the specified tasks if he/she were willing to do so given his/her level of perceived pain?" Though a qualified response, this represents an extremely important step forward, as it is essentially equivalent to the type of information generally available to the physician when making a determination about physical capabilities after extremity injury. The crucial factor in extremity medical practice appears to be the unanimity of opinion among multiple physicians based on their independent medical evaluations, something that rarely occurs in low back disability examinations. Given uniform, predictable results of standardized physical capacity testing, well understood by these examining clinicians, considerably greater uniformity of opinion may be anticipated in the future. The subject is further discussed in Chapter 19 dealing with disability impairment evaluation.

In conducting the various task performance tests, it is still felt to be a useful to obtain a Global Effort Rating from the therapist after each test. A patient may do well on certain tests, but not on others. For example, a worker injured in a fall may climb poorly, but put good effort into lifting tests. A global summary of all effort measures by the therapist has proven empirically to be a useful and reasonably reproducible assessment. As a single factor, it is easier for the clinician reviewing the report to digest than multiple effort factors.

Ultimately, we anticipate simplifications of both performance and effort scores. Just as grade point averages sum up multiple grades to give a measure of a student's performance, so can performance and effort be graded by averaging "percent normal" scores on multiple tests. Such sophistication will hopefully be developed in the near future.

WHAT CAN'T WE DO?

We have come to the end of our exploration of methods of physical capacity assessment in the low back. New technology certainly grants us a great many opportunities to provide relevant tests for those aspects of the deconditioning syndrome that limit lumbar and whole body function in patients with low back pain. However, short of actual observation of the patient, we are not presently able to quantify factors such as fatigue resistance throughout an 8-hour day, the coordination to do repetitive tasks in an efficient way, and other factors affecting the patient's ability to perform in a competitive work environment. Lest we be too concerned about this problem, we should note how sports medicine physicians have handled this in the extremities. It has been repeatedly observed that even following ideal rehabilitation of extremity joints in sports medicine centers alone, a return to optimal athletic performance was almost never possible. Instead, simulation followed by progressive return to the specific activity to be performed was necessary, be it pitching a baseball, running with a football, or dunking a basketball. Many ingenious ways have been devised to simulate the sport by breaking down the components of the activity and training to increase tolerance to segmented activities first. Ultimately, these segments are combined into a "return to the sport" itself. While the ability to perform these segmented activities can be observed but not objectively quantified, this technique has proven effective in returning the extremity-injured athlete and worker to the highest level of performance that can be anticipated. Currently, this represents the limit of physical quantification for the extremities, and will have to suffice for the low back also. The "sport" to which the injured worker returns is a job. The transition from rehabilitation program to job may be another difficult step, but one which can dependably be taken by most motivated patients.

In summary, it appears that a combination of the psychophysical lifting protocol and Liftask isokinetic and isometric testing can provide the clinician with a global view of lifting capacity, endurance, and effort. We must await the development of additional dynamic lifting devices to judge whether the present unique technology will stand the test of time. Obstacle courses and other new methods for assessing positional tolerance await commercial development and standardization.

CHAPTER REFERENCES

Arnold J, Rauschenberger J, Soubel W, et al.: Validation and utility of a strength test for selecting steelworkers. J Appl Psych *67*:588–604, 1982.

Asfour S, Ayoub M, Mital A: Effects of an endurance and strength training program on lifting capability of males. Ergon *27*:283–290, 1984.

Ayoub M, Mital A, Bakken L, Asfour S, Bethea N: Development of strength and capacity norms for manual materials handling activities: the state-of-the-art. Human Factors *22*:271–283, 1980.

Bigos S, Spengler D, Martin N, Zeh J, Fisher L, Nachemson A, Wang M: Back injuries in industry: a retrospective study II. Injury factors. Spine *11*:246–251, 1986.

Bigos S, Spengler D, Martin N, Zeh J, Fisher L, Nachemson A: Back injuries in industry: a retrospective study III. Employee-related factors. Spine *11*:252–256, 1986.

Caldwell L, Grossman E: Effort scaling of isometric muscle contractions. J Motor Behav *11*:5–11, 1973.

Carsloo S: With what degree of precision can voluntary status muscle force be repeated? Scand J Rehab Med *18*:1–3, 1986.

Chaffin B: Human strength capability and low-back pain. J Occup Med *16*:248–254, 1974.

Chaffin D, Andersson G: Occupational Biomechanics, New York, John Wiley & Sons, 1984.

Chaffin D, Herrin G, Keyserling W: Pre-employment strength testing: an updated position. J Occup Med *20*:403–408, 1978.

Harber P, Soohoo K: Static ergonomic strength testing in evaluating occupational back pain. J Occup Med *26*:77–82, 1984.

Jackson A, Osburn H, Laughery K: Validity of Isometric Strength Tests for Predicting Performance in Physically Demanding Tasks. Proceedings of Human Factors Society, 28th Annual Meeting, San Antonio, TX, October 22–26, 1984, pp. 451–454.

Jackson J: Biomechanical hazards in the dockworker. Ann Occup *11*:147–153, 1968.

Kamon E, Kiser D, Pytel J: Dynamic and static lifting capacity and muscular strength of steelmill workers. Am Indust Hyg Assoc J *43*:853–857, 1982.

Keyserling W, Herrin G, Chaffin D: Isometric strength testing as a means of controlling medical incidents on strenuous jobs. J Occup Med *22*:332–336, 1980.

Kishino N, Mayer T, Gatchel R, Parrish M, Anderson C, Gustin L, Mooney V: Quantification of lumbar function Part 4: Isometric and isokinetic stimulation in normal subjects and low-back dysfunction patients. Spine *10*:921–927, 1985.

Kondraske G: Towards a standard clinical measure of postural stability. In Proceedings of the 8th annual conference of the IEEE Enginering in Medicine and Biology Society (Kondraske G, Robinson C, Eds.) *3*:1579–1582, 1986.

Kondraske G, Potvin A, Tourtellotte W, Syndulko K: A Computer-based system for automated quantification of neurologic function. IEEE Trans Biomed Eng *31*:401–414, 1984.

Kroemer K: An isoinertial technique to assess individual lifting capability. Human Factors *25*:493–506, 1983.

Marras W, King A, Joynt R: Measurements of loads on the lumbar spine under isometric and isokinetic conditions. Spine *9*:176–1988, 1984.

Matheson L, Ogden L: Work Tolerance Screening. Trabues Canyon, CA, Rehabilitation Institute of Southern California, 1983.

Mayer T: Using physical measurement to assess low back pain. J Musculoskel Med *6*:44–59, 1985.

Mayer T, Barnes D, Kishino N, Nichols G, Gatchel R, Mayer H, Mooney V: Progressive isoinertial lifting evaluation, Part I: a standardized protocol and normative data base. Spine, 1988, in press.

Mayer T, Barnes D, Nichols G, Kishino N, Coval K, Piel B, Hoshino D, Gatchel R: Progressive isoinertial lifting evaluation, Part II: a comparison with isokinetic lifting in a disabled chronic low-back pain industrial population. Spine, 1988, in press.

Mital A, Channaveeraiah C, Fard H, Khaledi H: Reliability of repetitive dynamic strengths as a screening tool for manual lifting tasks. Clin Biomech *1*:125–129, 1986.

Pope M, Frymoyer J, Andersson G, Occupational Low Back Pain, New York, Praeger Scientific, 1984.

Pytel J, Kamon E: Dynamic strength test as a predictor for maximal and acceptable lifting. Ergonomics *24*:663–672, 1981.

Reilly R, Zedeck S, Tenopyr M: Validity and fairness of physical ability tests for predicting performance in craft jobs. J Appl Psych *64*:262–274, 1979.

Schultz A, Andersson G, Haderspeck K, et al.: Analysis and measurement of lumbar loads in tasks involving bends and twists. J Biomech *15*:669–675, 1982.

Snook S, Campanelli R, Hart J: A study of three preventive approaches to low back injury. J Occup Med *20*:278–481, 1978.

Snook S, Irvine C: Maximum acceptable weight of lift. J Am Indust Hyg *9*:322–329, 1967.

Spengler D, Bigos S, Martin N, Zeh J, Fisher L, Nachemson A: Back injuries in industry: a retrospective study I. Overview and cost analysis. Spine *11*:241–245, 1986.

White A, Gordon S: Synopsis: workshop on idiopathic low-back pain. Spine *7*:141–149, 1982.

Chapter 12

Psychosocial Assessment of Chronic Low Back Pain

As we noted in Chapter 4, with the introduction of the gate-control theory of pain in 1965 by Melzack and Wall, the scientific community came to accept the importance of central, psychologic factors in the pain perception process. As a result, there has been a great deal of research attempting to isolate psychologic characteristics associated with low-back pain patients. For example, the Minnesota Multiphasic Personality Inventory (MMPI) has been widely used to delineate these psychologic characteristics. This early work attempted to differentiate "functional" low-back pain from "organic" low-back pain. However, as was pointed out in Chapter 4, Sternbach (1974) challenged the utility and validity of attempting to make a functional-organic dichotomy when dealing with chronic low-back pain. Moreover, from research conducted with patients participating in the PRIDE program, Barnett (1986) found that elevation of scores on tests such as the MMPI of chronic low-back pain patients significantly *decreased* to lower levels after successful treatment. Thus, elevations in these scores are most likely due to the trauma and stress associated with the chronic disabling condition and not due primarily to some stable psychologic traits.

Chronic pain is a complex and interactive psychophysiologic behavior pattern that cannot be broken down into distinct, independent psychologic and physical components. In the functional restoration approach, psychologic assessment is not used to try to differentiate "organic" from "functional" causes. Rather, the assessment is directed at evaluating the important psychologic characteristics of each individual patient in order to help guide the treatment process, as well as to help predict therapeutic outcome. This psychologic assessment evaluates not only the patients' self-reported pain, but also evaluates overall psychologic functioning in order to help therapeutic team personnel to effectively integrate each patient into the intensive treatment program. Quantified changes in many of these measures are used to document therapeutic improvement.

In this chapter, we will provide an overview of the various psychologic assessment devices used in the functional restoration treatment approach. Currently, a wide variety of diverse tests are used because there has not been a comprehensive instrument developed specifically for chronic low-back pain. We are currently in the process of developing such a psychometrically sound test, which will hopefully be available for use in the near future. As will be emphasized, a comprehensive psychologic assessment of each patient is essential to "guide" the patient effectively through such an intensive treatment regimen, and to evaluate the patient's cognitive-psychologic resources that may affect response to treatment.

PSYCHOLOGIC TESTS

Minnesota Multiphasic Personality Inventory (MMPI)

This inventory is one of the oldest and most frequently used tests of psychologic functioning. Often in the past, however, it was used simply because "everyone else uses it." By itself, it does not offer much help in choosing among treatment options. However, in a comprehensive evaluation using several types of assessment tools, the MMPI can add valuable information regarding psychologic functioning.

Of the 10 major clinical scales by which the MMPI responses are classified, the Hysteria (Hy), Depression (D), and Hypochondriasis (Hs) Scales are the most important when evaluating a chronic pain patient. Elevation of the Hysteria and Hypochondriasis Scales with a normal Depression Scale produces the so-called *Conversion V.* This test profile was thought to be associated with pain that has a large psychologic component. It generally flags patients who are neurotic and anxious, and who magnify their symptoms while remaining somewhat indifferent to the limitations of their behavior produced by these symptoms. They often have little insight into their own problems and often use denial as a defense against facing such problems. On the other hand, patients who have a *neurotic triad* (Hysteria, Depression, and Hypochondriasis Scales are *all* elevated) are more aware that their symptoms have a psychologic component and are better able to express their anxiety and stress.

As discussed previously, Barnett (1986) evaluated changes in MMPI profile scores before and after functional restoration treatment. Figure 12–1 presents these two profiles. As can be seen, there was a substantial decrease in the elevation of scales after treatment. It should be clearly noted that these figures represent *averaged* profile scores across many patients (104 at pretreatment and 69 at follow-up). There are wide individual differences whenever viewing any one particular patient profile.

Over the years, there have also been numerous other scales developed for the MMPI. The *McAndrew* scale, initially standardized on an outpatient population of alcoholics, helps one to recognize the patient with an alcoholic or drug-dependent personality type. Therefore, it can determine which patients are at high risk for drug abuse, before habituation occurs. Patients do not need to be actively taking drugs to have a positive score on the McAndrew scale, and even reformed substance abusers often score very high. This scale is useful in evaluating acute low back patients to select out those who may be particularly susceptible to long periods of hospitalization for bed rest and excessive intramuscular analgesic use.

Patients scoring high on this test scale also tend to be prolonged users of oral opiate analgesics and tranquilizing muscle relaxants as their pain becomes more chronic. Since the personality profile of the dependent drug abuser bears some resemblance to that of many chronic pain patients, abnormalities on this scale can raise a "red flag" for clinicians to beware of early adverse behavioral changes. In a later section, we will discuss the concept of "red flags" raised

PRETREATMENT MMPI

POSTTREATMENT MMPI

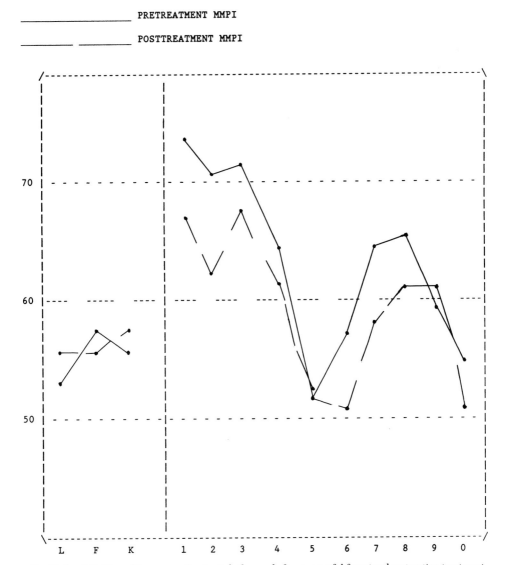

Fig. 12–1. MMPI profiles scores of patients before and after successful functional restoration treatment.

by psychologic assessment, and how they can be helpful in the treatment process.

The *ego strength* scale is another special scale that can help identify patients who have limited emotional resources. Patients who exhibit particularly low ego strength, along with other psychologic problems, are less likely to benefit from treatment regimens that demand motivation and personal responsibility than are patients who score higher on the ego strength scale.

In terms of the MMPI as a whole, there are certain practical drawbacks to the test. It is lengthy and somewhat disturbing for patients to take, often producing a conviction that their physicians think "it's all in my head." Efforts need to be made to convince patients that the reason they are being asked to take the test is to provide an overall "picture" of general psychologic functioning, and not to categorize them into any psychiatric pigeonholes. In addition, the test was standardized on a psychiatrically-disturbed population of English-speaking subjects, predominantly of Scandinavian heritage. Therefore, the test has substantial built-in biases based on race, national origin, language, and psychiatric disease.

It should be noted that, as an alternative to the MMPI, the SCL-90 can be administered. This test was developed to measure psychopathology in both psychiatric and medical outpatients (Derogatis, Lipman, Covi, 1973), and has been demonstrated to have a high degree of convergence with the MMPI. It takes only 20 minutes to complete, and provides an alternative to the much more time-consuming MMPI.

Millon Behavioral Health Inventory (MBHI)

Millon, Green and Meagher (1982) devised a 150-question true-false test based on 20 clinical scales that reflect medically related concerns, such as compliance with treatment regimens and reaction to treatment personnel. This test was intended as an alterative to the MMPI. Unlike the MMPI, however, which was originally designed for a psychiatric population, the MBHI was developed and standardized on an actual medical population. Since it is a relatively new test that has not yet appeared frequently in the literature, the 20 scales of the MBHI, as well as a brief summary of each, are presented in Table 12–1.

One advantage the MBHI has over the MMPI is that it requires only about 20 minutes to complete. Moreover, most patients find it to be less threatening than the MMPI because it includes questions related to medical care.

The Millon Behavioral Health Inventory is still too new to have substantial evidence to document its reliability. However, we find this inventory useful as part of our overall assessment of patients with low back pain. A number of scales have been found to be clinically meaningful. For example, we have generally found that subjects who score low on the cooperative style scale and high on the sensitive style scale demonstrate poor outcome. These individuals tend not to follow advice and can be unpredictable and moody. Obviously, such characteristics can be quite detrimental to the group treatment process. In contrast, patients scoring high on the cooperative and sociable scales demonstrate excellent outcome. We have also found that patients scoring high on the emotional vulnerability scale usually require additional psychologic help in dealing with their disabilities. Finally, some of our preliminary research has suggested that individuals scoring high on the premorbid pessimism and forceful style scales often seek out surgical treatment as an alternative.

Beck Depression Inventory (BDI)

The BDI consists of 21 items with a cumulative scoring system focusing on manifestations such as sleep disturbance, sexual dysfunction, weight change, and anhedonia. It was originally developed by Beck (1967) as a means of assessing the cognitive components of depression.

Depression, like anxiety, is a frequent concomitant of long-term back dysfunction. Although it is unclear whether depression precedes or follows the onset of low back symptoms in the majority of cases, knowledge of its presence can be quite helpful. Offering depressed patients pharmacologic treatment may

Table 12–1. Summary of MBHI Scales (Millon, Green and Meagher, 1982)

Introversive Style: High scorers are rather colorless and emotionally flat, tending to be quiet and untalkative. Health care professionals should give clear directions and not expect these patients to take the initiative in following a treatment plan.

Inhibited Style: High scorers tend to be hesitant with others and are often shy and ill at ease. However, they do seek understanding and attention; with a sympathetic attitude, one should be able to get them to cooperate.

Cooperative Style: High scorers tend to be eager to attach themselves to a supportive professional and will follow advice closely. These patients become very dependent and may resist when suggestions are made for referral to other doctors or clinics.

Sociable Style: High scorers tend to be outgoing, talkative, and charming. However, dependability is likely to be low.

Confident Style: High scorers act in a calm and confident manner. If these patients are impressed with the critical importance to their health of following the medical regimen, they will do so carefully.

Forceful Style: High scorers tend to be somewhat domineering and tough-minded. It will be necessary for the team to work hard to get these patients to follow the prescribed treatment course.

Respectful Style: High scorers are likely to be responsible, comforting, and cooperative. They do not like being sick since it signifies weakness and inefficiency.

Sensitive Style: High scorers tend to be unpredictable and moody. Rapport may be easy on some days but difficult on others.

Chronic Tension: High scorers on this scale are disposed to suffer various psychosomatic and physical ailments, notably in the cardiovascular and digestive system. Where feasible, the thought of reducing tensions and slowing down the rapid pace of life these patients pursue should be discussed.

Recent Stress: High scorers on this scale have an increased susceptibility to serious illness for the year following test administration. Regular and frequent contact with medical personnel would be advisable during this period to anticipate and avert the possibility of serious illness.

Premorbid Pessimism: High scorers on this scale are disposed to interpret life as a series of troubles and misfortunes and are likely to intensify the discomforts they experience with real physical and psychologic difficulties.

Future Despair: High scorers do not look forward to a productive future life and view medical difficulties as seriously distressing and potentially life threatening.

Social Alienation: High scorers are prone to physical and psychologic ailments and a poor adjustment to hospitalization is common.

Somatic Anxiety: High scorers tend to be hypochondriacal and susceptible to minor illnesses. They experience an abnormal amount of fear concerning bodily functions and are likely to overreact to the discomfort of surgery and hospitalization.

Allergic Inclination: High scorers among patients with allergic disorders—urticaria, dermatitis, asthma—experience emotional factors as significant precipitants of their disease process.

Gastrointestinal Susceptibility: High scorers among patients with gastrointestinal disorders—ulcers, colitis, dyspepsia—are likely to react to psychologic stress with an increase in the frequency and severity of symptomatology.

Cardiovascular Tendency: High scorers among patients with cardiovascular symptoms—hypertension, angina pectoris—are susceptible to a significant increase in complaint symptomatology under conditions of psychic tension.

Pain Treatment Responsivity: High scorers on this scale are similar in their results to patients whose management with a traditional medical treatment program was less than satisfactory.

Life Threat Reactivity: High scorers who are currently suffering a chronic or progressive life threatening illness are likely to deteriorate more rapidly than is typical among patients with a comparable physical illness.

Emotional Vulnerability: High scorers facing major surgery or other life-dependent treatment programs are vulnerable to severe disorientation, depression, or frank psychotic episodes.

encourage greater patient motivation and compliance with therapy. Indeed, the adjunctive use of antidepressant medication has become increasingly popular in the treatment of chronic pain. The recognition that the antidepressants have an effect not only on the clinical depression frequently associated with chronic pain, but also on the pain itself (Ward, 1986), should not leave the unsuspecting clinician to conclude that there may still be a "magic pill" to "cure chronic pain." Antidepressants should be used only on a short-term basis with only a small number of selected patients.

The simplicity of the BDI also makes it attractive. Patients can complete the form in less than 5 minutes; scoring takes less than 1 minute. The BDI can also be repeated at subsequent visits to chart progression of the patient's depressive phenomenon and the effects of treatment programs.

When the test is used in conjunction with a psychosocial interview, grossly exaggerated or underplayed scores may give one significant insight into a patient's defense mechanisms and approach to pain, and may suggest the need for psychiatric or psychologic referral. For instance, patients who deny the existence of depressive symptoms (those with low BDI scores) but have considerable pain and functional impairment are often defensive about accepting any psychologic aspect of their illness. On the other hand, patients who have excessively high scores often are fragile psychologically. Those with a high BDI score, but low functional impairment, generally are dependent and feel overwhelmed by all stressors.

Table 12–2 presents the means and standard deviations of the BDI at the initial assessment before functional restoration treatment and at a 3-month follow-up assessment after treatment. As can be seen, there is a decrease in depression after successful treatment for both males and females.

It should be noted that the BDI primarily measures cognitive factors in depression. For careful evaluation of vegetative signs of depression, the Hamilton Rating Scale for Depression can be used (Hamilton, 1960). The major drawback of this scale is that the interviewer has to administer it verbally.

SELF-REPORT MEASURES

Quantified Pain Drawing

Mooney, Cairns and Robertson (1976) developed the pain drawing as a nonverbal assessment of pain location, severity, and subjective characteristics. The pain drawing allows the patient to express freely all of his/her symptoms on a plain front-back drawing of a person. In a later modification, a 10 cm line for indicating intensity of pain was also added to the drawing. A carefully constructed overlay has been designed at the University of Texas Southwestern Medical Center at Dallas to quantitate the pain display. Boxes that are bilaterally

Table 12–2. Means and Standard Deviations (SD) of the BDI at Admission and the 3-Month Follow-Up Evaluation for Males (M) and Females (F)

	Admission		Follow-up	
	Mean	SD	Mean	SD
Males	13.9	8.0	9.6	7.3
Females	16.5	8.1	11.7	8.6

symmetric and of approximately equal area cover the pain drawing, but also quantitate pain extending "outside the body" (Fig. 12–2). Two scores, one for the "trunk" and the other for "extremities," allow differentiation of localized mechanical and referred/radicular pain patterns. Maximum trunk and extremity scores are 72 boxes each.

Many factors involved in pain perception are assessed by the pain drawing. Anxiety, a major factor in chronic low back dysfunction, often leads to a more dramatic display and higher pain drawing scores. Pain that extends outside the body usually identifies a person as a pain magnifier. Rarely, "outside the body" pain is seen in a patient who is experiencing somatic delusions.

Changes in a patient's pain score can document the patient's changing pain perception and shifting pain pattern. However, comparisons of drawings for different patients are of little value, except in alerting the clinician that a patient may be exaggerating. Again, as a source of comparison, Table 12–3 presents the means and standard deviations of these pain drawing measures at the initial assessment and at the 3-month follow-up assessment after treatment in a functional restoration program.

Million Visual Analog Scale

Million, Haavik, Jayson et al. (1981) published a validated visual analog scale, consisting of 15 questions, describing both pain and disability (Fig. 12–3). Responses are expressed on a 10 cm line that spans the gamut of responses (for example, "Do you have a pain in the back? How severe is it?") A score for each of the 15 questions can be quickly derived using a ruler or grid superimposed on the paper. Visual analog scales are desirable because of their high degree of reproducibility and opportunity for nonverbal expression. Good correlation is found between the subjective analog scores and "objective" findings of the clinician. Since the test focuses primarily on pain and the functional limitations pain imposes, it can be used on multiple occasions to assess the patient's symptomatic improvement. In addition, markedly exaggerated responses that do not correlate with the physician's assessment of the patient may lead to further psychologic evaluation. Table 12–4 presents averaged figures on this scale found before and after functional restoration treatment.

Oswestry Scale

This self-rating scale was originally developed by Fairbank, Davies, Couper and O'Brien (1980). It can be administered and scored in less than 5 minutes, and illustrates the degree of functional impairment the patient is experiencing. This scale, however, has not yet been adequately correlated with objective findings or used in an analysis of therapeutic modalities. Therefore, it is used only as a global clinical index, integrated with other assessment measures.

The primary advantage of the Oswestry Scale is that it has only 10 questions, with responses for each scored from 0 to 5, providing a simple percentage score that can be compared with the scores of tests given on other occasions. Its grading scale categorizes the degree of functional loss. It also indicates a score above which symptom magnification has likely occurred.

A comparison of results on the Oswestry Scale and the BDI can sometimes offer an index of the patient's level of denial and indicates which patients are symptom magnifiers. Patients with high scores on the Oswestry (high functional

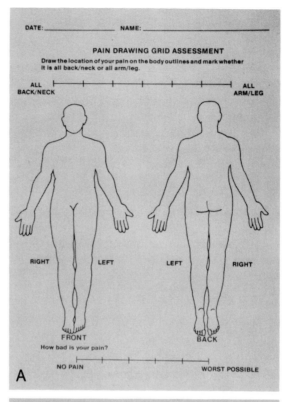

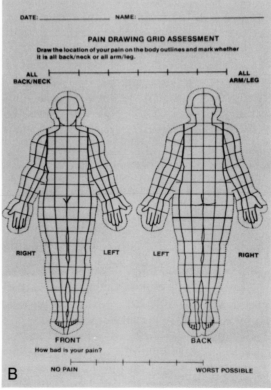

Fig. 12–2. The quantitated pain drawing (A) with the transparent grid overlay (B).

Table 12–3. Means and Standard Deviations (SD) of the Pain Drawing Measures at Admission and the 3-Month Follow-up Evaluation for Males (M) and Females (F)

		Admission		Follow-up	
		Mean	SD	Mean	SD
Males	Pain Drawing—Trunk	9.7	6.8	8.7	6.8
	Pain Drawing—Extremities	12.2	10.8	11.2	12.5
Females	Pain Drawing—Trunk	12.7	9.6	9.1	7.8
	Pain Drawing—Extremities	18.2	18.2	11.6	15.5

loss) and low scores on the BDI (low depression) are often patients who want to "receive a medical cure" and reject the possibility of an emotional component to their pain.

THE CLINICAL INTERVIEW

The most powerful clinical assessment tool is the psychosocial interview. In the functional restoration approach, this also holds true. In addition to the traditional areas evaluated in clinical history-taking, the following areas are explored:

Potential signs of depression

Patient and family mental health history

Patient and family history of substance abuse

History of head injury, convulsions, and impairment of function

Financial history, contrasting current income with past income and comparing these with current cost of living

Work history, including explanation of job losses and job changes

Any litigation that is pending for the patient's current medical problems

An important covert part of the interview is the determination of the patient's motivation for change. Patients with chronic back pain have often restricted their lives by avoiding any risk of pain, through immobilization and use of analgesics. Those patients who are not candidates for surgical intervention (for any reason), and who refuse to work toward active rehabilitation, clearly have suspect motivation which has to be carefully evaluated. Obviously, this motivation factor is important for potential success in the functional restoration program.

The clinical interview also allows us to contrast the patient's current psychosocial functioning with past functioning, and to compare the psychologic testing data with the interview data. One can then develop a reasonable judgment concerning the potential for getting the patient to change behavior in a positive direction.

OTHER SPECIFIC TESTS SOMETIMES USED

Thus far, we have reviewed asessment tests used for rating subjective complaints, function, depression, and personality characteristics. Coupled with the clinician's careful psychosocial history-taking, these data will be sufficient for evaluating the great majority of low back pain patients. However, in certain situations, further information may be needed to help answer specific ques-

DATE_____   NAME_____

PLEASE MAKE AN "X" ALONG THE LINE TO SHOW HOW FAR FROM NORMAL TOWARD THE
WORST POSSIBLE SITUATION YOUR PAIN PROBLEM HAS TAKEN YOU

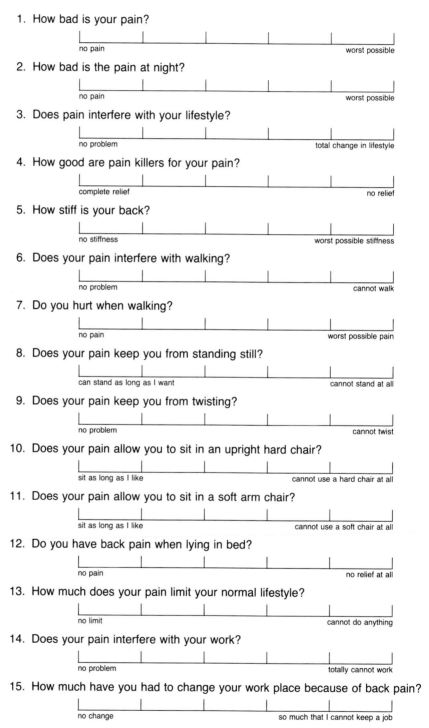

1. How bad is your pain?

no pain   worst possible

2. How bad is the pain at night?

no pain   worst possible

3. Does pain interfere with your lifestyle?

no problem   total change in lifestyle

4. How good are pain killers for your pain?

complete relief   no relief

5. How stiff is your back?

no stiffness   worst possible stiffness

6. Does your pain interfere with walking?

no problem   cannot walk

7. Do you hurt when walking?

no pain   worst possible pain

8. Does your pain keep you from standing still?

can stand as long as I want   cannot stand at all

9. Does your pain keep you from twisting?

no problem   cannot twist

10. Does your pain allow you to sit in an upright hard chair?

sit as long as I like   cannot use a hard chair at all

11. Does your pain allow you to sit in a soft arm chair?

sit as long as I like   cannot use a soft chair at all

12. Do you have back pain when lying in bed?

no pain   no relief at all

13. How much does your pain limit your normal lifestyle?

no limit   cannot do anything

14. Does your pain interfere with your work?

no problem   totally cannot work

15. How much have you had to change your work place because of back pain?

no change   so much that I cannot keep a job

Fig. 12–3. The Million visual analog scale. The scores for each line are added together. The highest possible score is 150; the lowest possible score is 0.

Table 12–4. Means and Standard Deviations (SD) of the Million Analog Rating Scale of Admission and the 3-Month Follow-up Evaluation for Males (M) and Females (F)

	Admission		Follow-up	
	Mean	SD	Mean	SD
Males	92.3	21.1	73.9	28.2
Females	97.0	19.0	70.8	25.3

tions. There are several additional assessment tests that we sometimes use on a referral basis. These are reviewed below.

Schedule of Recent Experiences

For those patients who actively deny depression or other psychologic problems, the Schedule of Recent Experiences (Homes, Rahe, 1967) can detect major life stressors such as divorce, job change, and major relocation. Although this test has not been found to reliably predict how low back pain patients will respond to treatment, it does have another major function. Patients may view attempts to identify psychologic factors accompanying their low back pain with some degree of suspicion. The suggestions that there may be an important psychologic component to their pain may be met with open resistance. This scale will help convince patients that significant stress is present in their lives. The relationship of this stress to muscle tension (and thus back pain) is often a simpler one for patients to accept. This test can therefore serve as a useful bridge to assist in attempts in obtaining patient cooperation for the various interventions involved in functional restoration.

Trail Making Test

This test provides a global screening method for possible neuropsychologic dysfunction. Gross forms of organic brain dysfunction produced by drugs, alcohol, or head injury may accompany persistent low back symptoms and are suprisingly common, particularly when cervical strain and postconcussive syndrome accompany low back injury. Unusually bizarre behaviors should trigger the clinician to use this screening test. Moreover, even minor head injuries can account for various forms of maladaptive and disruptive behavior. If results show any subtle signs of abnormality, then more sensitive neuropsychologic tests can be given by a psychologist with neuropsychologic training. A structural neurologist may provide careful physical examination findings coupled with structural tests such as EEG, CT scan, or MRI for additional information.

Wechsler Adult Intelligence Scale (WAIS-R)

Adequate intellectual functioning is important for patients to effectively perform and integrate the various facets of functional restoration. Whenever there is a question concerning such function, an intelligence test such as the WAIS-R should be administered. This intelligence test must be administered by an experienced psychologic tester. The results of this test can be helpful in several regards. First, it can assist the physician in understanding the degree of comprehension available to his or her patient. Those patients with limited cognitive resources frequently are unable to integrate anything but the most simplistic of treatment regimens (coincidentally, people with limited resources are the most common source of heavy labor and therefore are an extremely high back-pain risk population). The second way the WAIS-R can be useful is in corroborating equivocal data on neuropsychologic functioning. It can provide further behavioral data related to coping style and basic psychologic functioning.

Wide Range Achievement Test (WRAT)

The WRAT is a test of academic, school achievement. Three basic subjects around which most school studies revolve are tested—reading, spelling, and arithmetic. The range of school levels tested extends from kindergarten to college. This test provides important information concerning the school grade ratings of these basic skills that correlate well with general intellectual functioning. When a comprehensive intelligence test such as the WAIS-R cannot be administered, then the WRAT can serve as a substitute means for a global determination of intellectual functioning.

Projective Tests

Projective tests, such as the Rorschach inkblot test, also must be administered by someone experienced in psychologic testing. They are particularly valuable tools to assess emotional resources, and as a guide to understanding individual personality dynamics. Although they are unproven as predictors of response to any type of low back disability treatment, they can be valuable adjunctive tests to use with particularly problematic patients for whom it has been difficult to fully evaluate and comprehend psychologic functioning. For example, in patients who show severely disorganized thought processes on the Rorschach, chances are quite good that they will not be able to make a firm commitment to treatment and stick to it.

INTEGRATION OF ASSESSMENT DATA

As we have noted, a comprehensive psychologic assessment of each patient is essential to "guide" the patient effectively through the intensive functional restoration treatment regimen, as well as to evaluate the patient's cognitive-psychologic resources that may affect response to treatment. No one psychologic test can reliably be used for this assessment process. Indeed, one of the major misapplications of psychologic measures in the field of medicine has been the assumption that one psychologic instrumemt can be used as a sole conclusive predictor or descriptor variable. As Gatchel and Mears (1983) note in their discussion of the field of personality psychology, such data should be viewed as just one source of information to be used with other types of information in helping to make a probability statement concerning the prediction of some behavior. It is extremely rare to be able to make a totally accurate prediction of some behavior based upon a single psychologic instrument.

An experienced clinical psychologist is needed in the functional restoration approach to integrate the various pieces of assessment data that we have reviewed. This assessment can then be communicated to other staff team members in guiding the treatment process.

COMMON CLINICAL OBSERVATIONS

The above review of tests should not be viewed as an exhaustive list of potential assessment instruments that can be used with a chronic low back pain population. They are simply the tests that we have come to find useful in the functional restoration approach where an assessment of psychologic and intellectual functioning is important for involvement in the treatment regimen. As noted earlier, we are in the process of developing a more time-efficient test battery developed specifically for a chronic low-back pain population which will hopefully be available for use in the near future.

Using these assessment methods, we have developed better psychologic profiles of typical chronic low-back pain patients which we will briefly review in this section. This review will serve as a "springboard" into the next chapter which will discuss how these psychologic data are integrated into the overall functional restoration treatment program.

We believe that most cases of chronic low back pain involve some degree of somatization, *not* malingering (which implies conscious, sociopathic behaviors). For these patients, somatization represents an exaggerated fear of reinjury or a way of expressing a repressed fear, anxiety, or depression that has been provoked by one of many real or imagined losses (this can include the subconscious awareness of the loss of function caused by normal or premature aging). In general, these patients have spent a lifetime either ignoring the emotional component of their lives or being overwhelmed by that emotional component.

Indeed, the MMPI profile of a patient can add insight into this emotional factor. As we noted earlier, the *Conversion V* pattern generally depicts individuals who magnify their symptoms while remaining somewhat indifferent to the limitations produced by these symptoms. In females, when this pattern is in combination with a *V* pattern on scales 4, 5 and 6 (elevation of the sociopathy and paranoia scales and a low masculinity-femininity scale), then there is usually a great deal of anger, acting out, and paranoia that accompany their high somatization. These individuals are usually extremely difficult to work with in a treatment program. Additional efforts are usually required by the treatment staff.

It is not uncommon in an outpatient population to find histories of alcoholism that is now under control, heavy use of tobacco, or clinical obesity that occasionally has been controlled by multiple gastric bypass surgical procedures. If patients use these coping mechanims to avoid depression and anxiety, then it is not surprising that these same people will somatize when their emotional life becomes too difficult to handle.

In terms of general psychosocial indicators derived from the clinical interview data, individuals who have a "welfare mentality," in the sense of viewing the state as needing to take care of them, usually display poor treatment outcome. Moreover, there are a number of additional variables related to poor outcome: individuals with a poor prior work history; individuals with a great deal of social isolation (no support groups and close family system); individuals who refuse or resist completing all of the required paperwork and testing (this obviously reflects their lack of motivation to get involved in the program); individuals displaying a great deal of "external locus of control" (i.e., the view that they cannot directly control what happens to them). An example of this latter variable is the person who elects to undergo gastric bypass surgery in order to lose weight because he perceives that he cannot lose weight on his own.

As patients recover from chronic disability and notice that their function returns, their stamina increases, and their discomfort diminishes, fairly predictable changes often occur. In patients who rely heavily on denial as a defense mechanism (such defense mechanisms will be discussed more thoroughly in the next chapter), there will be little change in their basic personality characteristics (as assessed by the MMPI), but their self-rating scales of function (the Million visual analog and the Oswestry scales) will improve.

In patients who can admit to their depression, BDI scores usually decrease, as will MMPI scores on the first three clinical scales. However, because these patients often become more sensitive to their own emotional issues, many of the scales on the Millon Behavioral Health Inventory will increase. This can be a good clinical sign. However, in patients who consistently deny their depression, but have elevations in self-reported pain and disability, some difficulty and resistance to the overall program can sometimes occur.

Finally, in the few malingerers we have seen, there are no changes in the various measures, particularly on the functional scales. In most cases, this is accompanied by a progressive increase in reported impairment. Such a pattern is extremely rare if an individual is actually working towards rehabilitation. These patients usually do not take a chance of being "discovered" in a rehabilitation program, and will find one excuse or another for not participating such as "no transportation" or "no child care."

CHAPTER REFERENCES

Barnett J: The Millon Behavioral Health Inventory and the Minnesota Multiphasic Personality Inventory Compared as Predictors of Treatment Outcome in a Rehabilitation Program for Chronic Low Back Pain. Ph.D. Dissertation, Division of Psychology, University of Texas Health Science Center at Dallas, 1986.

Beck A: Depression: Clinical, Experimental and Theoretical Aspects. New York, Harper & Row, 1967.

Capra P, Mayer TG, Gatchel RJ: Using psychological scales to assess back pain. J Musculoskeletal Med, July 1985:41–52, 1985.

Derogatis LR, Lipman RS, Covi L.: The SCL-90: An outpatient psychiatric rating scale. Psychopharm Bull, *9*:13–28, 1973.

Fairbank JC, Davies JD, Couper J, O'Brien, JP: The Oswestry low back pain disability questionnaire. Physiotherapy, *66*:271–273, 1980.

Gatchel RJ, Mears FG: Personality: Theory, Assessment, and Research. New York, St. Martin's Press, 1982.

Hamilton M: A rating scale for depression. J Neurol Neurosurg Psychiat, *23*:56–62, 1960.

Holmes IH, Rahe RH: The social readjustment rating scales. J Psychosomatic Res, *11*:213–218, 1967.

Million R, Haavik K, Jayson MIV, et al.: Evaluation of low back pain and assessment of lumbar corsets with and without back supports. Ann Rheumat Dis, *40*:449–454, 1981.

Millon T, Green CJ, Meagher RB: Millon Behavioral Health Inventory. 3rd ed. Minneapolis, Interpretive Scoring System, 1982.

Mooney V, Cairns D, Robertson J: A system for evaluating and treating chronic back disability. West J Med, *124*:370–376, 1976.

Sternbach RA: Pain Patients: Traits and Treatment. New York, Academic Press, 1974.

Ward N: Tricyclic antidepressant for chronic low back pain: mechanism of action and predictors of response. Spine, *11*:661–665, 1986.

Chapter 13

Integration of Physical and Psychosocial Assessment Data to Guide the Treatment Process

The overall philosophy of the functional restoration approach emphasizes focus on function rather than pain, and the quantification of this function to guide treatment and monitor progress. As such, it becomes extremely important to integrate the physical and psychosocial assessment data in order to maximize this process. In general, in the functional restoration program as conducted at PRIDE, the assessment results are reviewed at a general staff meeting during the start of the treatment program, at which time any modifications of the basic program are formulated for each patient. Subsequent weekly staff meetings then evaluate progress of each patient and intiate any modifications if needed. Table 13–1 presents the cardinal purposes of these assessments and weekly staffings.

THE ROLE OF THE PSYCHOLOGIST

Treatment issues in a functional restoration approach tend to deal with the present and recent past, focusing specifically on overcoming physical and psychosocial difficulties, and returning to a productive, functional lifestyle. Within this framework, an awareness of important psychologic issues is imperative. It falls to the psychologist to sort out the contribution of psychologic factors impacting on patients, and alerting the remainder of the staff to patient characteristics that may not respond well to a short-term approach. As we discussed in the last chapter, important psychologic issues, such as the overall emotional functioning of an individual, can be comprehensively assessed with the various assessment tests at the clinician's disposal.

In passing, it should be emphasized that because of common misconceptions regarding psychology, because many patients in the past have often been told "the pain is in your head," it is imperative that patients be properly educated about the role of psychologic services in the functional restoration program. It should be acknowledged to the patient that treatment is being administered because he or she has had an injury and has legitimate physical problems. Nonetheless, as with any ongoing chronic medical condition, these types of injuries lead to pressures and changes in lifestyle that most people find unpleasant at the very least. These types of unplanned and unwanted changes lead to stress, which makes persons feel worse than they ever anticipated, and which can actually interfere with their physical recovery. It is helpful to explain

Table 13–1. Cardinal Purposes of Assessment

Identify correctable deficits in physical capacity

Identify psychosocioeconomic barriers to functional restoration

Establish level of patient effort

Guide physicians and therapists in establishing treatment goals

Document patient progress to feed back information to patient and clinicians

Provide reassurance to patients to participate in reconditioning which may occasionally require "working through pain"

Document patient physical capacity, work tolerance, and motivation to overcome structural lesions upon completion of rehabilitation

this in terms of a cycle wherein the injury and the changes it brings leads to stress, which leads to increased pain, which leads to increased stress, etc. Figure 13–1 presents a summary of factors involved in this cycle. The role of psychology, then, is to assist patients in dealing with *stress-related issues* while they are also working on their physical problems. The terms psychologic problems and psychopathology should be avoided. When assistance is presented in this light, most patients are relieved, and consequently more open to the availability of psychologic assessment and intervention.

It should be noted that there is a great deal of overlap between psychology and occupational therapy when dealing with these work-related and psychosocial issues. As will be discussed in Chapter 16, occupational therapy plays a pivotal role in the process of integrating psychologic functioning, physical symptoms, and socioeconomic factors bearing on the patient's loss of productivity. Because of their external communication and contacts with attorneys, insurance companies, and employers, the occupational therapist has access to information that can provide important insight into specific barriers to recovery and "hidden agendas" that the patient may have. Such information is necessary to develop the most comprehensive understanding of the various stress-related issues that may arise.

Even when psychologic services are presented in the framework emphasizing stress-related issues, many of the patients in this chronic pain population may

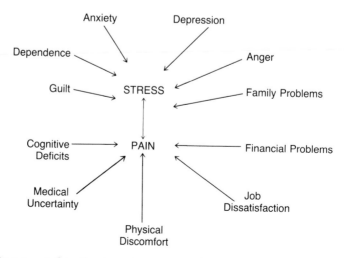

Fig. 13–1. Factors magnifying the stress-chronic pain cycle.

be resistant to psychologic assessment interventions. There are several reasons for this. Sociologically, in the PRIDE program at least, most of these individuals come from physically oriented, blue-collar backgrounds (of course, this may vary widely from one treatment facility to the next). Therefore, their approach to stressors and problem-solving tends to be action-oriented, rather than verbal and reflective. Moreover, chronic pain patients tend to use denial, projection, and somatization as primary defense mechanisms. That is to say, they will attribute any problems they are having to physical problems or external factors and not even partially to their own inability to adequately cope psychologically with their current condition. Table 13–2 presents a brief summary of common primary defense mechanisms.

In past treatment programs, when presented with the availability of psychologic services, and confronted with the assumption that they were experiencing psychologic distress, patients would generally say nothing was wrong psychologically. Moreover, they would protest and insist that they were "here for my back and not for my head." Furthermore, a few of these patients are in treatment more to avoid the repercussions of refusing rehabilitation services than to actively seek to improve their physical/psychosocial situation. On the other hand, many of these patients are in a great deal of psychologic distress, and are relieved to hear that this is a natural part of a chronic illness pattern, and that services to deal with these problems are available. Thus, the psychologist must be sensitive to these issues as a first step in the integration of patients into the treatment program. One of the major advantages of the functional restoration approach is that patients are exposed to careful quantified evaluation which clearly communicates the fact that rehabilitation of their physical disability is the major goal of treatment.

BARRIERS TO RECOVERY

An important concept in the functional restoration approach is that of *barriers to recovery*. These barriers include psychologic, physical, financial, legal, social, and work-related issues that can significantly interfere with the patient's return to full functioning and a productive lifestyle. Psychologically, these

Table 13–2. Common Psychologic Defense Mechanisms

Denial:	One of the most primitive defense mechanisms in which there is a rejection or nonacceptance of some aspect of reality because the psyche perceives a strong internal or external danger that it can neither escape nor attack
Projection:	Attributing the cause of some discomfort or conflict to another individual, a group of individuals, or external events
Repression:	A strong anxiety-provoking thought or conflict is forced out of conscious awareness, resulting in the individual not having any immediate knowledge or understanding of it
Resistance:	The conscious or unconscious censorship or opposition to a therapist's suggestions and requests
Somatization:	The physiologic expression of certain psychologic states or emotions that are prevented from being conscious because they are unacceptable or conflicting

barriers include traditional concepts such as secondary gain (e.g., the chronic disability may be allowing the individual to avoid an unpleasant job situation); symptom magnification (an increased sensitivity and concern about physical symptoms as a means of justifying continued disability); and resistance to change. At other times, real interfering circumstances may be used as "smoke screens" or excuses for sub-optimal performance and failure to adhere to the treatment regimen.

Staff members must also be alert to potential secondary gains of continued disability, whether legal, financial, job-related, or familial. It is important that members of the treatment team be knowledgeable of all psychosocial issues while the patient is in rehabilitation. This knowledge allows staff members not only to better understand and serve the patient, but also to be more effective in problem-solving when the patient is not physically progressing as expected. Indeed, failure to progress physically generally represents psychosocial barriers to recovery, since there is no way the muscles and joints will fail to respond if they are being exercised and trained as planned (unless rare denervation or ankylosis has occurred).

These *barriers to recovery* issues must be effectively assessed and brought to the attention of the entire treatment team. Steps can then be taken to understand their origins and avoid their interference with treatment goals. These issues are discussed below.

General Psychologic Issues

As the reader should be aware of by now, chronic pain and back dysfunction are more than just physical phenomena. One can safely assume that the majority of patients who are in a chronic pain population (and are not working and/or are receiving compensation) are depressed and demoralized by their present physical, psychologic, and socioeconomic status. Only a small percentage of patients are consciously malingering or "faking" for personal gains. By the time most patients reach a comprehensive rehabilitation program, their lack of progress has left them frustrated, discouraged, with low self-esteem, and almost always with significant severe financial hardship. Most patients have been to several physicians, often receiving conflicting information in the process, resulting in frustration and distrust of medical systems. In addition, adversarial interactions in the work place or with insurance companies may have left many patients feeling betrayed and cheated. Furthermore, longstanding work, family, and self-esteem issues come into play when the patient is injured and not fulfilling his or her usual social roles. All of these experiences can lead to psychologic barriers to recovery. These barriers must be directly dealt with, once assessed, through a variety of interventions. Such interventions are made not only by the psychology department, but through sensitive interactions and education efforts of all staff members.

Compliance/Resistance Issues

Unlike athletes, who usually have to be held back from doing too much quickly, chronic back-disabled patients tend to be reluctant to "work through" their pain. Often this is related to fears of reinjury, depression, or other psychosocial barriers to recovery. In the early stages of treatment, when fear and trust are usually major issues for the patients, noncompliance or failure to progress is dealt with in a supportive and educational manner. A great deal of time and effort is put into explaining the treatment rationale to the patients and working with them in a collaborative manner. At the same time, however, staff members establish their roles as trained and experienced professionals who are expert in the functional restoration approach so that they can "push" patients to greater physical activity.

Financial Disincentives

A major set of barriers to recovery revolves around financial disincentives. Such disincentives serve as secondary gains for not getting better. Most patients entering a functional restoration program are receiving some type of financial supplement, which will cease once the patient is no longer medically restricted from working. When the amount of the supplement approaches the patient's usual earnings, or is sufficient to support the patient's lifestyle, the economic incentive for returning to work is often removed. Patients may be involved in some type of injury-related litigation, which may or may not be affected by appearing "disabled" and in pain. An anticipated monetary settlement may alter the patient's customary behavior patterns, slowing recovery and increasing pain complaints. In many cases such behaviors, if not arrested early, may lead to "illness behaviors" that are difficult to reverse.

Other financial disincentives or secondary gains for not getting better include: *(a)* hoping for early retirement; *(b)* having loans paid by disability insurance; and *(c)* hoping for a new or better job based on the patient's being too "disabled" to perform the old job. The specifics of these financial issues vary, depending on state laws and whether the patient is involved in state, federal, Social Security, long-term disability, or FELA compensation systems. These issues are discussed in more detail in Chapter 16 when reviewing the role of occupational therapy. While the occupational therapy department is primarily responsible for uncovering and addressing these issues, all staff members, especially those involved with psychology, need to be aware of financial disincentives for each patient, since these issues have a major influence on motivation, pain reports, and adherence to treatment.

Somatization/Symptom Magnification vs. "Malingering"

As a result of multiple *barriers to recovery,* progressing the patient towards full physical functioning may at times be difficult. Moreover, psychosocial influences may lead the patient to be irritable, dependent, passive, or noncompliant, all of which may significantly tax the patience of health care professionals. There is a temptation at these times to view these patients as malingerers and "fakes." In order to maintain a sense of respect for the patient that is vital in this type of intensive treatment, it is important to understand that these individuals use their physical symptoms as a way of dealing with, and communicating about, their emotional lives (*somatization*). That is to say, physical symptoms may be easier to accept as causing current unhappiness and discontent than admitting that some psychologic reason is contributing to it. Only rarely is a patient consciously "faking" disability, although many times symptoms may be exaggerated consciously or unconsciously. Symptoms may also be magnified as a way of "saving face" and "justifying" continued disability after such a long period of dysfunction (i.e., *symptom magnification*). These processes are most apparent in the realm of self-report pain measures. It is essential for the psychologist to carefully delineate such issues and develop an appropriate strategy to effectively deal with them.

General Behaviors Suggesting Barriers to Recovery

Table 13–3 presents a list of behaviors that may indicate some of the "Red Flags" or psychosocial barriers to recovery that we have been discussing. As will be noted, they represent a wide array of different behaviors that may be observed in different situations. This again highlights the fact that constant communication and coordination among treatment staff is essential for the effective functioning of the treatment program.

These behaviors will need to be dealt with actively in order to ensure that patients will progress through the treatment program. At times, because these barriers cannot be adequately dealt with, a particular patient may have to be removed from the program in order to avoid demoralizing the other patients.

GENERAL EMOTIONAL REACTIONS

There are also some general emotional reactions that can be expected in most chronic low back pain patients. The intensity of these reactions needs to be adequately assessed for all patients because it can greatly affect the treatment process. That is why the assessment devices reviewed in the last chapter are essential for developing a comprehensive clinical picture of a patient. Indeed, adequately assessing and dealing with the emotional fallout of the patient's upheaval in lifestyle is important in every treatment approach, including functional restoration. The following describes these important emotional reactions.

Table 13–3. Red Flags

The patient is agitating the other patients with behavior disruptive to the treatment milieu

No work plan/changing work plan

Patient receiving/applying for Social Security, long-term disability

Opposition to presence of psychology, or refusal to fill out forms or answer questions

Florid psychosis

Significant neuropsychologic/cognitive deficits

Excessive anger at individuals involved in the case

Current substance abuse

Family resistance to patient recovery/return to work

Patient with young children at home and short-term work history done primarily for financial reasons

Continual complaints about facility, staff, program, and accommodations ("smoke screen" issues) rather than willingness to deal with physical and psychologic issues

Patient continually late to activities and other cases of noncompliance, with excuses that do not "check out"

Patient continues to focus on pain complaints in counseling sessions, rather than dealing with psychologic issues

---

Depression

Almost all these patients will be depressed to some degree (whether they can acknowledge these feelings or not) due to the multiple losses they have sustained. Besides material and financial losses, these patients have lost jobs, family roles, important sources of their self-image and self-esteem, and in some cases their belief in "the system" (medical and otherwise). A severe, debilitating level of depression may have to be temporarily dealt with through antidepressant medication. This will have to be carefully evaluated and monitored by the medical and psychologic staff.

Anxiety and Fear

Along with depression, almost all patients are experiencing some degree of anxiety and fear. There is often a great fear of reinjury which may significantly affect effort in the physical reconditioning component of the program. This is a good example of an issue which needs to be dealt with across all departments—psychology, physical therapy, and occupational therapy—in a coordinated fashion.

In terms of general anxiety, this emotional state is hardly surprising given the current level of disruption patients are experiencing in their lives. Furthermore, lack of closure regarding the long-term effects of their injury on finances, careers, relationships, and physical capacity adds to their concerns. The active physical component of the program will often gradually decrease this anxiety level. Also, stress-management and biofeedback procedures, which will be discussed in Chapter 17, are included to deal with this negative emotional state.

Anger

Reactions involving anger are perhaps the most obvious among this population. There is usually a great deal of anger at the workplace, which may be longstanding, or may result from real or perceived mistreatment since the injury. By the time most of these patients reach a comprehensive rehabilitation program, they have also developed an adversarial relationship with their insurance company, leading to an intensification and generalization of anger. Frustration with the lack of physical progress and lack of consistency in medical treatment can produce dissatisfaction with medical systems in general. This same lack of progress leads to anger at family and friends, who may imply that they are faking their injury because of the invisible nature of the physical handicap. It is important for staff to be sensitive to this anger and to defuse it whenever possible.

Entitlement

Along with their sense of anger, patients often have a sense of entitlement. This comes not only from longstanding psychologic issues mentioned earlier, but from a sense of feeling misunderstood, cheated, and betrayed. The financial and material losses they have sustained add to the belief that someone (or everyone) involved in the compensation process "owes me." Again, this emotional reaction needs to be adequately assessed since it can seriously jeopardize progression through the physical functional restoration component of the program.

ASSESSMENT, THEN TREATMENT

These general emotional reactions are common clinical states that a well-trained psychologist can effectively deal with in the majority of cases. Quite often, when there is suboptimal effort being shown in physical therapy or occupational therapy, these reactions are prevalent and need to be addressed. When the physical or occupational therapist reports suboptimal effort on testing, then the various barriers to recovery that we have reviewed, including fear, somatization, etc., need to be carefully evaluated by the psychologist and a treatment strategy developed to deal with them. In Chapter 17, we will discuss various psychologic treatment techniques that have proven successful in the overall context of the functional restoration team approach. These techniques, like the philosophy of the overall program, are quite active and goal-oriented. As will be seen, weekly staff meetings are extremely important for making a coordinated treatment team decison concerning what techniques will be used to address these important psychologic issues in order to ensure that patients successfully progress through the program.

Part III

Functional Restoration Treatment

Chapter 14

An Overview of Functional Restoration Treatment: The Basic Issues and the Therapeutic Team Approach

As the reader should be aware by now, the philosophy of the functional restoration approach is that almost all patients suffering from spinal pain and disability can be returned to a productive lifestyle, regardless of chronicity. This approach differs from other past treatment approaches in that the primary goal for each patient is restoring high levels of function, rather than eliminating pain. That is not to say, however, that patients will fail to experience varying degrees of significant pain relief. This functional restoration is accomplished through an aggressive individualized physical reconditioning program patterned after "sports medicine," not through traditional passive treatment modalities. Furthermore, as we have reviewed in Part II, treatment is guided by quantified measurement of function instead of subjective pain reports. Quantification not only allows the reconditioning to proceed safely, but provides quantifiable documentation of compliance, effort, and eventual success.

In addition to physical rehabilitation, functional restoration uncovers and addresses psychologic, financial, legal, and work-related complications that exist for each patient. These psychosocial issues are called "barriers to recovery;" they have been discussed earlier in the text, and will be discussed in more detail in the various chapters in this section. Throughout treatment, patients also receive a great deal of education about self-care in an effort to decrease future reliance on health care providers. Given the complex issues involved in treating chronic spinal pain/disability patients, an interdisciplinary team of health care providers is required to successfully implement the functional restoration program.

In this chapter, we will provide an overview of the conceptual issues and practices that make up the basic framework of this functional restoration treatment approach. These include physical issues, barriers to recovery, pain issues, medication issues, and the coordination of the interdisciplinary treatment team. Subsequent chapters in this part of the text will provide a more detailed discussion of them as they relate to each of the major treatment disciplines that make up this approach—physical therapy, occupational therapy, psychology, and medical/nursing professionals.

PHYSICAL ISSUES

There are a number of important physical issues that need to be addressed in this approach. Although these issues usually become most apparent in physical therapy, the other disciplines will also encounter them and will often need to address them.

The Deconditioning Syndrome

As we have earlier discussed, deconditioning is a progressive process whose onset cannot be defined easily. When the spine is injured, persistent pain often follows, and bedrest is generally recommended during the acute phase. Healing may be delayed by internal factors such as poor blood supply or external ones like cigarette smoking. Although deconditioning is likely to be induced more slowly in the spine than in an immobilized extremity, extended periods of inactivity and restricted motion take their toll on functioning. The effects can include stiff, hypomobile joints, muscle atrophy, loss of endurance, tightening of connective tissues, inhibition of neural outflow, and eventual loss of cardiovascular fitness. Because atrophic muscles are more irritable and subject to overload, recurrent spasm or deformities are often produced. These symptoms may then be misinterpreted as "new injuries," with continued bedrest following, which perpetuates the disuse phenomenon.

Scar Tissue

The formation of scar tissue is an additional problem. Even in patients who have not had surgical treatment, some amount of scarring may be presumed as a result of tearing of the tissues at the time of injury. In patients who have undergone surgical procedures (particularly more than one), formation of scar tissue becomes an even greater hindrance to functioning. Besides the stiffness and adhesions this scarring produces, nerve entrapment may take place as well. Postoperative neurologic findings are generally the result of epidural fibrosis, and not of acute nerve root impingement that would necessitate surgical intervention or epidural injection. While modern imaging techniques still reveal little of soft tissue structure, the intricate coupling mechanism of the spinal 3-joint complex makes it reasonable to hypothesize biomechanical aberrations as a result of injury.

Physical Progression Issues

In the past, continued pain and disability in the back-injured patient was treated by passive means only with extended "conservative care." However, the use of bedrest after a sufficient healing period only amplifies the secondary and deconditioning problem. Traction, heat, massage, ultrasound or lasers, and purely psychologic techniques are unlikely to provide prolonged benefit, and may actually produce deleterious changes in connective tissues. Furthermore, such treatments tend to teach the patient to rely on medical professionals to "fix me," rather than actively engage in his or her own treatment. This not only leads to excessive reliance on health care systems, but may start the patient spiraling into a sense of helplessness and hopelessness.

In order to address these issues, functional restoration treatment adopted a "sports medicine" approach involving the gradual physical progression of the patient to normal, or even above normal, functional capacity. The quantitative methods now available to measure back mobility and strength have made this system possible. Not only does quantification allow for strenuous, yet safe, conditioning, but it gives objective feedback to the patient and therapist alike. As in sports medicine rehabilitation, the training regimen often results in temporary pain increases. Among many patients, this may initially be perceived as injury, and heightens their fears about reconditioning. Furthermore, continued pain is often misinterpreted as a sign of failure to progress, leading to discouragement and decreased adherence to treatment. The objective quantification of the patient's progress helps overcome these hindrances. By seeing progress in spite of pain, the patient is encouraged, develops a sense of mastery over fear and pain, and begins seeing himself or herself as functional again. Although the primary goal is to restore function rather than to eliminate pain, the vast majority of patients do experience significant pain reduction once they have achieved normal mobility and above normal levels of strength and endurance in the spinal musculature.

Stages of Progression

As we have pointed out earlier in the text, when discussing functional restoration of the spine, it is helpful to think of the spine as a "lifting chain," with the legs, buttocks, lower back, upper back, shoulders, and neck forming the links of the chain. Although physical reconditioning focuses on rehabilitating the most dysfunctional links in the chain, occupational therapy focuses on the entire lifting chain, as related to daily living activities.

In the initial stages of functional restoration, the main goals are to increase the patient's flexibility and mobility. Through stretching and range-of-motion exercises, the patient is able to stretch scar tissue, tight muscles and contracted connective tissues. A full range of motion is essential to attain maximal benefit from the subsequent strengthening exercises.

Based on the initial functional capacity (as determined by a quantitative functional evaluation), the patient enters a strengthening program. The purpose of this program is to increase overall physical strength and endurance in all parts of the body, but particularly in the damaged areas. The beginning points and rate of progression of this program are based on several factors. Simultaneously, the patient is engaged in activities designed to increase cardiovascular endurance. Also, as strength increases, musculoligamentous coordination and endurance are emphasized. Coordination and endurance exercises build on the foundation of strength and flexibility, assisting the patient in returning to the functional positions and activities encountered in daily living. Finally, throughout all of these steps, the patient trains for specific tasks as well as general overall body fitness.

Failure to Progress

Failure to progress physically generally represents psychosocial barriers to recovery, since there is no way that muscles, joints, and ligaments will fail to respond if they are being exercised as planned in the absence of systemic disease or specific drugs. Quantitative data represent objective evidence that non-physiologic influences are impeding progress. As we shall see, when used in a sensitive, yet authoritative manner, this information is powerful "ammunition" in dealing with psychosocial issues and lack of compliance. Additionally, by requiring the patient to attain minimal daily increases in repetitions or weights, therapists can use quantification as a means of measuring adherence and success.

BARRIERS TO RECOVERY

Physical issues are not the only ones that need to be systematically addressed. As we discussed in Chapter 13, an important assessment issue in functional restoration is that of *barriers to recovery.* Barriers can include psychologic, social, economic, or work-related issues that interfere with a smooth return to a functional and productive lifestyle. This concept of *barriers to recovery* encompasses, but is not limited to, traditional concepts, such as secondary gain, symptom magnification, and psychologic resistance, as well as financial disincentives. These barriers may be conscious, unconcious, or some combination of the two. They may range from intervening life events that impede treatment (e.g., car problems, no money for child care), to more subtle emotional issues (e.g., depression, anger in the work-place), to conscious attempts to manipulate the system (although these are usually rare). At other times, real interfering circumstances may be used as "smoke screens" or excuses for suboptimal performance and failure to adhere to the treatment regimen. All staff members must also be alert to potential secondary gains of continued disability whether legal, financial, job-related, or familial. It is important that members of the treatment team be knowledgeable of all psychosocial issues while the patient is in rehabilitation. This knowledge allows staff members not only to better understand and serve the patient, but also to be more effective in problem-solving when the patient is not progressing as expected.

PAIN ISSUES

As we thoroughly reviewed in Chapter 4, pain complaints are "subjective" phenomena. They represent a central, cognitive interpretation of multiple events such as peripheral stimuli, psychologic patterns, and effects of endogenous and exogenous neurotransmitters (such as medications or endorphins). However, most patients recognize only a "direct link" between a peripheral stimulus and its central expression as pain, localizing all pain patterns as if they were noxious external stimuli. This layperson's conception brings the patient into rehabilitation with several pre-established attitudes. First of all, the patient is rarely able to consider causes for the perceived pain other than a single, pain-producing lesion somewhere in the back. It is often difficult to educate a patient about basic concepts such as referred pain/nerve root compression. Furthermore, the patient has been conditioned by the accomplishments of the past generation, embellished by the media, to expect that this lesion can be identified by state-of-the-art diagnostic technology, and then be excised by the skillful surgeon. Another misconception concerning pain is that the connections from the back to the central "switchboard" are such that the patient is able to distinguish the exact location and type of problem by its perceived quality (e.g., the pain "is deep in the bone" or is "right at this level in front of the spine"). Ample evidence exists of the lack of sensory specificity in the low back region, making most health care professionals aware that the patient's perceptions are often inaccurate. Finally, and most significantly, pain is a profoundly frightening problem, raising the prospect of a life-threatening or disabling disease. Once the patient has been reassured that this is not the case, however, the impact on the patient's lifestyle becomes the major source of anxiety. Thus, while the patient intially compels the clinician to focus on subjective pain complaints, ultimately the loss of function is the greater concern.

Pain Versus Function

The emphasis on function rather than pain relief as the primary goal sets the functional restoration approach apart from other spinal rehabilitation programs. The patient's pain is always acknowledged as real, since an injury was sustained at some point in time and structural damage, with or without an identified pain source, cannot be denied without impugning the veracity of the patient. However, the staff does not focus on pain, and the overriding goal is to restore functioning, not to produce a totally pain-free individual. As in sports medicine rehabilitation approaches, the patient must "push through" pain in order to obtain the benefits of stretching and strengthening exercises. Patients must understand that decrease in pain perception is ultimately proportional to increases in physical capacity in the normal range. Waiting for the pain to go away first will guarantee failure to progress physically, as well as failure to obtain any pain relief at all.

Hurt Is Not Equivalent to Harm

One of the most difficult concepts to impart to patients is that pain does not equal harm or injury once pain has become chronic. The patients are taught that they must learn to distinguish between acute pain that signals new tissue damage, and chronic pain that gives them no new information regarding their physical condition. Furthermore, they must understand that increased pain with increased activity, including the acute pain of breaking down scar tissue, is actually a sign of progress. Quantification of function becomes extremely important at this point since it shows patients that, in spite of how they feel subjectively, they are in fact progressing physically as evidenced by increasing quantitated strength and mobility measurements.

Addressing Pain Issues with the Patient

In helping the patient negotiate the sometimes unpleasant rehabilitation process, the staff must balance its efforts in trying to keep the patient as comfortable as possible, emphasizing function rather than pain, and in decreasing the patient's reliance on health care professionals. It is important that staff members listen to pain complaints in a concerned, and open-minded fashion. They are taught to support the patients' new pain treatment tools, including the use of stretching, ice, relaxation, and anti-inflammatories. By consulting with the physical therapist and comparing the patient's current pain reports with the initial pain reports, one can determine if the problem represents the normal side effects of the physical progression, or in fact represents overtraining or a new injury. Because of the acute fear of reinjury experienced by these patients, it is essential that staff members share their diagnostic and treatment rationale with the patient at these times. Moreover, sharing this information helps the patient learn to distinguish between chronic pain, "flare-ups," and acute muscle pulls or strains.

MEDICATION ISSUES

Along with continued use of bedrest after the acute phase of injury has passed, the chronic use of opiates or semi-synthetic analgesics may contribute to the patients's increasing disability. Besides their central pain-relieving effects, these medications have a substantial hypnotic effect that adds to the patient's deactivation. They also reinforce the patient's passive reliance on external sources of relief and "cure," and the addictive potential must also not be ignored.

The use of opiates, semi-synthetic analgesics, muscle relaxants, and sedatives is basically incompatible with a functional restoration approach. Patients need to be alert and physically responsive in order to derive full benefits from a functional restoration program. Furthermore, patients need to be aware of kinesthetic and proprioceptive feedback that takes place during exercise. Since most of the patients tend to be emotionally depressed, eliminating the central nervous system depressant effects of these medicines helps them to begin to break out of their depression. The avoidance of "pain medication" also reinforces the program emphasis on functional restoration, rather than pain relief as the end goal.

During the initial phase of treatment, the usage of the above types of medication is gradually tapered. The rationale for tapering off is clearly explained to the patient, using the points emphasized above. In place of these medications, anti-inflammatories and antidepressants may be substituted. Anti-inflammatories are used because they reduce inflammation rather than block pain perception centrally, which is particularly important as patients increase their physical activity. Since a majority of the patients are depressed by the time they reach the functional restoration system, antidepressants are often used. Patients who are experiencing vegetative signs of depression, particularly sleep disturbance and low energy, will have a difficult time participating fully in strenuous conditioning programs. Coupled with individual counseling, the antidepressants will also help the patients' mood and outlook improve, which is important in their overall recovery. Furthermore, there are indications from recent research that in some patients, antidepressants have a pain-relieving effect. Psychologists work closely with the nursing/medical staff in monitoring the patient's response to antidepressants, his or her compliance, and any need to adjust dosage and type.

THE INTERDISCIPLINARY TREATMENT TEAM APPROACH

With these above issues clearly in mind, we can now discuss the treatment team approach to functional restoration. It should be apparent from the discussion so far that the functional restoration approach encompasses all aspects of the complex physical and psychosocial interaction impinging on the back-disabled patient. The success of this approach lies in the coordinated efforts of the interdisciplinary treatment team. The use of the team allows the staff to thoroughly address the numerous issues facing each patient. Furthermore, patients are treated in a consistent manner by staff members who share a unified philosophy and reinforce the importance of each of the other departments. The functional restoration system involves physical therapy, occupational therapy, psychology, and medical/nursing professionals.

Department Responsibilities

The physical therapy department is responsible for the instruction and supervision of patients in their individualized physical therapy programs. They focus on the retraining of the specific injured area of the body, and treating the spine as a functional unit. The occupatonal therapy department also supervises physical reconditioning, but focuses on functional task performance (i.e., lifting capacity, positional and activity tolerance) through work hardening and work simulation. Additionally, the occupational therapy department is involved in addressing the financial, legal and work-related barriers to recovery that might interfere with the ultimate return to work goal for each patient. The psychology department addresses the psychologic, psychosocial, and behavioral issues that affect the patients during this time of upheaval in their lives. These issues are dealt with through a cognitive-behavioral, crisis intervention approach, rather than through long-term, traditional psychotherapy. Individual counseling, group meetings, and educational classes provide the vehicle for this interaction. The nursing department functions as an extension of the program physican, assessing and dealing with the patient's physical/medical needs. It acts as a triage without direct physician involvement as much as possible to avoid "over-pathologizing" the patients. The nurse serves as an extension of the physician, with responsibilities such as checking and ordering medications, injections, and initial evaluations of any medical problems affecting a patient's ability to engage in the physical reconditioning program. The nursing department also serves an an important conduit of information between the physicians and the other members of the treatment team.

Interdepartmental Communication

In this approach, it is essential that the treatment orientation of each department "dovetails" with that of the other departments. Staff members also support the authority, expertise, efforts, and rationale of the other departments. Members from each department must work together in tailoring their approach to meet the individual needs and idiosyncrasies of each patient. Some patients will attempt to sabotage their treatment by giving different information to different staff members, or by attempting to play one department against another. If conflicting messages have been given out to the staff, the information needs to be clarified, and a unified message given to the patient. In situations where the patient appears to be fabricating miscommunication as a diversionary tactic, a short meeting with all parties present will reinforce to the patient that the staff works in unison. In formulating a treatment plan and tailoring it to the individual, staff members from each department should be available for consultation with members of the other departments.

Clear communication between the departments is vital not only regarding the treatment of a specific patient, but in the maintenance of the overall treatment environment as well. Inconsistencies between departments are confusing to the patients at the very least, and can escalate into disruption in the treatment environment since the patients then perceive the staff as disorganized. Staff members also need to be sensitive to the disruptive effects of rumors and disgruntled patients. In any of these situations, immediate interdepartmental communication is required to formulate an appropriate course of action for maintaining a positive treatment environment.

Importance of Education

Besides direct treatment, a great deal of education by each department takes place as part of the functional restoration approach. This is in keeping with the philosophy of involving patients in their own treatment and increasing their self-reliance in long-term physical well-being and pain management. Furthermore, many of these patients are skeptical and/or distrustful of medical systems by the time they arrive at a comprehensive program. By having the staff openly explain the treatment rationale, patients not only increase their understanding, but tend to become more trusting and therefore more likely to adhere to the treatment recommendations. The goal of increased independence requires that patients take what they have learned in the program and enact changes in their lifestyle, usually on a permanent basis.

This educational process takes place in several ways. A great deal of the education, particularly in early treatment phases, takes place in one-to-one interactions when the patient is meeting individually with staff members from each department. This is when the patient is first introduced to concepts of sports medicine, the deconditioning syndrome, the interaction of psychologic with physical functioning, and the use of new pain control techniques. This same information, as well as specific stress management and work issue classes, is taught formally when the patient enters a treatment group (to be reviewed below). For example, a class is taught which provides basic education about the spine and how it functions (Fig. 14–1). Individual educational efforts also continue during this phase of treatment. By answering questions, suggesting alternate exercises and activities, sharing personal experiences, openly discussing the meaning of symptoms and complaints, and sharing the rationale for treatment, the staff in all departments creates an atmosphere of learning.

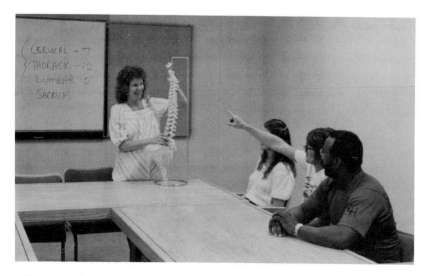

Fig. 14–1.   Spine education class.

The repetition of information and its consistency across departments is important, since at any given point in time an individual patient may not be ready or able to hear the message, for whatever reason.

Treatment Program Time Format

The program typically consists of four phases, as presented in Table 14–1. As noted in the table, each program is divided into a variety of comparable phases. The comprehensive program focuses on the most important and expensive chronically disabled cases; i.e., those generally unable to work. Under certain circumstances, working patients may be admitted into the comprehensive program, as will be discussed below.

In the preprogram phase, issues of pain and barriers to functional recovery, specifically those related to compliance and willingness to get well, are focused on. In Phase II, the major portion of the program, a 10-hour/day, 3-week program is usually participated in by the patient. The follow-up phase is of variable length, based primarily on such factors as patient proximity to home, degree of deconditioning, and ergonomic demands of the patient's anticipated work. Finally, there is an outcome tracking phase involving periodic quantified functional evaluations (QFEs) to assess maintenance of physical capacity. Patients are referred back to their original physicians, generally return to a productive lifestyle, but are also followed at length to be sure that treatment goals are maintained in various outcome areas. This program may involve using structured telephone interviews at specified intervals.

Eligibility and Program Placement

Table 14–2 presents the basic comprehensive program eligibility requirements. These requirements are designed so that excessive or unnecessary treatment is not administered, but that appropriate opportunity for rehabilitation is given. Certainly, some candidates are more likely to be successful in a comprehensive functional restoration program than others, and this is part of the assessment in Phase I of the program (the preprogram phase). These selection criteria choose only those who should be given *an opportunity* for entering such a program. It is then up to the patients' motivation and level of participation as to how much they will obtain from the treatment process.

The primary selection criterion relates to time after injury. It is known that

Table 14–1. Phases of Treatment Programs

	Phases	Comprehensive Program	Outpatient Programs
I.	Pre-program	4–8 sessions (may begin with QFE)	1–2 sessions
II.	Core (intensive) program	3 weeks (full day)	6–24 sessions, over 3–6 weeks
III.	Follow-up	0–20 sessions, over 0–6 weeks	1–2 sessions Home program instruction
IV.	Outcome tracking	Physician re-referral Periodic repeat QFEs Structured telephone interview annually	

Table 14–2.   Selection Criteria for Comprehensive Program Admission

1. *Minimum* 4 months after disabling injury (program entry usually not before 5 to 6 months)
2. Surgery "ruled out" (i.e., all appropriate structural diagnostics have been performed)
3. English-speaking (non-English-proficient patients may participate in outpatient programs)
4. Funding available

---

by the time 3 to 4 months have passed since an industrial accident, more than 90% of patients will have returned to gainful employment. They may continue having pain, but their disability issues will have been overcome for all practical purposes. On the other hand, of those remaining, more than half will remain disabled at the end of a year without functional restoration intervention. This is the group for whom the cost and effort inherent in a comprehensive program can be justified, since it will prevent prolonged disability costs, and in a certain percentage of patients, avoid unnecessary surgery, medication usage, and habituation to disability. There is no limit on the length of disability that can be addressed in such a program, but it is generally true that patients disabled for more than 2 years will present exceedingly difficult rehabilitation obstacles.

The question of ruling out surgical treatment is a diffcult one. Surgical rates and approaches are extremely variable from one community to another. For instance, disc surgery rates per lost time injury vary from 1.5 to 5% within the United States itself; rates drop as low as 0.5% in some European countries. For fusion surgery there are far wider swings, with few clear-cut indications to guide practitioners in the performance of such procedures. Therefore, while surgery can never be truly "ruled out," we are still obligated to make every effort to be certain that no reasonable passive alternative has remained unexplored prior to program participation. The technique for achieving this must also vary from one locale to another. It is basically the medical director's responsibility to evaluate the patient on the basis of previous diagnostic testing and physical examination findings. He or she then orders other appropriate structural diagnostic tests as necessary to evaluate any previously missed pathology. Finally, consultation may be required from surgeons familiar with practice patterns in the community to finally determine whether a surgical procedure might be indicated. The patient has a great deal of importance in this evaluation, since a patient still motivated by a surgical "magic wand" may be unable to place his or her full attention on a functional restoration program or avoid subsequent "doctor shopping" when unrealistic expectations for complete pain relief are not met.

Even though all "necessary and reasonable" medical care is generally provided for under workmen's compensation statutes, this may not always be the case in practice. Such is the adversary relationship regarding spinal rehabilitation that many third-party carriers will make every effort to block nonoperative care of the chronic patient. A great deal of education is still required among employers, attorneys, and the insurance community before such programs can achieve their rightful place. Quality assurance is the key to providing the necessary confidence.

The comprehensive program consists, in its major portion, of about an equal division between physical training and education/counseling. A patient not understanding English simply is unable to obtain the requisite information from such a program. Moreover, if attempts are made to translate for this individual, it generally creates a disturbance within the treatment milieu that is counterproductive for other patients. Foreign language-speaking patients can often be accommodated in other programs, as noted below.

Partial programs are sometimes arranged for partially disabled workers. Patients meeting all criteria for a comprehensive program, but who have returned to work in a "light duty" capacity, may be eligible for a partial program. Since the last week of the program frequently focuses on occupational issues which are also dealt with during the follow-up period, such patients may participate in a 2-week comprehensive program with little or no follow-up. The average cost for these patients then becomes only about one-half that of a full comprehensive patient with follow-up. Furthermore, these patients are generally receiving no or minimal compensation relative to the totally disabled patients, and this also leads to lower costs and fewer disincentives to functional return.

Other patients are handled in different ways. Chronically disabled, foreign language-speaking patients may be appropriate for a reconditioning program, since this focuses primarily on physical activity with much less emphasis on education. Individual training problems can be handled by therapists skilled in the foreign language common to a given area, such as Spanish in the southwestern portions of the United States. Similarly, patients failing to meet these selection criteria for the comprehensive program are eligible for less intensive reconditioning and work-hardening programs. Postoperative patients may participate in a short reconditioning program as part of their rehabilitation within a few weeks after surgical procedure on an outpatient basis concurrent with their return to gainful employment. It is the presence of *disability issues* which determines the need for comprehensive management. Finally, the patient with an acute recurrence is definitely not a comprehensive candidate at that time. An adequate healing period appropriate to the new injury should be made available prior to comprehensive program participation. A patient, once having gone through such a program, should not require another full program, even if disability issues arise once again. Instead, a brief outpatient reconditioning or follow-up program should be sufficient to handle his or her problems.

Chapter 15

The Role of the Physical Therapist: Active Sports Medicine, Not Passive Modalities

A HISTORICAL PERSPECTIVE

The traditional physical therapy approach, like that of medicine, is to address the underlying condition or pathophysiologic abnormality. In many cases, the physical therapist confronts conditions which cannot be corrected, and like the physician, then focuses on amelioration of symptoms. Since by far the greatest number of visits to both physicians and and physical therapists involve a chief complaint of pain, the traditional focus quite naturally involves altering the patient's pain perception and self-report. Rarely does the physical therapist consider advocating modes of therapy that involve activities that either induce or maintain a painful stimulus. In fact, pain of any kind is generally a limiting factor for performing a recommended activity. Instruction in this principle is often a major part of the education provided by the physical therapist (and physician) to the patient.

Physical therapy can be broken into two broad areas: active and passive. The latter involves those things done to the patient, including modalities, manipulation, passive exercises, etc. Active treatment usually involves exercise, in which the physical therapist is acting as an educator in demonstrating pain-relieving techniques. Just as in most surgical specialities, most of the prestige and economic incentive is related to passive, not active, treatment, be it invasive surgery and injections or hot packs, mobilization, or lasers. Education and training usually become adjunctive to these primary treatment objectives. The patients also contribute to this imbalance by generally valuing the things given or done to them much more highly than what they are told; this issue forms the basis of many current medical controversies, not the least of which involves reimbursement discrepancies between groups of physicians (i.e., psychiatrists versus internists versus surgeons).

Fortunately, in the last few years, automated equipment facilitating both testing and training (Cybex, Lido, Kin-Com, etc.) has become available for strengthening. Initially available only for extremity use, but now useful in the spine as previously discussed, this equipment allows therapists the luxury, generally unknown to the physician, of more equitably distributing effort from passive to active treatment. Over the past quarter-century, sports medicine training has added considerably to the luster of the physical therapy specialty.

Observers have noted a persistent shift of emphasis into this area, contributing to growth of the specialty and male:female ratio, involvement with exercise physiologists and athletic entertainers, improved patient education, and alteration in reimbursement patterns.

Yet, in the lumbar spine area, these changes have progressed only slowly. Hampered, until recently, by inability to measure physical capacity, the therapist has relied on passive modalities, traditional exercise protocols such as William's and cautionary education based on inferences poorly drawn from validated research. The net result has been physical therapist complicity in maintenance of approaches that encourage rest and inactivity long after anticipated healing periods have run their course. In the chronic back pain situation, as we have seen, such approaches are counterproductive.

Another barrier to functional restoration inherent in present physical therapy patterns is also noteworthy. The growth of sports medicine in the extremities has involved an acute phenomenon. Conservative care and rehabilitation are generally closely meshed, since healing periods in the extremities are relatively short and visually observable. Thus, many active treatment programs are instituted within 2 to 6 weeks following injury or surgical procedure. They are often completed in a matter of 4 to 6 additional weeks. Few psychosocial barriers to functional recovery develop in this time frame, and thus the traditional physical therapy one-on-one relationship to the patient can be maintained.

However, this is an unusual model when considered in the context of musculoskeletal and neurologic rehabilitation. While "conservative care" soon after acute injury is often handled within a hospital or outpatient program by a single physical therapist, rehabilitation has involved a "team approach" for many years. One need only consider the interdisciplinary team involved in rehabilitation of stroke, head injury, spinal cord injury and amputation to recognize that those entities which can be structurally expected to heal only incompletely are generally restored to function by a team, not an individual. In the spine, this team approach concept was applied by the pain clinic pioneers in the early 1960s, as they recognized the psychosocial barriers to recovery. The physical therapist, dealing with the generally unrecognized physiologic components of the chronic back pain process, were generally relegated to a supportive role by psychosocially oriented therapists.

This historical perspective sets the stage for a phenomenon already being noted in the functional restoration approach to back pain. Reconditioning and "work hardening" programs, generally dominated by the physical therapy specialty, are rapidly sprouting up as adjuncts to physical therapy practices. These follow the traditional single physical therapist, non-team approach model to the physical deconditioning noted in back pain patients. While this may be appropriate in the acute and subacute stages (less than 4 months after injury) of a back pain episode, they are inadequate for dealing with the relatively small percentage of patients with chronic back and neck pain. Because those patients who will have relatively short-term problems form the overwhelming majority, these reconditioning programs probably serve a worthwhile function. However, since the chronic 10% of the back pain group produces 80% of total costs, society will ultimately demand a team approach dealing with all psychophysiologic and disability issues. If this is to be achieved, some physical therapists must be willing to work in an interdisciplinary group.

PHYSICAL PROGRESSION ISSUES

At this time it will be helpful to review some of the physical progression issues generally dealt with primarily by the physical therapist members of the functional restoration team: the deconditioning syndrome, scar tissue, progression of physical activity, and barriers to progression of exercise.

The Deconditioning Syndrome

As we have noted previously, deconditioning is a progressive process related to disuse whose onset cannot be precisely documented. Some factors are clearly mechanical, as related to maintaining static postures, brace wear, and prolonged, excessive bedrest. Others are more difficult to define, such as the relationship between a painful peripheral stimulus altering muscular tone through a set of neurologically mediated processes. Changes in the spinal reflex arc may reflect one such mechanism, while higher centers may also be involved in the process. What is clear is that if the deconditioning process is not terminated, the process becomes a progressive vicious cycle in which lower physical capacity predisposes to pain recurrence with lower and lower levels of physical activity. The pain induced by increased activity may be perceived by the patient as a "new injury," leading to renewed efforts to find a solution through the medical care system. Mental passivity, dependence, and depression accompany the physical changes.

Scar Tissue

By now we should recognize our level of ignorance regarding the actual cause of the peripheral painful stimulus in most chronic low back pain cases. Our complex imaging procedures document the cause of the problem in only a small percentage of patients who have surgically treatable disorders. In the vast majority of unoperated patients, or in those operated patients in whom surgical treatment has not been successful in relieving symptoms, an unknown process continues to produce pain even after a reasonable healing period. At this time, the most plausible explanation for this pain is the postulation of a soft tissue injury in disc anulus, ligament, joint capsule, tendon or muscle, which heals routinely with scar. This less pliable and more easily injured tissue adversely alters the spinal biomechanics with the process complicated by subsequent deconditioning. Activity and training reverse the process, but its effects are limited by the location, amount, and maturity of the scar tissue. Subsequent tearing of scar or instability produced by hypomobility in some contiguous segments, and hypermobility in an injured one, may lead to pain during the training process, which must be overcome or "worked through" if functional restoration is to be achieved.

Progression of Physical Activity

Persistent pain and disability in the back continue to be treated in a majority of facilities with passive modalities and minimal stretching programs suitable primarily for acute back care. Passive processes such as traction, heat, massage, ultrasound, diathermy, TENS or lasers, may have several detrimental effects.

By producing temporary pain relief through the relaxation of collagenous tissue stiffness, these processes may give the patient a false sense of well-being. Continued reliance on these techniques, generally provided only at the direction of the therapist, places the patient's treatment responsibility on the medical care system rather than on the chronically disabled patient. Finally, these processes are unlikely to provide any long-term benefit. In fact, they may actually produce deleterious effects in connective tissues since the removal of applied heat often reduces tissue pliability and increases local swelling. The dependence engendered by these passive processes may also accentuate the feelings of helplessness and hopelessness the patient is already experiencing.

The sports medicine approach involves a progression of physical activity in a graduated fashion. How to provide this process to minimize pain complaints, but to also provide sufficient tissue response to produce increased joint mobility and muscle strength/endurance, is the heart of the conundrum. These choices are generally made on an empirical basis, using information obtained from treating large numbers of patients. As one might expect, in the chronically disabled back pain patient, progression tends to be slow in the majority of patients unless they are cajoled by the therapist. However, in a minority of patients, a combination of impulsiveness and lack of coordination predisposes them to recurrent injury if they are not carefully watched and kept within the limits of a graduated program. These "accident-prone" individuals are at the opposite end of the spectrum. The subacute, work-motivated executive or professional person usually falls somewhere in between.

The critical aspect of progression is that it cannot be permitted to occur in a haphazard manner. The therapist, most important of all examiners, must recognize the limitations of relying on patient complaints and therapist visual and palpatory skills alone in making judgments. The therapist must learn to place increasing reliance on objective functional capacity assessment technology for mobility, strength and endurance with tests being performed at multiple intervals through the treatment process. Furthermore, a generic program designed for all, like Williams' exercises, is inappropriate since the type and degree of deficits vary greatly from one patient to the next. Therefore, treatment programs must be individualized from the beginning, and modified as necessary based on the progression that the patient actually demonstrates.

As in other training regimens, progressive resistance above the subject's current capabilities may produce a painful episode that is interpreted by the patient as a "new injury." In actuality, the patient has merely exceeded his or her pain threshold which has generally been reduced to a low level by disuse, depression and drugs. Such episodes are not merely common, they are nearly universal and must be dealt with promptly and effectively if the patient's confidence and willingness to participate in rehabilitation is to be maintained. Since we have already seen that chronic back disability may often select a somatizing and often cognitively limited individual, the need for education provided by the therapist to constantly validate the progression procedures in the patient's mind cannot be overemphasized.

The interrelationship between pain and progression is a fascinating one. Continued pain (the only perception the patient really has of back function) is often misinterpreted as a sign of failure to progress leading the patient to become discouraged and decreasing adherence to training regimens. The physical therapist must be not only diligent in education on pain relief maneuvers consistent with the training, but also prepared to perform physical quantification tests as pain is increasing in order to restore confidence to the patient. By seeing progress on physical capacity in spite of pain, the patient is encouraged, develops a sense of mastery over fear and pain, and begins seeing himself or herself as more functional and on the road to recovery once again. While the primary goal of rehabilitation is to restore function, the diminution of pain is a secondary goal which receives the therapist's highest priority. Since the patient is already well acquainted with the fact that pain can be relieved, albeit temporarily, by inactivity and passive modalities, it requires all of the therapist's skill to keep the patient's "eye on the ball" of functional restoration.

Stages of Progression

Therapists and patients are encouraged to think of the body as a series of "functional units" or "links in a chain," involved in supporting the head, body or arms in a variety of positions and activities. Although functional restoration focuses on the most deficient links in the chain, prolonged inactivity always leads to potential dysfunction in other areas. Thus, as the patient's back becomes more mobile and strong with training, certain activities may lead to new pain complaints common to musculoskeletal specialists, such as shoulder tendonitis, "tennis elbow," or patellofemoral dysfunction. These areas also fall within the purview of the physical therapist to treat.

The initial stages of functional restoration focus on mobility with the goals being to increase flexibility and joint motion through stretching tight connective tissue and scar. As full a range of motion as possible is essential to attain maximal benefit from subsequent strengthening programs. Strengthening proceeds through a progressive resistive exercise program based on the quantitative assessment of function and certain critical modifiers such as age, gender, and body weight. Since endurance involves both a muscular and cardiovascular/aerobic component, strengthening protocols involve both maximum resistance and repetitive low load exercises. The cardiovascular component to endurance is developed through the use of aerobic training devices. Improvement of agility and coordination with other body parts is extremely important in any sports medicine program, but is generally assigned to the occupational therapist as part of their training in specific task performance. However, learning to perform the task at a variety of speeds, resistances, and ranges of motion is a part of the physical therapy training process.

Barriers to Progression in Physical Training

As we have seen, a multitude of barriers to functional recovery exist, usually falling into psychosocioeconomic categories. The identification of increases or decreases in these barriers is critical to allow members of the team to deal with escalating problems and encourage calming influences. The failure to progress in physical training areas is perhaps the single most important indicator of insurmountable or increasing barriers to recovery. Quantification data represent objective evidence that nonphysiologic influences are impeding progress. When this information is presented to patients in a sensitive, yet authoritative manner, it provides powerful ammunition in subsequently dealing with psychosocial issues and noncompliance. By requiring the patient to attain minimal daily improvements in repetitions, resistance, or quantitative test data, the therapist can use the measurements as a means of judging program adherence and success and provide a powerful reinforcer to the patient's involvement in the program. When patients persist in resisting progression, "small group staffings" are generally called (these are described subsequently).

As we discussed previously, the barriers to functional recovery are manifold. Fear of injury, depression, demoralization, lack of trust, frustration, loss of self-esteem, anger at physicians and employers and financial stressors are only some of the conscious and unconscious factors which may limit a patient's motivation to return to productivity. However, such attitudes are dynamic, not static. As we will see, in the functional restoration program, they are subject to change with appropriate training, education and counseling. It is the therapist's ability to recognize when these barriers are operating, and then to deal with them through the interdisciplinary team approach, that characterizes the therapists who are competent in providing functional restoration services.

Pain Issues

We have discussed the fact that pain complaints are "subjective" phenomena, representing a central, cognitive interpretation of multiple events. These may include peripheral noxious stimuli, psychologic patterns, and effects of exogenous and endogenous neurotransmitters, such as opiates and endorphins. However, most patients only recognize a "direct link" between a peripheral stimulus and its central expression as pain, localizing all pain patterns as if they were external stimuli. It requires a great deal of education to help a patient understand the delicate interplay of such issues as stress and depression in the pain process in order to overcome the patient's multiple pre-established attitudes. In practice, the therapist is responsible for educating the patient about basic concepts such as referred pain, nerve root compression, or epidural scarring. Second, the patient must be reassured that passive treatments designed to alter the natural history of the pain process will be attempted before the patient is expected to undergo any pain attendant upon physical active training. Further, the patient must be taught that the quality, location and intensity of the pain is not necessarily a reflection of underlying disorder, nor is it often useful to the therapist in making judgments about alteration in the treatment approach. The patient must constantly be reminded of a reasonable healing period within his or her past experience. Inspiring the patient with confidence in the therapist's ability to deal effectively with painful situations, should they arise, is one of the most critical aspects of the "bonding" which takes place during the early portion of any treatment program. While attempts have been made to do this in "back schools," these programs have generally lacked the hands-on contact only afforded by the therapist, or the coherent conceptual framework necessary for patient understanding and shifting of beliefs, as part of a rehabilitation process.

Emphasis on functional restoration rather than pain relief as the primary goal of the rehabilitation program sets this apart from other spine rehabilitation programs previously practiced. The patient's pain is always acknowledged as real, since it is unlikely to be "internally created" (i.e., a delusion). However, the staff does not focus on pain, nor is an unrealistic goal of a complete "cure" of pain held out to the patient. By the time the patient has been chronically disabled, this can usually be well understood. In fact, the patient who insists that he or she must be "pain-free" before resuming any level of productivity is putting up one of the most significant socioeconomic "red flags" the therapist is likely to encounter. Education is necessary to help the patient "push through" pain in order to achieve the benefits of the reconditioning exercises.

One of the most difficult concepts to impart is that pain does not equal harm or injury once it has become chronic. The patients are taught that they must learn to distinguish between acute pain, which can potentially reveal new tissue damage, and chronic pain which informs them only that they have exceeded low levels of physical capacity to which they have fallen. It is also necessary for the patient to understand that increased pain related to increased activity, the stretching of scar and immobile joint capsules, is not only harmless, but is actually a sign of beneficial progress. Again, quantification of function assists the patient in understanding this process despite his subjective report of how he feels.

Finally, the therapist must constantly guard against falling into the same unjustified prejudices that have prevented solutions of chronic back disability in the past. While it is true that many chronic patients are unconscious somatizers and symptom magnifiers, and some may be abusing the disability system in their desperation to hold on to some level of economic security, these excesses usually do not occur in a fraudulent or dishonest manner. Patients may be faced with difficult choices as part of their rehabilitation, and their response to these changes may not always be predictable. This is the nature of a treatment approach dealing with this group of patients, and is illustrated by its lack of universal success. Yet, the "true malingerer" generally does not make it into a functional restoration program. These individuals are generally bright, pleasant, self-satisfied sociopaths who will usually find any manner of excuse to avoid participating in a rehabilitation program which will alter the course on which they have embarked. They usually have specific financial goals they are seeking to attain, and will be satisfied only when their financial motivation has been addressed by negotiations involving the legal system. Thus, the therapist must constantly keep in mind that every patient willing to participate in rehabilitation will obtain some level of motivation to improve his life status. In summary, refusal to participate in functional restoration is a problem of patient "secondary gain" for illness behavior, while failure to succeed is primarily due to the balance between structural/functional deficits and barriers to recovery within the rehabilitation system.

Muscle Atrophy Versus Inhibition

Patients will enter the program with muscular deficits of widely varying degree. The physical capacity between 50 to 80% of normal is commonly seen associated with good or excellent effort. Those with low physical capacity, including some who produce no force at all on strength tests, usually show variable and inconsistent curves and suboptimal effort. Low strength levels are generally *not* a sign of severely advanced muscle atrophy in producing extreme loss of muscle bulk or fatty replacement. Rather, these deficits generally represent other factors including fear of injury, neuromuscular inhibition, and alteration of neural input to the muscle from higher centers.

It is important to the therapist to keep in mind that changes brought about by factors other than structural loss of muscle bulk may be reversed quickly by training, and dramatic increases in measured trunk strength may be achieved during a short intensive training program. These changes are usually due to enhanced cooperation and confidence, rather than to alteration in muscle bulk. Strength changes based on alteration of muscle size are much harder to achieve and take considerably longer. Thus, some persistent physical capacity deficits following intensive training are the rule rather than the exception in chronically disabled back patients. It is critical that the patient continue to improve physical capacity utilizing a home maintenance program of exercise. These programs may be assisted by a variety of home devices or regular attendance at a fitness center or health club provided the appropriate variable resistance equipment is available. Ultimately, progressive change in muscle circumference may be demonstrable by single cut CT scans or magnetic resonance imaging.

OUTPATIENT TREATMENT MODELS

Reconditioning Programs for Subacute, Chronic Episodic or Postoperative Patients

A large group of patients may be treated in a simpler and less expensive manner than that employed in a comprehensive program following a customary therapy model. This program is generally reserved for patients beyond the acute post-injury stages of back pain, but before development of major psychosocial barriers to functional recovery. Most of the patients in this category are *not* disabled from work or, if they are postoperative, soon to return to the job. In these outpatient programs, treatment follows a simpler therapy model, without the need for complex staffings or interaction between groups of therapists. Psychology and nursing are generally not involved, while physical and occupational therapists may provide treatment alone or in tandem. Like other programs, however, quantification of function technology is at the core of the decision-making process. An initial Quantitative Functional Evaluation (QFE) is followed by a physical therapy assessment and basic introduction to training methodology. The primary program involves a series of 12 to 24 sessions over a 4 to 6 week period ending with a repeat QFE. Follow-up consists of instructing a patient in a home program for continued development of mobility and strength, while follow-up is on a p.r.n. basis only, should the patient require additional testing and instruction at some point in the future. As part of the program, a series of educational sessions are interspersed to provide "back school" education as a contained module. Because of its brevity and intensity, this program can handle much larger numbers of patients bringing the essence of functional restoration physical reconditioning to bear without undue emphasis on disability management issues. However, it is inappropriate to use this approach for the disabled patient as a high degree of failure can be expected in this group without comprehensive intervention.

Acute Programs

Our survey would not be complete without some discussion of acute programs. This is the most controversial area, with up to 80% of the population at one time having an episode making them potentially eligible for some medical intervention. Of course, only a small fraction of this group ever seeks medical attention for these problems, with many others utilizing chiropractic care, home remedies, or self-medication. A wide variety of alternating and often conflicting methodologies have been advocated for this purpose, generally with little scientific basis (Deyo, 1983; Deyo, Diehl, Rosenthal, 1986). Most are familiar with the variety of medically sanctioned treatments for the acute back pain process, which generally include rest, heat and medication. Bedrest lasting from 2 days to 6 weeks has been advocated, while a variety of medications including anti-inflammatories, muscle relaxants, and opiates, are commonly given. Physical therapy modalities including heat, massage, ultrasound, diathermy, and lasers, are used in an attempt to promote increased circulation to the injured area, often accompanied by massage, traction or mobilization/manipulation. Back school education and specialized exercise programs, such as suggested by McKenzie or Williams, are commonly applied. The eclectic nature of this treatment is well known, but the effectiveness of such treatment is greatly dependent on the "bonding" between the therapist and the patient. Effectiveness is almost impossible to evaluate because the time course of acute back pain is so rapid in most cases that the effects of treatment cannot be statistically evaluated.

THE COMPREHENSIVE TREATMENT PROGRAM

Phase I: Pre-Program

The first phase of program participation is the most important in determining whether a patient is really ready to get well, and the physical therapist is the key individual during this process. This period utilizes the physical therapist's talents for one-on-one hands-on physical treatment and education to invest the patient with a sense of trust and confidence in the arduous treatment process on which he is embarking. Besides dealing with issues of trust and skepticism concerning staff and the program, the physical therapist also must be the primary evaluator of compliance, being sure to give the patient every opportunity to participate. Excuses concerning "transportation," "child care," "my check was late," are commonplace and are often merely an expression of irrational fears about the rehabilitation process. Helping patients overcome this fear through individual therapy is extremely rewarding. Finally, the exercise progression process must begin by mobilizing stiff soft tissue and scar. A stretching regimen with education in a frequently performed home exercise program is essential.

A potential trap for the physical therapist is to focus solely on the patient's probable specific structural pathologic condition without appreciating the multiple factors contributing to current physical functional deficits. When dealing with a chronic pain problem, a therapist must understand there is an actual disorder whether or not it can be isolated. There are many dysfunctions in the deconditioned patient that can be treated specifically without spending undue time looking for a certain structural cause. The therapist must be confident that the medical director and previous physicians have isolated and identified what causes they can, and that these are encapsulated in their reports. If the therapist does not feel confident, he or she must so inform the physician at the earliest possible time, preferably after the initial physical therapy evaluation. From then on, the knowledge of the structural disorder serves only as a focus for educating the patient as to specific problems for which his or her program must be individualized, but for which no "surgical fix" is available. The physical therapist must be confident that regardless of how numerous the previous diagnostic tests or surgical procedures are that have been done in the past, the patients are ready to enter a functional restoration program once they have been cleared by the program physician.

The Quantitative Functional Evaluation (QFE) is performed early in Phase I to set a baseline for physical capacity. The most important elements focused on at this stage are the patient's effort, the "grade" or cumulative score on testing, and the range of motion. This sets the stage for progression of the exercise program which gradually seeks to push the patient's physical capacity to normal or above normal levels relative to a normative database, regardless of the degree of underlying structural disorder. This is the "football knee" concept in which, despite prior knee surgery and instability, a sports medicine approach designed to mobilize and strengthen the articular and peri-articular structures can allow for high levels of performance in spite of the fact that stability and complete pain relief can never be attained. The patient, having applied effort to reach a desired end point, makes a definitive decision on what risk and activity level to tolerate, and what minimal maintenance training levels to continue. The major goal of this initial phase is greater flexibility and mobility, not only in the peri-articular capsular structures, but also in supporting ligaments and presumed scar in soft tissue. As has been shown (Pearcy, Sheperd, 1985), the problem in a pathologic condition of the spine is generally *hypomobility.* Therefore, the stiff spine is more like a rusted chain than an excessively mobile one. Hypomobility can add to problems when dealing with an unstable segment or biomechanical link in that immobility above and below an unstable segment thrusts increased loading upon the injured segment. Thus, the need to evaluate instability only when mobility has been re-established in adjacent, generally flexible joints (Pearcy, Sheperd, 1985; Pearcy, Portek, Sheperd, 1985).

Interesting work done in the past on soft tissues can give us some guidelines to appropriate stretching methodology. Recent work on soft tissue healing demonstrates that the strongest and most pliable soft tissue healing occurs in response to early motion and stress (Gelberman, Manske, Akeson, Woo, Lundberg, Amiel, 1986). Basically, it was shown that early passive motion created a scar whose collagen fibers were aligned along the lines of stress, whereas immobilized repaired tendons developed a bulbous scar with fibers oriented in random directions, with considerable adherence to adjacent tissue that limited subsequent mobility. The strength of the bulbous scar was only a fraction of that of the passively mobilized repair. In essence, this theory represents a "Wolff's Law of soft tissue" in which, just as in bone, the collagen fiber aligns itself for maximum strength along the lines of stress if appropriate mechanical stimuli are applied.

Other evidence is based on work done on rat tail collagen (Russek, 1976; Sapega, Quenfeld, Moyer, et al., 1982). The conclusions are that frequent moderate stretches just beyond the point of elastic deformation create the most substantial gains in mobility. Heat can assist this process by loosening the collagenous bonds temporarily, but if stretch is not maintained while the tissue is cooled down, the tissue contracts back to original levels. Cooling the tissue in the stretched state presumably "locks in" the gains ascribed to tissue heating.

Thus, a frequently performed home stretching program is advocated to patients in phase I. Their compliance with this program is part of the monitoring that is performed principally by the physical therapist, with the effort demonstrated through the relationship of hip mobility to straight leg raising (Keeley, Mayer, Cox, Gatchel, Smith, Mooney, 1986; Mayer, Tencer, Kristoferson, Mooney, 1984) which assesses the patient's willingness to progress through the initial phases of a reconditioning program in spite of some discomfort.

The accompanying figures demonstrate the basic generic stretching programs which patients are taught initially (Fig. 15–1). All efforts to strengthen are eliminated during this initial phase while the patient focuses on a frequent stretching program. Because a pan-hypomobility is customarily present, all exercises are taught. However, the program is individualized for specific deficits identified on the QFE. An aid to regaining mobility is a prototype CPM (continuous passive motion) device produced to induce slow sagittal mobility. This device (Sutter Biomedical, San Diego, CA) is not only helpful during the initial mobility processes in fearful individuals, but also to deal with spasm that occurs during the strengthening phases of the program.

Phase II: Intensive Treatment Phase

Phase II consists of the portion of the program involving the major contact with and supervision of the patient. During a 3-week comprehensive program, approximately 150 contact hours occur, about 50% in physical training and another 50% in education/counseling. This is the critical phase in the program, in which a patient is given every opportunity to participate in rehabilitation, but is confronted with difficult psychosocioeconomic issues in attempting to restore function. It is anticipated that 7 to 10% of those who enter the program will "drop out" or be expelled for disruptiveness to the treatment environment or a variety of noncompliant behaviors.

From the point of view of physical progression, it is anticipated that most mobility issues have been resolved prior to program entry, and the comprehensive program can focus on strength, endurance, and aerobic capacity. Strengthening of the injured body part, often the trunk extensors, is usually the primary issue and must be done gradually and carefully. Constant re-education and "first aid" for muscular discomfort/spasm is necessary, involving modalities such as ice, stretching, and/or lowered resistance. The basic principles of progressive resistive exercises have been well described previously and should be familiar to the reader (DeLorme, Watkins, 1951; Gould, Davies, 1985). Various variable resistance machines are used to strengthen the basic functional units as shown in Figure 15–2. The trunk extensor functional unit, consisting of trunk extensors, gluteii and hamstrings is usually trained in counterpoint to sagittal flexors: the recti, hip flexors and quadriceps. Combined machines such as a leg press are also useful. The variable-resistance equipment is produced by several companies and is easily found in multiple fitness centers and YMCAs, where it can be very useful in maintenance programs after comprehensive education of the patient. However, it should be used with extreme caution in the absence of functional quantification.

Maximal exercises are performed, as well as repetitive contractions against considerably lower resistance to improve muscle endurance. Simultaneously, the patient is trained aerobically using exercise bicycles to increase cardio-

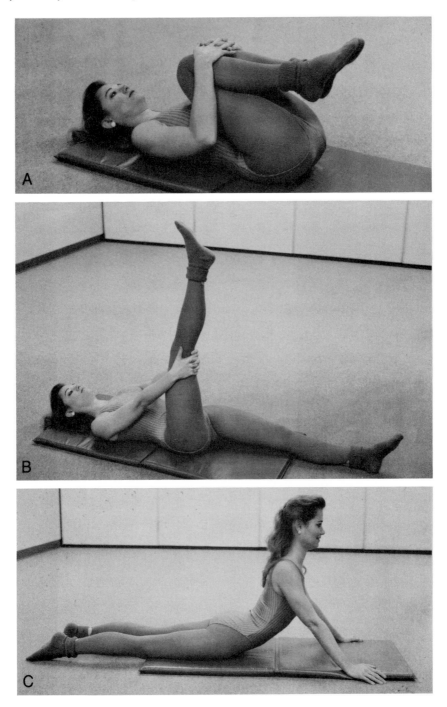

Fig. 15–1. A, Stretch to increase true lumbar flexion. B, Stretch for SLR. C, Stretch for true lumbar and hip extension. *(Continued on following pages.)*

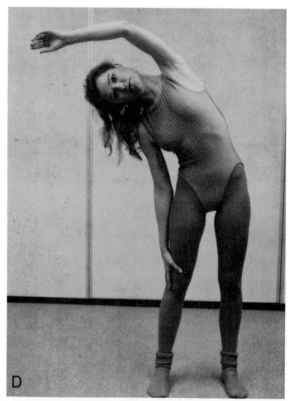

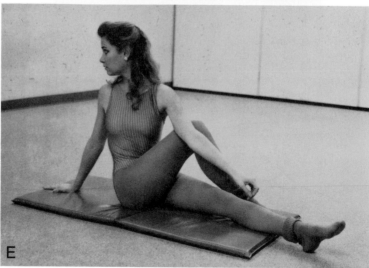

Fig. 15–1 (Cont.). D, Stretch for lateral bend, E, Stretch for torsion. *(Continued on following page.)*

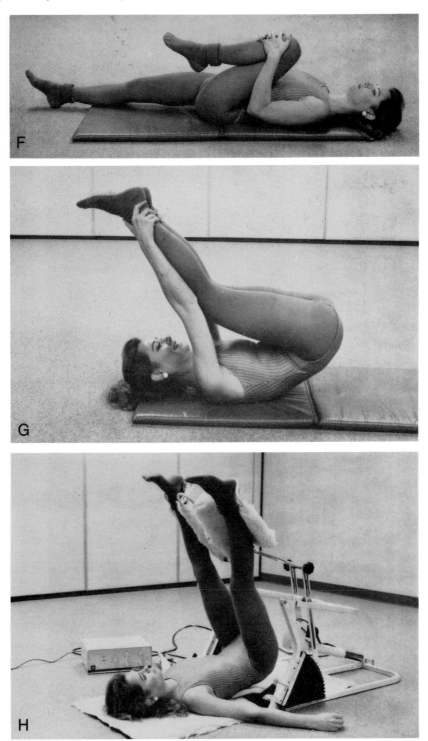

Fig. 15–1 (Cont.). F, Stretch for hip flexion (flex one hip up). G, Advanced true lumbar flex when hip mobility is near normal. H, Use of continuous passive motion (CPM) prototype for regaining sagittal mobility.

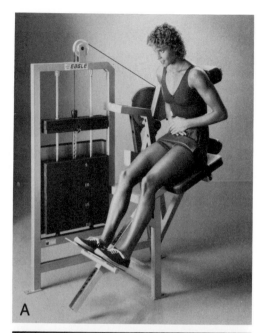

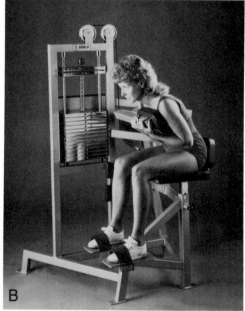

Fig. 15–2.   A, Back extension machine. B, Abdominal flexor machine. *(Continued on following pages.)*

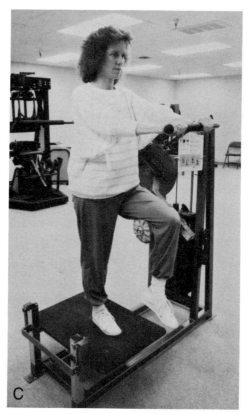

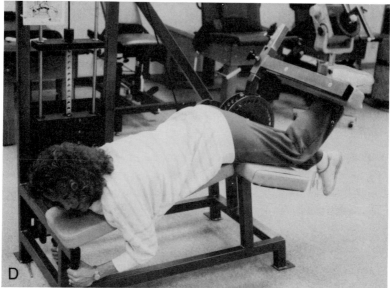

Fig. 15–2 (Cont.).   C, Hip machine for strengthening hip extensors, flexors, abductors, and adductors depending on machine positioning. D, Hamstring "leg curl" exercise. *(Continued on following page.)*

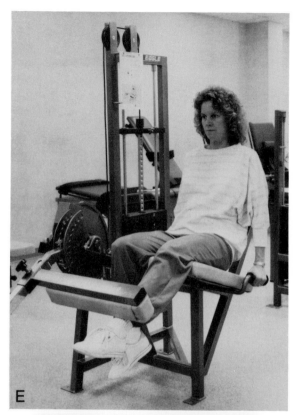

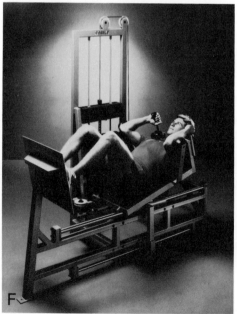

Fig. 15–2 (Cont.). E, Knee/leg extension quadriceps strengthening machine. F, Leg press for combined knee and hip extension, essentially performing a squatting maneuver. (A, B, and F courtesy of Cybex, Division of Lumex, Inc.)

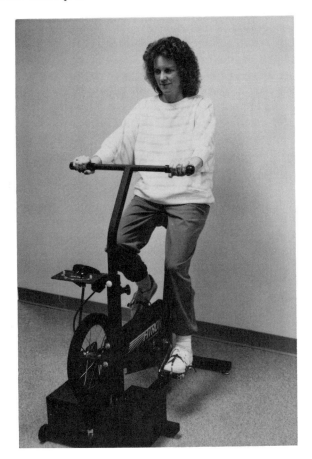

Fig. 15–3.　Patient on exercise bicycle is performing aerobic training.

vascular endurance (Fig. 15–3). This not only improves overall physical function, but also increases sufficiency of nutrient flow to the muscles. Many factors modify the progression in a given individual, including age, weight, gender, previous surgical history, length of disability and initial quantitative testing. In fact, the onset of Phase II is marked by a second QFE to "reset" the appropriate exercise level. Hopefully, if significant mobility deficits were identified on initial Phase I testing, these have improved during the Phase I program, as have any deficiencies in measured effort. However, trunk strengthening is generally a frightening activity for patients, often abetted by bad advice from friends, relatives, and co-workers, and education must succeed in progressively improving effort during this 3-week comprehensive program.

Repetitive exercises can help in developing fatigue resistance, and this can now be measured utilizing a variety of endurance and recovery protocols on strength testing devices. One of the most difficult areas, however, is in measurement of coordination and agility. Development of programs for neuromuscular facilitation is still in its infancy, but basic principles include exercise at physiologic loads and a variety of speeds, with particular emphasis on simulating common tasks related to the injured body part, such as bending or twisting. Just as in most sports medicine programs, there is a gradual progression with some overlap of mobility, strength, endurance, and neuromuscular training. There is also a combined emphasis on training for specific tasks, as well as generalized overall body fitness. A set of floor exercises, combining mobility, aerobic aspects and specific agility tasks, can be a helpful adjunct to the portions of the program already mentioned (Fig. 15–4). During Phase II, the patient continues building trust and confidence in the program and staff.

Generally, maximum weight begins to increase dramatically around the middle of the program as fear of injury and neuromuscular inhibition are gradually erased, with concomitant improvement in effort measures. A lack of improvement in all of these areas during the middle of the program signifies the fact that psychosocial issues are limiting the patient's improvement. This failure is often accompanied by markedly increased pain complaints without underlying physical findings to support them, and these issues must be addressed by the entire treatment team. This is one of several critical times, when attention to the psychosocial issues can often break down the barriers and help the patient turn failure into success. Failure patients will generally display continued noncompliance, slipping attendance, and perhaps even escalating disruptiveness or undermining of the treatment milieu.

Physical appliances and modalities are generally inconsistent with the philosophy of a functional restoration program. This is not to say that certain modalities may not help in the pain relief process, but they have become so familiar as "dependency producers" and they provide such an opportunity for the patient to demand inappropriate individual attention, that they are best not used at all. Similarly, appliances such as casts, braces, or support devices also should not be used in the chronically disabled patient as they generally unduly limit function without countervailing evidence of improved stability. There may be exceptions, as in the case of supports for unstable knees or as a means to allow a patient to continue exercising in the presence of patellofemoral dysfunction. Naturally, braces used for true paralysis, such as a drop-foot, ankle-foot orthosis, would not fall into this category. However, these are extremity braces for back-related extremity disorders. Axial braces have not been found

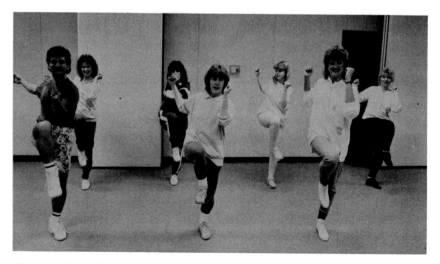

Fig. 15–4.   Aerobic and agility training utilizing floor exercises.

to be beneficial in the functional restoration process. TENS units may also be a possible exception, as they are under direct patient control, but have the negative effect of acting as a "magic black box," distracting the patient from the goals at hand. If used, they should be monitored with considerable caution.

Because the physical therapist has specialists in stress management and relaxation training available to him or her, pain control can be aided by utilizing these techniques. Physical therapists should be trained in these skills, or utilize the services available in this area during the Phase II program. Ice and stretching should also be used. The techniques can be facilitated by individual attention, actually performing the exercises with the patient when he or she has a spasm, is having a "bad day," or is requiring reassurance concerning pain while engaged in a physical activity. The continuous passive motion device appears promising in offering patient assistance in this area also. Finally, the therapist should be certain that the patient has an appropriate anti-inflammatory medication available and is complying with instructions for its use.

While the physical therapist generally does not treat psychosocial issues directly, these may have a considerable impact on performance of the patient's exercise and report of pain. The physical therapist should keep two critical questions in mind when evaluating poor performance, increased pain, noncompliance, or disruptiveness: (1) what, if any, is the physical component of the new pain?; (2) what psychosocial issues is the patient facing at this time? Increased pain complaints may represent either physical inflammation caused by the demands of physical training and/or psychosocial issues related to emotional, financial, legal, or employment issues. The physical therapist should not take a merely mechanistic approach to these problems, but keep in close consultation with other staff members, particularly through staffings and small group meetings, to "get to the bottom" of the pain exacerbation. When the psychosocial issues manifest themselves in noncompliance or disruptiveness, the physical therapist cannot fail to recognize these processes. In these situations, the therapist deals with the patient in an authoritative but supportive manner, avoiding power struggles and a punitive or authoritarian stance.

The therapist must establish his or her position as a trained and experienced professional who is an expert in progressing exercise with patients with chronic back problems. Confidence and trust in the functional restoration approach must be re-established. While a great deal of time and effort is put into explaining treatment rationale, the quantified testing, and the previous structural diagnostics to the patient, it cannot be emphasized too strongly that this time is well spent. It may need to be done on multiple occasions in a collaborative manner with a therapist in charge of both exercise progression and education. The patient must understand that certain aspects of the program may be modified temporarily if certain symptoms appear, but only rarely are exercises completely eliminated (and then only temporarily). After a short period of modification, patients will be returned to their normal progression as symptoms abate or appropriate healing is anticipated.

Initially, it is anticipated that effort will be limited by fear of injury, skepticism, and confusion about the physical demands of this activity. Frequently, the requirements of functional restoration will conflict with what the patient has been told in previous "back schools," or modality-oriented physical therapy where education has been aimed at the acute, not the chronic phase. Such re-education requires a period of trust-building prior to any reasonable likelihood that the new information will be accepted by the patient. As the patient begins to see progress occurring, and noting that the goals that have been set are being met or exceeded, often counterpointed against failures of previous modes of treatment, confidence is established and compliance is gradually obtained. However, under certain circumstances, confrontation becomes necessary.

Phase III: Follow-up Phase

The follow-up phase, which is of variable frequency and duration, is planned around both the outstanding psychosocial issues and the degree of improvement attained in physical training. In most cases, by the end of the comprehensive Phase II, patients have dramatically overcome fear of injury, immobility, and neuromuscular inhibition issues. However, depending on the degree of damage to soft tissues, issues of strength, endurance, and agility may be only partially resolved. Post-surgical patients may have a considerably more difficult time, as there is considerable potential for biomechanical laxity, due to severed posterior ligamentous complexes, capsular laxity, or denervated musculature. Any or all of these problems may arise asymmetrically, producing unilateral or unpredictable bilateral effects. It is one of the unfortunate aspects of spine surgical training that, until recently, respect for soft tissue integrity following surgical procedures has not been a high priority in our teaching programs. Anterior lumbar surgery is not immune to these effects, as it is accompanied by a high pseudorarthrosis rate. Excision of large portions of disc anulus replaced by amorphous scar may subject the unfused segment to rotatory and translational strains not generally noted after posterior surgery. Furthermore, partial psoas denervation may affect, probably asymmetrically, control of true lumbar spine mobility.

Exercise progression issues during follow-up usually focus on dealing with the slower process of dealing with actual muscle atrophy. Heavier weights may be involved, with more repetitions. Because the "weak link" is no longer grossly below standards of the remainder of the body, other musculoskeletal complaints may arise, which may need to be dealt with. Total body conditioning and strengthening now become of greater importance.

At the same time, the patient is returning to a home environment that may be less than fully supportive. Much of the responsibility for ongoing exercise is now on the shoulders of the patient, who may regress to previous levels of irresponsibility in some cases. Coincident with the follow-up program, therefore, it is essential to develop a feeling of patient accountability for maintaining a regular home program with use of floor exercises, home training devices, and/ or use of a YMCA, fitness center, or gym on a regular basis. For some individuals, whose jobs are primarily sedentary or light, development of positional tolerance for sitting, standing, etc., is the primary occupational requirement. In these individuals, subnormal levels of physical capacity can be tolerated, though patients remaining at these levels tend to report higher pain levels in general. Whether this relationship between high pain report and low physical capacity, even after a training program, is a predetermined personality characteristic, or represents a true physiologic cause of relationship, cannot be ascertained at this time. What is clear, however, is that, on a statistical basis, patients with the highest physical capacity scores tend to have the lowest pain report.

In terms of dealing with pain and psychosocial issues, the patterns of management are essentially unchanged. The physical demands of more vigorous reconditioning may precipitate other symptoms, but these can generally be easily dealt with as customary training overuse syndromes, whose management is familiar to every physical therapist and athletic trainer. In patients with heavy job demand categories who must achieve high strength levels, such problems are commonplace. Particularly susceptible to these problems seem to be the smaller men and women, with less muscle mass, who must achieve a higher percentage of their total potential in order to perform the same tasks as larger individuals. Supernormal functional capacity is often demanded of these individuals, and the achievement of this may prove to be challenging. In general, these patients have mastered adversity related to their size in the past, and are also able to achieve it under these conditions.

The sudden reappearance of symptom magnification, disruptiveness, non-compliance, or regression in test performance or effort may be dramatic during this phase. This usually implies that major psychosocial issues have reached a critical stage and are exerting a profound effect on the patient's behavior. Typical problems at this stage have less to do with physical difficulties than with outstanding legal, employment, compensation, drug dependence, or family difficulties. Supportive counseling, gentle education, and continued focus on vigorous physical training are the key elements in assisting patients through this time.

Ideally, at the completion of the follow-up phase, the patient not only performs, but *understands* the need for continued maintenance of a physical program and the major elements included therein. The patient will be alert to problems that may arise from time to time, how to deal with them, and when and where to reconnect to the medical care system. The patient will have been returned to the care of the original referring physician, who will usually be prepared to deal with new acute problems that may arise. The results of the first follow-up QFE will have been explained to the patient and compared to previous tests. Specific recommendations to the patient on dealing with deficits still noted complete the process. Changes in cumulative scores of a typical QFE are shown in Figure 15–5.

Phase IV: Outcome Tracking Phase

The long-term tracking phase is not primarily a physical therapy responsibility. Patients may be retested at intervals of 3, 6, and 12 months post-program, but attendance typically drops off as patients become more familiar with functional restoration and their return to a productive lifestyle. It is gratifying to note, in follow-up studies, that the use of the medical care system declines dramatically in a 2-year follow-up after the disability management program (Mayer, Gatchel, Mayer, Kishino, Keeley, Mooney, 1987).

CUMULATIVE TEST SCORE	PT	OT
This Test	92%	103%
Last Test	89%	99%
Initial Test	57%	48%

Fig. 15–5. Portion of QFE done post-program, showing cumulative scores for patient on the follow-up test, as well as changes from initial and discharge testing done previously.

Relatively minor recurrences or reinjuries may be profoundly frightening to patients when they occur after a hiatus of many months. The process, though physically similar to what the patient may have experienced during supervised program phases, reminds the patient of the extreme life changes that occurred during the period of disability from a previous injury. The anxiety produced by these memories may be truly terrifying to the patient, and in some cases lead to another disastrous round of "doctor-shopping," renewed disability, occupational alienation, and ineffective treatment. A close and trusting relationship developed between the patient and physical therapist goes a long way toward fostering a willingness on the part of the patient to return for re-evaluation when commonly used learned techniques have been exhausted.The patient who has left the treatment program with the recognition that the physical therapist is capable of flexible responses to new situations will be most likely to seek help again when new difficulties arise.

CHAPTER REFERENCES

DeLorme T, Watkins A: Progressive Resistance Exercise: Technic Medical Application, New York, Appleton-Century-Crofts, Inc., 1951.

Deyo R: Conservative therapy for low back pain: distinguishing useful from useless therapy. JAMA *250*:1057–1062, 1983.

Deyo R, Diehl A, Rosenthal M: How many days of bedrest for acute low back pain? N Engl J Med *315*:1064–1070, 1986.

Gelberman RH, Manske PR, Akeson WH, Woo SL-Y, Lundberg G, Amiel D: Kappa Delta Award paper: flexor tendon repair. J Orthop Res *4*:119–128, 1986.

Gould J, Davies G (eds.): Orthopedic and Sports Physical Therapy, St. Louis, C.V. Mosby Co., 1985.

Keeley J, Mayer T, Cox R, Gatchel R, Smith J, and Mooney V: Quantification of lumbar function Part V: reliability of range-of-motion measures in the sagittal plane and an *in vivo* torso rotation measurement technique. Spine *11*:31–35, 1986.

Mayer T, Gatchel RJ, Mayer H, Kishino N, Keeley J, Mooney V: A prospective randomized two year study of functional restoration in industrial low back injury utilizing objective assessment. JAMA *258*:1763–1767, 1987.

Mayer T, Tencer A, Kristoferson S, Mooney V: Use of noninvasive techniques for quantification of spine range-of-motion in normal subjects and chronic low-back dysfunction patients. Spine *9*:588–595, 1984.

Pearcy M, Sheperd J: Is there instability in spondylolisthesis? Spine *10*:175–177, 1985.

Pearcy M, Portek I, Sheperd J: The effect of low back pain on lumbar spinal movements measured by three-dimensional x-ray analysis. Spine *10*:150–153, 1985b.

Russek A: Biomechanical and physiological basis for ambulatory treatment of low back pain. Orthop Rev *5*:21–31, 1976.

Sapega A, Quenfeld T, Moyer R, et al: Biophysical factors in range of motion exercise. Phys Sports Med *9*:57–64, 1982.

ADDITIONAL REFERENCES

Deyo R, Diehl A: Measuring physical and psychosocial function in patients with low back pain. Spine *8*:635–642, 1983.

Wiesel S, Cuckler T, DeLuca F, Jones F, Zerole M, Rothman R: Acute low back pain: an objective analysis of conservative therapy. Spine *5*:324–330, 1980.

Chapter 16

The Role of the Occupational Therapist: Back to the Roots

A HISTORICAL PERSPECTIVE

Even in use of the terms, the relationship between work and occupational therapy is fundamental to the occupational therapy field. The basic concept of the profession rests on the understanding that man naturally needs activities and mastery over his environment, and will seek assistance in achieving the highest potential his body and mind are capable of, with illness seen primarily in the context of its interference with self-actualization. Philosophically, improved physical capacity as a means of increasing the quality of life is essentially synonymous with this specialty. A *handicap* (or injury) may impair the individual's ability to perform work, thus producing a *disability*. The occupational therapist attempts to restore *ability,* even in the presence of a persistent handicap.

Historians of occupational therapy (Bing, 1981; Hopkins, 1983; Harvey-Krefting, 1985) indicate that, beginning in the late 18th century, a "moral treatment" approach was taken with asylum inmates. Whereas they had previously been considered to be demonically possessed and were frequently treated as animals, they were soon to be treated as rational beings for whom activity and discipline were required. Work in and around the asylum became a favored means of achieving regularity, bodily action, improved attention, and distraction from symptoms. The initial use of this system for disabled individuals occurred in workshops for the blind in the late 19th century, after the introduction of Braille allowed experiments in the therapeutic use of work combined with demand for productivity among all members of society. It is clear from this historical development that the approach to work is conditioned upon both social attitudes and economic factors present in any era.

In the United States, beginning in the 1900s, many chronic diseases were treated with isolation and prolonged rest. With an absence of gainful employment, patients were often assisted by therapists to perform productive activities that under other circumstances would be considered leisure activities. Patients with poliomyelitis, tuberculosis, arthritis, and cardiac problems were supplemented by disabled soldiers following World War I, leading to organization of the field. Inherent to the process, however, was the concept that patients would generally not be able to return to competitive employment. Therefore, the concept of "arts and crafts" grew up as opposed to vocational rehabilitation, which was felt to be beyond the scope of occupational therapy.

Since the 1950s, with additional emphasis on a medical model and a restoration of physical function, occupational therapy has gone through several major changes, with its rules still somewhat undefined. Emphasis on physical restoration in the upper extremity and work evaluation/adjustment efforts have also resulted, to a great extent, in territorial skirmishes with other professions. This is because occupational therapy has developed involvement in a number of areas. From a physical point of view, the occupational therapist is not confined to a specific part of the body. Rather, he/she takes the responsibility for the "final honing" of the patient's skills, coordinating the "weak link" physically restored by the physical therapist, and developing skills in specific functional task performances. Subsequently, the occupational therapist coordinates efforts with external groups involved in the "disability system" in efforts to prepare the patient for a return to work. Only if the patient is unemployable under specific conditions of physical limitations, age, cognitive function, or level or vocational skills, is vocational evaluation and rehabilitation called for.

As noted before, it must be emphasized that the occupational therapist is a member of a team including physical therapists, psychologists, nurses, and physicians. As part of this grouping, the occupational therapist has come to hold a truly pivotal role: he or she must deal almost equally with physical and psychosocial issues. While physical therapists are most oriented toward physical progression issues, and psychologists toward the psychosocial ones, the occupational therapists must bridge the gap between these two areas, integrating most program aspects into a coherent plan for disability management. For this to be successful, the occupational therapist must have the unique understanding of the interplay between physical symptoms, personality, and socioeconomic factors bearing on the individual patient's loss of productivity.

Though this unique role developed over the years has also created a formidable task for them, we have learned that the background of occupational therapists provides them with many aspects of the training necessary to effectively perform it. In effect, the occupational therapist functions as an advocate for the patient in dealing with these individuals and the difficult disability issues they represent. A great deal of individual counseling is utilized with the patient in conjunction with the work-hardening and work-simulation aspects of developing productivity-oriented attitudes and behaviors once again.

IMPORTANT PROGRAM ISSUES

Physical Progression

Unlike the physical therapist, whose physical progression program is aimed at more general levels of fitness and physical capacity, the occupational therapist's progression is aimed at more specific goals of daily living. Normal or supernormal levels of physical capacity using a sports medicine work-hardening approach are to be attained. This type of strenuous rehabilitation is made possible by recently developed methods for quantification of occupational capacity, including lifting capacity and tolerance of a variety of positions and activities, such as squatting, bending, climbing or balancing. The quantification not only allows reconditioning to take place efficiently and safely, but permits documentation of effort. As in the case of other musculoskeletal testing, effort factors based on cardiovascular response and curve consistency are integral to measurement of physical progression, and they guide the occupational therapist in recognizing when psychosocial issues are interfering with physical improvement. By returning patients to high functional capacity levels, the occupational therapist helps the patient engage in normal daily activities, reduce the risk of future injury, and, in most cases, experience significant reduction in pain during daily task performance once physical progression has been completed.

The pattern of physical progression is similar to that followed by the physical therapist. In general, involvement of the occupational therapist is phased in slightly later than that of the physical therapist, since coordination and total body fitness, with which the occupational therapist is involved, follow early mobilization and strengthening of the injured part. Similarly, emphasis on work hardening and simulation parallels efforts in coordination and agility which characterize the later stages of any sports medicine program. Just as the returning baseball pitcher or football player must get the functional units of his body "into the groove" once again, the specific task performance emphasis leads up to the concluding aspects of the functional restoration program. Throughout all of these steps, the patient trains individual functional units as well as overall physical fitness. During this training, the physical progression takes place utilizing equipment and techniques designed to parallel, as closely as possible, the patient's real-life activities.

Lifting methods have frequently been taught as part of job safety and "back school" programs. Ergonomic analysis and biomechanical modeling suggest that it may be desirable that an individual be trained in "proper lifting" techniques for safety. This has been carried to extreme levels in physician and therapist advice to patients with back injuries. Depending on the perceived level of injury, patients are told either never to lift again, or to lift only limited loads, usually based only on the deconditioned patient's perception of what his or her limitations are. The physician usually functions merely as a scribe to document what the patient reports, usually regardless of critical factors such as age, gender, and body weight. In an example definitely not unique in our experience, a fireman was seriously advised by his surgeon, after a spinal fusion, "Never lift more than a beer can, and when you do that be sure to keep your elbow bent so the beer can stays close to your body." The patient followed his instructions to the letter, with an ensuing 5 years of disability, dependence, and dysfunction caused primarily by a literal interpretation of unreasonable medical advice. Following functional restoration, the patient has returned to active work in a fire department both on fire engines and as a paramedic on ambulances.

Concern over lifting techniques must be balanced by common sense and awareness of all factors involved in the lifting process. A considerable body of knowledge concerning isometric, isokinetic, and isoinertial lifting has evolved, much of it covered in an earlier chapter (Kishino, Mayer, Gatchel, Parrish, Anderson, Gustin, Mooney, 1985; Kroemer, 1983; Snook, Campanelli, Hart, 1978; Chaffin, Andersson, 1984; Pope, Frymoyer, Andersson, 1984). Certainly, when dealing with particularly heavy loads, it is advantageous to shorten the lever arm by holding the object, insofar as it is possible, close to the body. This principle must be considerably modified by age, body weight, size of object, lifting level, etc. Moreover, lifting with the back in neutral or extension removes the biomechanical advantage of taut posterior ligamentous complexes, forcing the muscles to act to transmit the lifting loads through the lumbar spine to the pelvis. This is an inefficient but generally "safer" lifting method because muscular feedback appears to be better than that from the ligament complex.

However, the reader need only watch a group of individuals lifting repetitively to recognize the fallacy of insisting on such lifting techniques for all tasks under all conditions. The body naturally seeks the most efficient lifting methodology, and the straight back, bent leg, squat position is definitely not the most efficient. Most patients lifting at floor level with light to medium loads will individually *select* a posture with slightly bent knees and a flexed spine and hips, particularly if there is lateral movement involved (Fig. 16–1). In this way, the body actually acts as a crane, efficiently "hanging on its ligaments" and allowing the length of the upper torso to "swivel" the load in a wide arc around an axial plane. There is no concrete evidence to suggest that we have acquired the wisdom to correct a technique developed through thousands of years of evolution through the limited understanding of back pain gained in the last 50 years. In fact, when not carefully observed, "back school-trained" individuals will invariably return to their older, more efficient lifting methods.

Under circumstances of very heavy loads, the patient's normal feedback

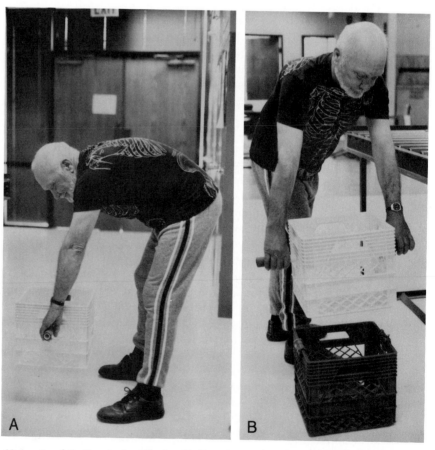

Fig. 16–1. A and B, Commonly utilized, self-selected method for lifting light to moderate loads with subject's body "hanging on its ligaments," permitting lifting and 180-degree translation in the axial plane.

mechanisms generally advise him or her that greater prudence is essential. Any subject will "test the weight," attempt to straddle the object, and straighten the back to decrease the lifting moment. Naturally, the more deconditioned the individual is, the lighter the acceptable loads at which he or she will self-select this lifting style. However, if this is the only method ever utilized, the patient loses the capacity for regulating his or her capacity for light bending and twisting, and becomes susceptible to pain exacerbation simply attempting any self-selected lift. The critical occupational therapy training issue involves communicating this information to patients, and assisting their transition from rigid constrained lifting to a situation in which they can be confident in their ability to self-select the most efficient technique.

In addition to general physical reconditioning and lift training, each patient must also work on specific activities of daily living related to positional tolerance and work activities. The tasks of work simulation and hardening are designed to duplicate, as closely as possible, the physical demands of the patient's workplace and home that will be encountered after leaving the functional restoration program. An obstacle course that includes bending, crawling, twisting, squatting, climbing, and pushing-pulling assists in quantifying these capacities and building functional tolerance. Indeed, this is a creative area for involvement by the occupational therapist in helping to devise new and alternate methods of work simulation in the individual facility.

Work Feasibility and Job Readiness

The ultimate outcome of the patient's physical progression in a sports medicine disability management program is returning to work, just as the injured athlete returns to his or her sport. Job readiness is assessed quantitatively through physical performance on the quantified functional evaluation (QFE), as well as daily progress in work simulation. It is always desirable for the patient to progress in physical readiness to a point beyond that required by the job demands. In this way, fears related to inability to perform and re-injury will be greatly diminished or eliminated, regardless of the degree of pain relief afforded. We have observed empirically that when a patient fails to achieve physical capacity sufficient to demonstrate mastery over work in a structured, supervised rehabilitation program, the chances for that patient to successfully return and remain on the job are significantly decreased. In most instances, however, the psychosocial, financial, and legal issues affecting the patient will usually have a greater bearing on the pain complaints, job readiness, and feasibility issues than the patient's true physical capacity.

Specific problems related to feasibility of employment are discussed with patients individually and in groups. Punctuality, appearance, attitudes towards employers and fellow employees, and teamwork are some of the factors in successful employment to which patients are introduced, occasionally for the first time.

Psychosocial Issues

While every department must be aware of psychosocial issues and barriers to functional recovery for each patient, the occupational therapy department tends to focus its efforts on covering and addressing the financial, legal, and work-related barriers. Because of their external communication contacts with attorneys, insurance companies and employers, the occupational therapist also has access to information that can provide insight into specific barriers beyond the functional restoration system, and any specific "hidden agendas" that the patient may have.

One important factor that the therapist must recognize is the difference between symptom magnification or somatization, and "malingering" or "faking." As we have noted before, because of the legal, financial and employment ramifications of back injuries involving compensation or negligence complicating the physical problem of the patient, there is often a tendency to label patients in a pejorative manner. However, only a small percentage of patients turn out to be consciously malingering. These patients are generally unconcerned about their disability predicament. They will either go to great pains to avoid participating in rehabilitation, or they will manipulate the milieu by doing their best to undermine the team's efforts with other patients during the program (disruptiveness). Following the program, they frequently return to referring physicians, attorneys, and insurance adjusters with lurid tales of mistreatment and staff incompetence. Sometimes the efforts can be comical, as in the case of a patient who felt unable to give up the generous long-term disability and workmen's compensation payments provided by his employer. After exhausting every "doctor shopping" alternative to demonstrate surgical disorders, he went to great efforts to contact patients with whom he had been acquainted in the functional restoration program to enlist them in signing a petition to have the rehabilitation process investigated by *60 Minutes,* a popular, sensation-oriented television news weekly. His efforts included multiple visits to patients in their homes, places of employment, and the hotel where out-of-town patients are housed. In this process, he customarily drove 300 miles in a round trip from his home once or twice a week. While he failed to collect many signatures, he certainly demonstrated his physical capacity to perform many types of work, including traveling salesman, messenger, census taker, or medium-haul truck driver, all of which he was qualified for by virtue of previous training and education.

In most situations, however, patients tend to express their emotional lives through physical changes, and with the underpinnings of their lives upended by their back disability, they begin magnifying symptoms dramatically. In some cases, patients have been strong somatizers prior to their back injury, as often demonstrated by histories of multiple surgical procedures, excessive medical visits, and for a variety of gastrointestinal, gynecologic, or musculoskeletal symptoms. Every primary care physician is aware that a significant part of his or her practice is made up of only a small percentage of the general population whose somatization magnifies their concerns about their physical well-being out of proportion to that of other societal members. A long period of disability may also predispose patients, consciously or unconsciously, to justify their continued disability and to "save face" in light of continued reinforcement of the psychosocial component of their lack of productivity. In keeping with the overall functional restoration philosophy, occupational therapists deal with patients based on their physical problems, but with the understanding that there is often an extensive interaction between symptoms and psychosocial stressors.

The occupational therapist has a need for a unique therapeutic relationship.

In order to have the most impact on a patient, the therapist needs to build a relationship that functions in an individual as well as a group environment, conveying support, concern and respect. From the beginning, the therapist must work to gain the patient's trust and confidence and to establish rapport. This may be difficult, since many of the patients are mistrustful of medical systems, particularly when they have had little choice in ongoing treatment and prior negative medical experiences. As a result of this lack of trust, patients may withhold information, attempt to avoid dealing with difficult psychosocial issues, and be resistant to progressing physically. Nonetheless, it is essential that the patient understand the therapist has his or her overall best interest at heart. To successfully engage the patient in treatment, then, the occupational therapist must utilize all available counseling skills, including being firm, authoritative, or even confrontational when needed.

Because the occupational therapist deals most directly with work and financial issues, interactions with the patient may become charged with intense emotion. Longstanding dissatisfactions in the work place, anger over treatment since injury, conflicts with insurance companies, financial losses and fears of reinjury or work return are dealt with daily. While the occupational therapist is not expected to provide intensive psychotherapy, he or she must be prepared to defuse these issues or channel them in a manner that is productive to the patient. This is an area where close interaction with the program's psychologist is helpful. The patient's psychologist can offer insights that are helpful in understanding the origins of the intense feelings, and in defusing more volatile impulses by devising a coordinated approach to treatment.

It is essential that patients be allowed to participate in treatment planning. They will frequently bring, from past medical experiences and miscommunications, a feeling of being manipulated by the medical/legal system, and will initially attempt to undermine their own rehabilitation. Conversely, they may interpret legal advice as counter to medical suggestions. Counseling thus must focus on collaboration and negotiation, with the patient encouraged to actively participate in, and even create, the critical planning and decision-making steps needed to resume productivity. On the other hand, the barriers to recovery that negatively influence the patient's decision-making processes should not be permitted to prevent the patients from moving forward. Naturally, the therapist must control and direct the treatment by such methods as the use of suggestion and reinforcement, the maintenance of self-esteem, and allowing the patient as much control as possible in the process. The therapist must also communicate that he or she has the patient's best interest in mind, and that this interest is constantly being taken into consideration.

Finally, barriers to recovery are often manifested in noncompliance with the treatment regimen, in both physical progression and attendance. If the occupational therapist is aware of the psychosocial issues, he or she can more readily generate hypotheses regarding the underlying reasons for the self-destructive behaviors that are occurring at any given time. In terms of actually addressing the problems, individual and small group staff meetings are generally used to focus attention on disruptive and noncompliant behaviors. Once the patient has had an adequate healing period, and all passive treatments have been exhausted, the patient's choices are really very few: (1) "Give in" to disability through premature retirement, or (2) face the difficult task of actively participating in his or her own rehabilitation. The patient must make the fundamental choice; the therapist can only assist the process.

Financial Issues

An understanding of each patient's financial issues requires an understanding of the patient's legal and employment situation as well. In general, one approaches financial issues by personalizing them. Upon entering functional restoration, most patients are preoccupied with immediate financial losses and stresses, as well as potential short-term gains. Rather than being "fakers who will get well as soon as they are paid off," most of these patients hold on desperately to their compensation and potential lump sum settlements as the "last life-line before drowning." Two-year follow-up surveys demonstrate that long-term disabled patients denied rehabilitation continue to fail to return to work in the majority of cases, and show a high reinjury rate (probably because deconditioning issues have not been adequately dealt with) when the termination of compensation forces them to resume employment in spite of lack of resolution of their symptoms (Mayer, Gatchel, Mayer, Kishino, Keeley, Mooney, 1987). In effect, in most cases, the socioeconomic system is manipulating the patient, instead of the other way around.

The therapist must help patients appreciate that the long-term financial implications of the decisions that they are making about rehabilitation are interrelated and may represent a "mixed bag." A great deal of education is usually needed, since most patients do not have a clear understanding of the long-term outcomes of their current legal and employment situations. As a part of the process, the therapist must help the patient assess future wage-earning potential, avoid additional financial losses in the short run, and focus on realistic financial expectation as related to the patient as a productive rather than a disabled individual. This can prove to be a delicate area of counseling, since patients usually cannot quarrel with improving physical well-being and resuming a productive lifestyle, but may well be concerned through interactions with friends, relatives, co-workers and attorneys that improved physical condition may adversely affect their financial/legal outcome.

It is an unfortunate but inescapable fact that society has evolved beyond traditional approaches, and social legislation now rewards disability. However, disability, as commonly understood by both the layperson and the professional, has two components: (1) the impairment produced by the physical damage to the body as a whole, be it paralysis, cerebral injury, amputation, or postoperative scarring and biological derangement of spinal anatomy; and (2) the disability produced by the preceding impairment or handicap. These issues are discussed further in Part IV of this text. For the purposes of this section, however, it is important to note two basic mechanisms for documenting a patient's entitlement to appropriate compensation: (1) Impairment is generally considered "permanent" in a legal sense, and is generally partial, with each legal system having a traditional range of accepted payments based on this degree of impairment. The therapist should not be placed in the position of "taking away" the impairment already established by surgery or diagnostic testing that has already been performed; (2) disability or lack of productivity is frequently equated with "proving" the degree of impairment. When financial disincentives to return to work exist, it accentuates the tendency of a disability system to encourage prolonged inactivity by giving the patient an opportunity to actively improve disability limitations without altering the underlying impairment. The therapist is giving patients an opportunity to "document" the fact that they are not merely attempting to maintain disability for financial secondary gain, but rather are willing to do their best to regain the highest level of physical capacity. Most disability systems will permit this to be done, once all aspects of the patient's financial situation, both long and short-term, are understood, without fear of jeopardizing any compensation to which the patient is legitimately entitled.

Disability/Compensation Systems

It is really beyond the scope of this text to discuss in detail the varying disability systems. The therapist must have an understanding of these systems and how they affect the individual patient with whom he or she is dealing in order to help find the best solution for resolving all outstanding disability issues.

Workmen's compensation systems exist in all 50 states and are generally administered by an agency of the state government. In addition, a large Federal workmen's compensation system, administered by the Department of Labor, exists for Federal employees. A few specialized systems with interesting histories, such as FELA and the Jones Act, cover specific groups of employees (Rockey, Fantel, Omenn, 1979). The therapist may also be dealing with personal injury litigation, in which partial disability may exist, with patients working for a prolonged period in a "light duty" situation. Alternately, they may be completely disabled and compensated through long-term disability payments. These situations, typically involving negligence or product liability, allow for compensation for pain and suffering, which is not usually permitted under workmen's compensation statutes. Again, however, the patient documenting his willingness to work through pain to decrease suffering and disability by his active efforts can, more often than not, be expected to favorably impress a jury of his peers that he has more in mind than financial "secondary gain."

The Social Security Disability System is currently most difficult to deal with. This "last-resort" compensation system is fraught with loopholes permitting claimants multiple attempts at receiving compensation, little long-term follow-through, and penalties in terms of loss of compensation for any level of work. Yet, there are few controls to prevent patients from "working under the table." As presently constituted, this system is a major incentive to "premature retirement," and the patient having received this entitlement is considerably more difficult to rehabilitate. However, there are hopeful signs that Social Security, under the pressure of ever-increasing disability payments decreasing the funding pool available for retirement (for which it was originally legislated), is considering reforms that may encourage rehabilitation rather than disability. Under 1980s political conditions, it has been difficult to obtain SSDI, but once a patient is on the rolls, SSDI becomes the "kiss of death" to patient motivation.

Regardless of the specific compensation system, there are a variety of "hidden agendas" with which many patients struggle, but are not necessarily willing to share with a treatment team. These include, but are not limited to:

1. *The Desire for Additional Surgical Treatment.* We have already discussed the "magic wand" hopes some patients bring to medical care, with ex-

pectations that they can be "cured" by their passive acquiescence to medical treatment. This is encouraged by medical systems and the media, but in the case of second or subsequent surgical procedures, the hope is simply not borne out statistically. Furthermore, ill-advised surgical procedures in the wrong population also have notoriously poor results (Dzioba, Benjamin, 1985). Moreover, injury from surgical treatment itself is recognized as adding scar and biomechanical derangement to the anatomy, and in the eyes of jurors documents the fact that "something must really have been seriously wrong." This situation leads to higher compensation for an operated patient than for a nonoperated patient, and disability ratings generally increase up to a limit with subsequent surgery. While an additional, previously missed pathologic condition is occasionally found in the rehabilitation process, socioeconomic causes are usually at the root of a patient's seeking additional surgical treatment following rehabilitation. These patients generally have rather typical personality profiles and patterns of behavior during a rehabilitation program, and tend to remain relatively unconcerned about surgical risks. It is interesting to note that a 2-year follow-up study of a "treatment dropout" group demonstrated a *50%* rate of surgery performed post-dropout. *None* of the operated patients returned to productive employment following surgery, in spite of the fact that they entered into the procedure putatively believing that the operation would "cure them" (Mayer, Gatchel, Mayer, Kishino, Keeley, Mooney, 1987).

2. *Private Disability Policies.* Patients may have supplementation of income or payments for specific possessions based on documented disabilities. Long-or short-term wage supplementation policies, or home/automobile disability payments, are typical. These protect the patient from substantial financial loss during times of disability, but when the total value of workmen's compensation and disability payments adds up to as much as or more than the patient previously earned on the job, these payments may cause substantial work disincentive.

3. *Lifestyle Adjustments.* The patient may, over a long period of time, have become habituated to disability. The patient's lifestyle may have been adjusted so that he or she can function on minimal income. Patients may actually enjoy the luxury and dependent role of becoming a disabled househusband or housewife, with little accompanying accountability for customary housework performance. Seasonal employment in rural settings may often go undetected, or illicit industries may provide untraceable and unreportable incomes. Such balancing satisfactions may make the patient even more hesitant to give up disability payments, even though those payments may be substantially lower than previous wage income. There may be fears that demonstrated improvement in physical abilities can jeopardize litigation outcome. Such litigation may have become viewed over the disability period as a bonanza of entitlement. This "sweepstakes" mentality is a gamble on which certain patients may place great emphasis.

4. *Job Insecurity.* This refers to the real or imagined fear that the promised job that is "being held for them" will be jerked away when they are returned to work, leaving them without job or compensation. This may

be true to a variable extent in different employment areas depending on employer enlightenment. It is generally strongly reinforced by other returning workers who have been terminated, even if those terminations have sometimes occurred for fully legitimate reasons totally unrelated to the industrial accident.

5. *The "Vacation Mentality."* This refers to the situation in which the patient recognizes that ultimate lump sum payments will be small or nonexistent, but that current compensation levels are quite favorable in relation to previous, taxed wages, and that "riding out" the compensation as long as possible is a reasonable alternative.

These and other "hidden agendas" may complicate the lives of the treatment team unless symptom magnification is recognized for what it is when it occurs: a cry for help through a difficult period in dealing with one of a number of complex issues.

Legal and Employment Issues

Although occupational therapists must be sensitive to legal issues and must clearly understand the compensation laws in their state, excessive involvement in the process breeds resentment. Attorneys are professionals just as are physicians and therapists, and may resent interference in their part of the process by groups they may perceive as inadequately trained interlopers. Thus, the therapist has primarily an educational role in making the patient aware of a variety of issues and alternatives, and informing attorneys of the progress and anticipated outcomes and prognosis of the rehabilitation program. The therapist must clearly avoid the temptation to act as a surrogate attorney or provide legal advice. In performing their educational role, however, therapists may serve as a catalyst for resolving litigation, since in most cases the functional restoration process brings to a close the treatment modalities available through the medical care system. The patient may not be "completely cured," but "maximum medical recovery" has probably been achieved. It is around this decisive determination that the legal system may draw its conclusions leading to case closure. The "external communication" with insurance companies, rehabilitation nurses/counselors, treating physicians and attorneys, as well as with the patient, facilitates this process. Keeping these groups informed about patient progress, when the chronic nature of the disease has allowed their file to "drift to the bottom of the pile," also serves to alert them to a complex problem in need of negotiation and solution. Documentation that these parties find particularly useful includes the patient's effort in physical progression, level of motivation, prognosis, impairment rating, and work limitations, either temporary or permanent.

Considerable effort must be expended in working with the claims representative of the insurance carrier. These harrassed individuals, half of whose caseload may be back-injured patients, have a difficult time sorting out the "legitimately injured" from the "malingering" patients. This labeling is an essential part of their training, and often personal experience. Moreover, they may have a difficult time separating the multitude of acute patients from the few high-cost chronically disabled ones, with concomitant difficulty in assigning priorities. Their skepticism about the effectiveness of spine rehabilitation may also impede communication. Nevertheless, communication is extremely important, both to assist the patient and to educate the claims representative regarding the policies and philosophy of functional restoration. Adjusters must understand that the rehabilitated, working patient is a far greater benefit to his or her company and society in general than the worker who has merely been "bought off" in a financial settlement. While this latter patient may not be able to work again for the previous employer, he or she may be forced to take the necessary steps to work for another employer insured by the same company, and may have a "new injury" a short time later. The therapist must be even-handed in documenting both good and bad information concerning the patient's motivation, compliance, effort, and physical performance to the other representatives of the Disability System. These interactions may also help in facilitating communication, through a rehabilitation nurse, with an employer who may previously have been negative or ambivalent toward accepting the injured worker back on the job.

Finally, major employment issues exist. Employers who would willingly hire a "handicapped worker" with visible stigmata, such as mental deficiency or amputation, will avoid the back-injured patient at all costs. While the Rehabilitation Act of 1973 and other pertinent legislation clearly defines the rights of handicapped citizens, the courts remain ambiguous on the relationship between handicap and back pain. Built-in prejudices, most based on information derived prior to the availability of functional restoration, continue to hinder re-employment prospects of back-injured patients. There is a general reluctance on the part of employers to hire patients with previous back injury because of reported high rates of reinjury. Once the patient has limitations and his or her ability to work is compromised, he or she is far less likely to be rehired because of fear that the morale of other employees will be adversely impacted. Unfortunately, during economic conditions with high unemployment, it is considered better business to "stonewall" such employees if at all possible. Usually, the adversary situation thus created actually ends up increasing the cost to the employer who believes he or she is acting in this way in his or her own self-interest. These costs, though borne by the insurance company, are ultimately passed back to the employer in the form of higher premiums (or administrative costs in the case of self-insured corporations).

While direct employment issues will be treated in greater detail later, it is *not* the goal of a functional restoration program to provide vocational rehabilitation services. In states where they are permitted, such services may be appended to the functional restoration program, or arrangements may be worked out with the state vocational rehabilitation or private rehabilitation agencies to carry this burden. Frequently, extensive services once thought necessary can be avoided, as patients' improved physical capacity allows them to re-enter the work force with confidence in their ability to work in areas in which they already have skills. The occupational therapist formulates a *work plan,* and it is the responsibility of the patient to carry this plan forward.

TREATMENT PROGRAMS

Acute Injury

The occupational therapist has a relatively small role in treatment of the acutely injured patient. This program is generally under the care of the physical therapist and is discussed in Chapter 15.

Sub-acute, Postoperative or Chronic Episodic Management Program

In these programs, physical and occupational therapists generally work together in a "therapy model." Instead of all patients being temporarily medically managed by the program physician, referrals may come from multiple physicians who continue to exert medical control, with the therapist acting under his or her prescription of services. This brief outpatient program is generally suited for a well-motivated group of patients with minimal psychosocial issues, and therefore contact by the occupational therapist with this group is primarily directed toward physical progression issues. These will be discussed in greater detail subsequently. Only when barriers to functional recovery affecting patient behavior become difficult to control will the occupational therapist be called upon to exercise his or her disability management skills. However, a good plan for restoring productivity is always the goal of such outpatient programs.

THE COMPREHENSIVE PROGRAM

Phase I: Pre-program

The involvement of the occupational therapist in pre-program is large, though not as primary a role as held by the physical therapist. Occupational assessment is done at the time of the QFE and initial occupational therapy interview, in which some of the psychosocioeconomic factors important in disability management are identified. Because mobility is usually such an early issue, physical training in the occupational therapist must be limited. In the latter stage of this phase, light bending and lifting activities are taught, but with emphasis on stretching rather than strengthening. Whole-body activities are encouraged, and education in goals of the comprehensive program takes place. The occupational therapist places great effort primarily on establishing trust and rapport, while getting to know the patient through attending to historical details of the patient's perception of his or her physical and occupational disability. Considerable attention is also paid to educating the patient about the expected initial effects of reconditioning. Compliance is carefully monitored, and the occupational therapist may become specifically involved in assisting the patient with those barriers to participation which are identified, such as "child care" or "transportation." When negative behaviors are particularly apparent, the occupational therapist is alert to hidden agendas or as-yet-unidentified financial, legal or employment dilemmas.

Phase II: Intensive Treatment Phase

As the patient enters the 150-contact hour comprehensive program, the occupational therapist assumes equal partnership as a member of the treatment team. The initial occupational therapy assessment consists not only of an admission evaluation, but also a full socioeconomic history.

In observing physical progression, occupational therapy functions very much as did physical therapy in its Phase II operations. Rather than focusing on "the injured part," occupational therapy is involved in specific task performance activities, specifically lifting training and tolerance of a variety of positions and activities such as bending, climbing, or crawling. Since lifting is one of the primary activities in manual handling techniques, a great deal of attention is placed on this activity. It represents the quintessential mechanism of transmitting load from the hands through all of the body's functional units down to a stable foot-floor contact. Even the neck is involved, as the body positions required for lifting involve the cervical spine supporting the head to permit vision, in a variety of postures.

As we discussed earlier, progressive resistive exercise in the form of increasing weights is the basic technique used for training, and can be done in a variety of ways utilizing free weights held on bars or a variety of containers. Activities are divided into those moving from floor to waist and those from waist to above shoulder, since the former involves lower extremities and lower trunk, while the latter involves arms and shoulder girdle primarily. Because patients have different capacities in these different ranges, and the site of injury and cervicothoracic and lumbar spines produces different "weak links" in the functional units, it is convenient to train these independently. Loads must be capable of rapid and easy adjustment according to present capacity and training needs, and a variety of adjustable heights can be used for training. One useful piece of equipment is produced by Work Evaluation Systems Technology, (WEST, Huntington Beach, CA), which permits lifting of specified weights through very specific ranges of motion (Fig. 16–2). By using the patient's job requirements as the ultimate training goal, the patient not only attains adequate functional

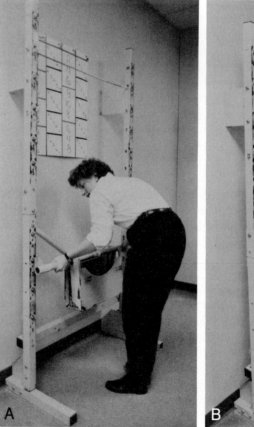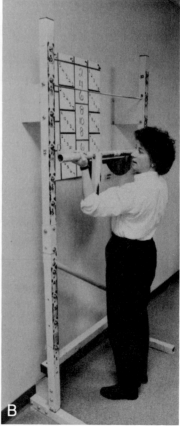

Fig. 16–2. WEST equipment being used in (A) lower ranges and (B) waist-to-above-shoulder range.

capacity specific to age, gender, and body weight, but is gradually desensitized to fears of lifting in the workplace. Furthermore, standardized protocols exist for using frequent lifting tasks as an assessment device, as has been discussed previously. Thus, the performance can be documented frequently, both on ultimate weight lifted and aerobic demand of the task, and compared to the normative database, as well as to the job requirements.

As a training tool, the Liftask device (Cybex, Ronkonkoma, NY) is as useful as it is as a testing device. The isokinetic technique allows training at specific speeds, to attain speed specific goals. Safety is a key factor, as the "accommodating resistance" of these machines is unmatched in any other lifting technique. This factor is probably more significant for testing than training. The isokinetic device removes the "acceleration factor" or impulse inherent in coordinated lifting. It can be used for the frequent, isoinertial lift training methods, and thus focuses entirely on the muscular strength aspects of the lift.

Since there is no anatomic stabilization, the patient can use any lifting style desired, but under certain circumstances specific deficiencies in lift can be identified and the patient trained uniquely in these involved postures. The computer curve analysis is particularly useful for this, since it can identify "pain dips" (small notches in the lifting curve at reproducible heights that are found consistently and identified by curve overlap). These generally occur at the point of engagement of facets as the lumbar spine begins to straighten out once hip extension is almost complete (usually at about 30 to 45 degrees gross flexion). By training through light loads at this level, whatever anatomic aberration appears to be causing this dip can often be "smoothed out," eliminating a potential situation for the back "giving out" in real lifting situations. Just as is done on isokinetic extremity equipment, the therapist can approach the pain notch lifting from below just to the point of the dip, and commencing again just above it until the notch is virtually erased.

While there are disadvantages to isokinetic devices, including inherent speed limitations and inability to "lower" weights, these disadvantages can be overcome with use of other simpler mechanisms such as variable resistance machines and free weights that are more suitable for training in this mode. Curve consistency is used as a measure of effort and persistence in training, and is frequently assessed through the training period. Similarly, endurance protocols to measure the dropoff on repetitive lifting capacity, and the recovery in a set period of time, identify this aspect of strength under the controlled conditions of an isokinetic lift, free of the confounding factors of agility inherent in the impulse or "acceleration factor" (Fig. 16–3).

Other training devices are designed to simulate as well as possible the physical demands the patient will experience after leaving rehabilitation. The obstacle course, described previously, is used for training as well as testing to develop improved task performance capacity. Training in climbing can be developed utilizing the Versa-climber (Heart Rate, Inc., Costa Mesa, CA), which operates on a hydraulic system with an adjustable resistance and pulse monitoring capability. Other devices involving pushing and pulling movements both in standing and overhead reaching positions can be used. Carrying blocks, climbing stairs, bending over bars, and projects involving both standing and sitting postures can be utilized to improve tolerance. Some of these are shown in Figure 16–4.

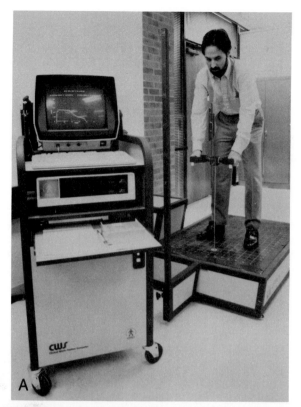

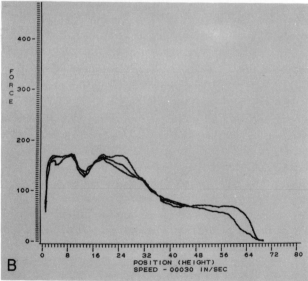

Fig. 16–3.   A, Liftask shown for use in training in a patient working through a "pain notch." B, Graph showing consistent "pain notch" in an otherwise strong individual.

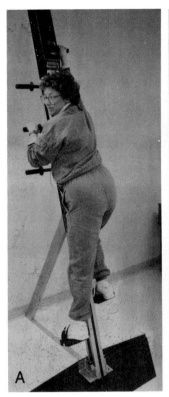 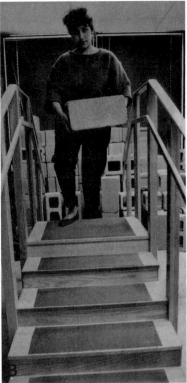

Fig. 16–4. A, The new OT climbing machine. B, Stairs with patient climbing, holding concrete blocks. (*Continued on following page.*)

As in testing on the obstacle course, training is performed utilizing demands of specific numbers of repetitions in set time periods. The patient's training is individualized to those tasks which are most specific to the patient's home and job requirements. For example, individuals functioning as steel workers on high buildings might emphasize such activities as climbing, balancing and carrying, though not to the exclusion of other positional tolerance activities. In this way, fears related to inability to perform specific tasks and activities of daily living can be greatly reduced or eliminated.

As is true in other parts of the program, pain may interrupt the patient's ability to perform these tasks, though the therapist needs to be persistent in educating the patient that training develops capacity to perform these physical tasks, just as it does the more general physiologic aspects of mobility and strength. For a variety of reasons related to structural damage, personality, emotional and socioeconomic factors, patients may feel a need to continue to enunciate pain complaints through the process. Most will acknowledge, however, after a period of training, that gradual improvement seems to be occurring, although there are still frequent "bad days." In evaluating the frequency and severity of pain complaints, the therapist must constantly be on the watch for barriers to functional recovery.

It is vital that the occupational therapy staff members understand enough about the treatment technique and rationale of other departments to reinforce

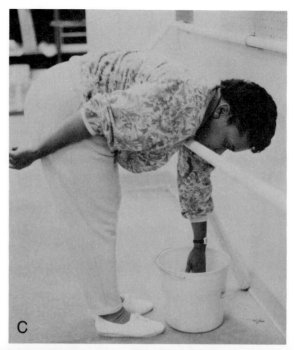

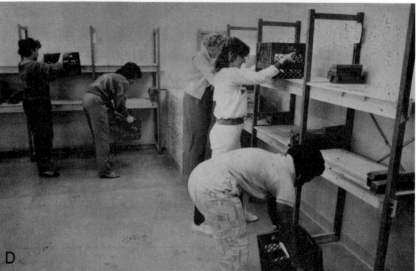

Fig. 16–4 (cont.). C, Bending bar. D, Lifting area.

their approaches with the patient's. While occupational therapists are not expected to perform as psychologists, physical therapists, or nurses, they should be alerted to the behavior and issues that affect the patient's performance in these departments. When the therapist becomes aware of problems relevant to other departments, this must be relayed to them. The customary way in which this is done is at the bi-weekly staffing conference, the major source for internal communication and discussion. However, on an "emergency" basis, the communication should take place directly between the involved parties, or perhaps even in a small conference with the patient.

Conversely, the occupational therapist receives a great deal of input from other departments. In some ways, occupational therapy sits at the fulcrum of the patient's physical and psychosocial functioning, binding physical reconditioning and disability management, as well as the patient's own unique contributions in these areas. Because of this position, the occupational therapist must rely on teamwork in order to avoid becoming overwhelmed with the multiple issues involving each patient. This situation becomes progressively more intense as Phase II reaches its completion, and a variety of employment and compensation issues must be dealt with.

Primarily during the second and third weeks of the comprehensive program, and then extending into the follow-up period, the employment and financial issues gradually assume greater importance to the occupational therapist, and to the staff as a whole. The experience at PRIDE is of particular interest, because the workmen's compensation environment supports the employer's reluctance to rehire a previously back-injured worker. Unions and job-preservation laws are in short supply, and thus the chronically disabled back-injured worker generally faces problems of unemployment compounding his or her re-entry into productivity.

It is noteworthy that, in spite of this environment, such a high percentage of return-to-work can be achieved in such a short time, albeit in many circumstances at lower wages with diminished security. Once back into the work force, however, the patient has an opportunity to "start over" in building a steady work record leading to enhanced future employment prospects. For the back-injured patient, the release to return to work is a fearsome prospect, since it usually correlates with an immediate cessation of weekly compensation benefits. Since he or she has hung on to this "last straw" so intensely for a prolonged period of time, the prospect of attempting to re-enter an alien workplace can be a significant stressor for the patient. It is the occupational therapist's responsibility to ease this transition to the greatest extent possible, through external communication and providing techniques in re-employment skills. Of course, if an old job is available, or if the even more ideal circumstance of temporary "part-time" or "light-duty" work is available in transition to the regular job, every effort is made to smooth any potential barriers between patient and employer. Recognizing the unemployment prospects of the majority of patients in the program, the patient who still has rehiring prospects with his or her old company generally appreciates this luxury and works toward overcoming barriers to the previous job.

When returning to work after having sustained an injury, patients experience an initial period of fear of reinjury and anxiety about ability to perform. These anxieties and fears are compounded by having to learn a new job, to form new work relationships, and to function in an unfamiliar setting. Furthermore, an 8- to 10-hour work day produces demands on a patient's strength, endurance, and agility which can never be completely prepared for in any work simulation and training setting. Just as the ultimate test for the injured athlete is the return to his or her original sport, the ultimate test for the disabled worker is the return to a job. Customarily, this reorientation period lasts anywhere from 2 to 8 weeks, depending on the factors above as well as the job demands. Warning the patient about this transition period, and assisting the process with supportive counseling, can greatly facilitate the process.

Dealing with employment issues and the patient's reaction to them is one of the most crucial and potentially volatile aspects of the occupational therapist's role. These issues go far beyond simply finding a job or returning to work. Longstanding employment dissatisfaction, self-esteem issues, and fears regarding interpersonal relations converge in the realm of employment. The atmosphere often becomes emotionally charged, particularly as compensation and financial issues are wrapped in the return-to-work problem, requiring a great deal of patient wisdom and skill on the part of the therapist.

Work issues are frequently motivating a variety of hidden agendas and other barriers to recovery to which the therapist must be alerted. As patients tend to focus on the recent conflicts they have been experiencing relative to the workplace, it is often fruitful to focus on the wider role of work. Work fills many needs and represents many things besides earning a living. For most people, work carries a certain amount of status, is a place to belong, a place to feel productive, and an important social network outside of the family. It is a place to experience feelings of self-esteem over a job well done, and a place to establish a self-image as a worker and producer. Most people lose sight of these important aspects of the workplace because of the recent conflicts they have been experiencing, but usually recognize some sense of loss regarding this part of their lives as the length of disability increases. Exceptions to this might occur in individuals who have never really established a firm work relationship, and this should be sought in the patient's history. The "habitual housewife," who has had only a few short-term or part-time jobs, or the individual probably involved in illicit industries who hides true sources of income, are examples of this group. It is generally useless to attempt to "reform" these individuals, who will be "failures" of treatment in one sense. However, disability management calls for an end to compensation issues and a return to some level of productivity within a societal framework, and thus partial success can generally be achieved.

Regardless of return to a new or old job, each patient must be re-established as a capable and functional worker. Interactions in this area must be handled sensitively, with a great deal of individual counseling, and often with the assistance of the involved psychologist as the intensity increases toward the end of Phase II. Quantification of function can be of special help during this time, since the therapist can use the patient's physical progression and performance to demonstrate that the patient will, in fact, be able to perform on the job in the future, thus allaying many of the realistic fears the patients bring to the process. This is also why using the patient's job demands to guide physical goals is so important. Similarly, external communication with employers, physicians, and attorneys can give the patient confidence that all members of his "disability/functional team" are working together to assist the return to productivity. Employers, initially dubious of the back-injured worker's motivation, and ambivalent about having them back even after long-term employment, may be amenable to education by occupational therapy.

When the treatment program and the rationale of the PRIDE system are explained, the employer may feel that these patients are no longer unacceptable risks. Even if the employer decides not to allow the patient to return to the job, this decisive information can then allow the therapist to prepare the patient for the arduous tasks of re-employment in setting other realistic job plans. In other words, re-employment issues are not "allowed to drift." As discussed previously, different compensation systems have different problems associated with them. However, they break down into two major groups: (1) workmen's compensation (whether Federal, state or specialized) in which medical care is linked to employment, and (2) personal injury/long-term disability systems in which no such linkage is present. In actuality, the second system is harder to work with, as the third-party carrier responsible for medical treatment is generally unconcerned about disability/employment issues. Because of this, their interest in funding rehabilitation is small. We have been surprised to note that, in some cases where different departments of the same large insurance carrier provide both the medical and the long-term disability coverage for a certain worker, they are unwilling to work together toward the goal of return to productivity. Another factor in this paradox is that the employer is generally unaware of this entire process, and therefore exerts no leverage on the insurance carriers.

In the situation where the previous job is unavailable, or where the patient's physical capabilities can simply not be raised to a level consistent with performing the previous task (due to age or degree of structural damage), alternate employment must be found. In facilitating re-employment, the therapist helps with a job return plan and supports the patient through this discouraging search. Strategies for overcoming employers' fear of hiring the previously injured worker are supplied. The therapist may additionally deal with prospective employers in a manner similar to when the previous job is available. Referrals are often made to state employment and rehabilitaiton agencies, to a "job club," or to rehabilitation nurses/counselors specializing in vocational assistance.

At the conclusion of Phase II, discharge QFE numbers are obtained. A solid job plan, return to work time, and potential impairment ratings are identified for the discharge report. A follow-up plan is set, and the patient embarks on the next phase.

Phase III: Follow-up Phase

In this phase, occupational therapy is the dominant department, as the length and frequency of follow-up are determined almost entirely by the remaining socioeconomic issues. The 3-week comprehensive program is usually sufficient to train patients with strictly physical problems to progress adequately in a home or fitness center program. However, the interrelated issues of job availability, previous training and skills, and anticipated job demands requiring higher levels of physical capacity are the follow-up determinants. For example, patients with a previous job to return to, and an employer who will permit a "light duty" transition to a previous job that is at or below the medium-heavy job demand level (see Tables 16–1 and 16–2), will often be able to return to work within a 1 to 2-week follow-up or an immediate return to work with a brief outpatient follow-up after work. Conversely, the unemployed patient, postsurgical with low skills and deficient functional capacity, may require a full 6 weeks of follow-up. Periods longer than this are usually counterproductive, as no follow-up program can assure compliance with necessary levels of physical activity as well as the actual return to the demands of the workplace. This is the "return to the sport" toward which all other activities are geared.

Bizarre behaviors, inconsistent with the patient's performance within the program, are sometimes observed during this time. Quietly compliant patients may "disappear" or display an astounding variety of excuses for terminating program participation at this juncture. In the chronically disabled back pain patient, however, they are all smoke screens.

The lack of firm, gentle guidance by the occupational therapist at this juncture, or absence of the active support of the program physician and other departments, may well result in the failure of this patient to carry through with discharge plans. Because the contact hours with patients drop off dramatically during this period, the therapists are forced to rely more heavily on the program physician for education and support. Physician visits every 2 to 3 weeks until the end of Phase III are usually necessary, and it is incumbent upon the occupational therapist to keep the physician well-informed about ongoing issues prior to scheduled patient visits.

While the program physician intends an early return to the orginal referring physician, it is important that he or she keep control of the case until the work return has been facilitated. It is at this point in the program that patients may

Table 16–1. Job Demand Categories Used by Rehabilitation Institute of Southern California (Matheson, 1986)

Level	Weight Lifted	Frequency of Lift	Walking/ Carrying	Typical Energy Required
Sedentary	10 lbs or less	Infrequently	None	1.5 mets
Sedentary-light	15 lbs	Infrequently	Intermittent self-paced	2.0 mets
	10 lbs or less	Frequently	No load	
Light*	20 lbs	Infrequently	2.5 mph no grade or	2.5 mets
	10 lbs or less	Frequently	Slower speed with 10 lbs or less	
Light-medium	35 lbs	Infrequently	3.0 mph no grade or	3.0 mets
	20 lbs or less	Frequently	Slower speed with 20 lbs or less	
Medium	50 lbs	Infrequently	3.5 mph no grade or	3.5 mets
	25 lbs or less	Frequently	Slower speed with 25 lbs or less	
Medium-heavy	75 lbs	Infrequently	3.5 mph no grade with 35 lbs load or	4.5 mets
	35 lbs or less	Frequently	115 lbs wheelbarrow 2.5 mph no grade	
Heavy	100 lbs	Infrequently	3.5 mph with	6.0 mets
	50 lbs or less	Frequently	50 lbs or less load	
Very heavy	In excess of 100 lbs	Infrequently	3.5 mph with	7.5–12.0 mets
	50 lbs to 100 lbs	Frequently	50 lbs or more load	

*Even though the weight lifted may be negligible, a job is considered "light" if it requires a significant amount of walking or standing or frequent use of arm and/or leg controls.

Table 16–2. Simplified Job Demand Categories Used at PRIDE

Classification*	Lifting Required	Duration of Vibration
Sedentary to light	0 to 10 lb frequently, or 10 to 20 lb occasionally	No vibration
Light to medium	10 to 25 lb frequently, or 26 to 50 lb occasionally	Up to 2 hours of vibration
Medium to heavy	25 to 50 lb frequently, or 51 to 100 lb occasionally	More than 2 hours of vibration combined with only sedentary to medium lifting
Very heavy	More than 50 lb frequently or more than 100 lb occasionally	More than 2 hours of vibration combined with medium to very heavy lifting

*Classify your patient's occupation by these levels if its physical demands include *either* the degree of lifting *or* vibration shown.

"doctor-shop" with the new symptoms, and the unwary outside surgeon may be misled into performing unnecessary additional diagnostic tests and even inappropriate surgical procedures. It is unfortunate that one of the inevitable outgrowths of a system designed to protect the injured worker is a situation in which a patient can be stimulated to manipulate others into performing procedures of potential bodily harm because of a misguided perception that this will provide greater short-term financial gain. However lamentable the scenario may appear, it is played over and over again on a daily basis as a by-product of the present workmen's compensation system. This situation can be expected to continue indefinitely until there is recognition, by the medical and legal establishment, codified into law, that increased financial rewards for patients to have surgical treatment will result in increased medical cost of unnecessary procedures.

The follow-up days end with the first post-program QFE. This initial opportunity for patients to demonstrate how well they have maintained or increased the physical capacity gains achieved during the comprehensive program should be carefully monitored and explained to the patient by the therapist and program physician. Significant decreases in physical capacity over this period are always a negative marker for potential future difficulties. Such patients should be given immediate attention with reinforcement and reinstruction in their home maintenance program. It is also essential that contacts be facilitated to ensure that promised home exercise equipment or prescriptions for unsupervised conditioning have been implemented.

The critical occupational therapy duty during this final phase is to be certain that the discharge employment plan is progressing smoothly. In many cases, changes in plans are necessitated by changes in direction on the part of the patient. Hidden agendas may rise to the surface, or employers may waver on previous commitments. As one plan decreases in feasibility, another must rise to assume priority. Though vocational retraining and/or education is a less desirable goal as it leaves the patient in a dependent "student role," such may be the only alternative available. Part-time employment may be necessary in conjunction with training or school. Additional assistance is usually required in these cases to maintain living standards during the retraining.

Finally, in rare cases, a patient may be too old, unskilled, or severely damaged by multiple operations or cognitive deficits to resume competitive employment. Given sufficient motivation, a wide variety of "home industries" are available, which can supply limited incomes that will decrease the burden to insurers or government for subsidizing this individual. We have constantly been amazed at the ingenuity of many of these patients in finding self-employment opportunity once conventional employment is recognized to be too difficult to attain. We must constantly reemphasize, however, that such compromises are rarely necessary. The patient may not be able to select his or her most desirable job initially, but is usually able to work up to a high level of employer confidence with renewed optimum levels of job performance.

Phase IV: Outcome Tracking Phase

Occupational therapy is likewise primarily responsible for the tracking phase of the program. Telephone contact is maintained with the patient at regular intervals, culminating in a twice-monthly follow-up conference led by occupational therapy. At this conference, the work, medical, and legal status of patients is discussed for at least 6 months, focusing primarily on "problem patients." During this period, the patient is expected to return for repeat QFEs on at least two occasions, at 3 and 6 months after Phase II. At this time, occupational therapy performs an extensive re-evaluation of socioeconomic outcomes and attitudes. These data do not merely provide information for quality assurance, but also provide valuable research material for publications and program modification. It is astounding how little medical attention has been paid to this area of major economic and social cost. The need for hard information in the area of disability management will continue to be in great demand for many years to come (Fig. 16–5).

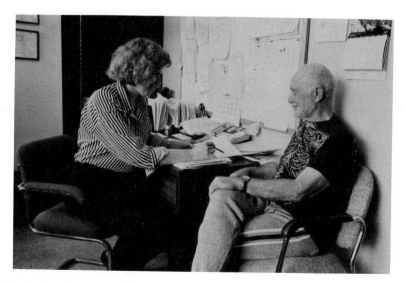

Fig. 16–5. Six-month occupational therapy interview with successful program completer reviewing final QFE.

CHAPTER REFERENCES

Bing R: Occupational therapy revisited: a paraphrastic journey. Am J Occup Ther *35*:499–518, 1981.

Chaffin D, Andersson G, *Occupational Biomechanics,* New York, John Wiley & Son, 1984.

Dzioba R, Benjamin J: Spontaneous atlantoaxial fusion in psoriatic arthritis: a case report. Spine *10*:102–103, 1985.

Harvey-Krefting L: The concept of work in occupational therapy: a historical review. Am J Occup Ther *39*:301–307, 1985.

Hopkins H: An Historical Perspective on Occupational Therapy. In *Willard and Spackman's Occupational Therapy,* 6th Ed, H Hopkins, H Smith, Editors. Philadelphia, J.B. Lippincott Co., 1983.

Kishino N, Mayer T, Gatchel R, Parrish M, Anderson C, Gustin L, Mooney V: Quantification of lumbar function Part 4: isometric and isokinetic lifting simulation in normal subjects and low-back dysfunction patients. Spine *10*:921–927, 1985.

Kroemer K: An isoinertial technique to assess individual lifting capability. Human Factors *25*:493–506, 1983.

Matheson L: Work Capacity Evaluation: Systematic Approach to Industrial Rehabilitation, Anaheim, CA, ERIC Publishing, 1986, pp. IV–6.

Mayer, TG, Gatchel RJ, Mayer H, Kishino N, Keeley J, Mooney V: A prospective two-year-study of functional restoration in industrial low back injury. JAMA *258*:1763–1767, 1987.

Pope M, Frymoyer J, Andersson G: *Occupational Low Back Pain.* New York, Praeger Press, 1984.

Rockey P, Fantel J, Omenn G: Discriminatory aspects of pre-employment screening: low-back x-ray examinations in the railroad industry. Amer J Law and Med *5*:197–214, 1979.

Snook S, Campanelli R, Hart J: A study of three preventive approaches to low-back injury. J Occup Med *20*:478–481, 1978.

Chapter 17

The Multimodal Disability Management Program

We have labeled the psychologic approach developed and refined at PRIDE as the *Multimodal Disability Management Program* (MDMP). It is based upon a cognitive-behavioral approach to crisis intervention, and focuses on overcoming physical and psychosocial difficulties that interfere with returning to a productive, functional lifestyle. Treatment issues deal with events in the present or the recent past, and patients are helped in understanding how thoughts contribute to feelings and behaviors. Within this framework, therapists also maintain an awareness of early learning experiences and longstanding psychologic issues that can affect reactions to recent life experiences. For example, many patients come from family backgrounds where there was some significant emotional deprivation. As a result, many experience chronic feelings of anger, depression, and low self-esteem. Relatedly, they also have a sense of entitlement stemming from a frustrated search for an idealized caretaker. These issues, along with the cognitions and emotions accompanying them, are rekindled quickly when the patients find themselves involved in a medical/compensation/disability system that fosters dependency.

It should be noted that this MDMP approach differs from many typical "pain clinics," of which there are now estimated to be some 2000 in the United States with a wide variety of treatment approaches. The early proliferation of pain clinics was stimulated primarily by a philosophy of focusing on "quality of life outcome criteria," rather than those having socioeconomic impact (Fordyce, Roberts, Sternbach, 1985). However, not only did such clinics proliferate in a nonstandardized manner, but when the rare scrutiny of treatment effectiveness has taken place, results sometimes no better than placebo results have often been observed (Fordyce, Roberts, Sternbach, 1985). Indeed, as Fordyce and colleagues (1985) indicate, the tendency of pain clinics to merely treat the experience of pain, and not the *disability* associated with pain behavior, has often led to unsuccessful treatment. Such overly narrow approaches were also frequently accompanied by the lack of recognition of physical capacity deficits such as the deconditioning syndrome, as well as the lack of technology to measure it. This lack of effectiveness has led to a general perception, particularly among third-party carriers, that rehabilitation for chronic back pain may be ineffective and, in fact, may be no better than placebo in attaining specific societal goals such as return to work (Mayer, Gatchel, Kishino, Keeley, Mayer, Capra, Mooney, 1986). The MDMP approach is an alternative to many of these

unsuccessful pain clinics, with the major focus being on the disability associated with the pain behavior, and not merely the experience of pain.

In this chapter, we will begin by reviewing the basic components of MDMP.
There are four major areas: (1) Individual and group counseling emphasizing
a crisis-intervention model (e.g., coping with family problems, unemployment).
Group counseling is conducted on a daily basis; the amount of individual
counseling is dependent on the particular needs of the patient. (2) Family
counseling, which is conducted on a weekly basis. During these sessions, family
members are encouraged to take an active part in the rehabilitation process
and are provided with information about the philosophy and specific details
of MDMP. (3) Behavioral stress management training that involves initial training in muscle relaxation, followed by exercises in guided imagery in which
patients practice relaxing while imagining themselves in various stressful situations. They also receive daily EMG/temperature biofeedback sessions during
which they refine their relaxation skills, with the understanding that these
skills will help them cope more effectively with residual pain and discomfort.
(4) Cognitive-behavioral skills training that includes instruction in assertiveness, rational versus irrational thinking, and the management of stress and
time.

INDIVIDUAL AND GROUP COUNSELING

Using a cognitive-behavioral approach to crisis intervention, treatment issues
deal with events in the present or recent past. They focus specifically on overcoming physical and psychosocial *barriers to recovery* that interfere with returning to a productive, functional lifestyle (we discussed the concept of *barriers to recovery* in Chapter 13). Within this framework, therapists also maintain
an awareness of early learning experiences and longstanding psychologic issues
that can significantly affect reactions to recent life experiences.

Because the primary goal of functional restoration is to return patients to
their previous productive lifestyle as quickly as possible, long-term, charac-
terologically oriented psychotherapies are inappropriate. A short-term cognitive behavioral approach has proved to be quite effective in helping patients
understand how thoughts contribute to feelings and actions and alter maladaptive thought patterns. Other psychologic issues are dealt with in terms of
their impact on present life circumstances, completing the program with the
most progress, and returning to a healthy lifestyle.

As was noted in Chapter 13, because patients often possess misconceptions
regarding psychology and have incorrectly been told "the pain is in your head,"
it is imperative that they be properly educated about the role of psychologic
services in the functional restoration approach. It is acknowledged that patients
were injured and have legitimate physical problems. Nonetheless, as with any
ongoing chronic medical condition, spinal injuries cause unforeseen changes
in lifestyle that most people find stressful. These stressors and the reactions
to them often lead to increased pain and can actually interfere with physical
recovery. It is helpful to explain this process to the patient in terms of a cycle
wherein the injury and the changes it brings lead to stress, which leads to
increased pain, which leads to increased stress, etc. An important role, then,
is to assist patients in dealing with stress-related issues while they are working
on physical rehabilitation. When psychologic services are presented in this

manner, most patients are relieved, and consequently more open to the availability of psychologic intervention.

There are also a number of other important psychosocial issues that need to be addressed. These are discussed below.

Resistance

Even when psychologic services are presented in the framework just reviewed, many of the patients in this population tend to be resistant to psychologic interventions. There are several reasons for this. Sociologically, most of these patients come from physically oriented, "blue-collar" backgrounds. Their approach to stressors and problem-solving tends to be action-oriented, rather than verbal and reflective. Moreover, chronic pain patients tend to use denial, projection, and somatization as primary defense mechanisms (these terms were discussed in Chapter 13). When presented with the availability of psychologic services, and confronted with the assumption that they are experiencing psychologic distress, many patients will claim that nothing is wrong psychologically. They will protest that "I'm here for my back and not for my head." Furthermore, a few of these patients may actually be in treatment more to avoid the repercussions of refusing rehabilitation services than to actively seek to improve their physical or psychosocial situation. On the other hand, many patients are keenly aware of their psychologic distress, are relieved to hear that this distress is a natural part of a chronic illness pattern, and appreciate services to deal with these issues.

A great deal of resistance to psychologic intervention can be avoided through thorough initial education about the purposes of psychology in the rehabilitation process. As in any counseling situation, the psychologist's skill in dealing with resistant patients is important. Because these patients have not sought out psychologic treatment specifically, some negotiation may need to take place to determine how the counseling sessions will be used. Often, the psychologist will deal with educational issues until the patient realizes he or she will not be forced to divulge any painful personal experiences and becomes more comfortable with therapy.

Support Issues

Supporting the patient throughout the rehabilitation process is another major function of psychology. The psychologist can help the patient in the overall rehabilitation process by assisting him or her in developing, clarifying, and attaining both long-term and short-term goals. The psychologist helps the patient make a commitment to the program, and maintain this commitment during times of frustration and difficulty. This includes motivating the patient to give 100% effort to all aspects of the program, regardless of the apparent worth or lack of short-term benefits.

Indeed, supporting the patients in their physical efforts often occupies the major portion of each session, particularly in the initial phase when pain is increasing, or in the latter phases when progress seems slow. The therapist must acknowledge the reality of the patient's pain and the frustration that accompanies increasing pain as he or she pushes ahead physically. Reinforcing the patient's functional gains, in spite of continued or increased pain, makes tolerating the pain easier for many patients. Besides supporting the patient's conditioning efforts, the psychologist also supports the patient in using new "tools" for dealing with pain (e.g., emphasizing the use of stretching and ice, as well as the biofeedback and relaxation skills the patient is learning in the program).

Frustration Regarding the Pace of Progress

Because of their present pain and functional limitations, most patients want to be fully recovered and pain-free as quickly as possible. This almost always leads to unrealistic expectations about the time involved in a functional restoration program. Part of the psychologist's responsibility is to educate the patient regarding a realistic time frame for rehabilitation. The psychologist must assist the patient in focusing on long-term gains, emphasizing that reduction in pain can come about only after function is restored and strength returns to above-normal levels. Short-term increases in pain and/or failure to quickly experience decreased pain levels will lead to discouragement unless the patient understands this time-frame and the relationship of pain to function.

"Smoke Screens"

In being supportive, however, the psychologist must not allow the patient to get caught up in complaints. Although the psychologist must be alert to legitimate complaints about the patient's physical condition, interaction with staff members, or treatment planning in general, he or she must be aware that these issues are often used as "smoke screens" to hide important psychosocial issues. The psychologist must be aware of these psychologic barriers to recovery, and clearly communicate about the issues behind the "smoke screens" to all other departments.

Specific Emotional Reactions

In Chapter 13, we discussed the specific emotional reactions that are common among low back pain patients and that will often have to be dealt with. These include depression, anxiety, anger, and entitlement. As was noted earlier, the amount of individual counseling needed to deal with these issues varies depending upon the particular needs of the patient. Group counseling, however, is conducted on a daily basis in order to focus on important issues that are most common across all patients. Table 17–1 presents a list of the common issues that are emphasized in this group counseling.

General Education Regarding Psychologic Issues

Besides educating patients about the nature, purposes, and potential benefits of the Psychology Department, psychologists must also educate them on the effects of stress and emotional changes on their physical functioning. Many patients do not realize that changes in pain, muscle tension, energy level, libido, appetite, sleep patterns, and sexual functioning are related to emotional changes from stress. Patients need to be educated about the effects these changes have on their self-image, self-esteem, and interpersonal relationships. One of the major education tasks is the teaching of new coping skills. This is accomplished in several ways. In individual counseling, the psychologist uses a wide variety of psychotherapeutic and educational techniques to help the patient overcome maladaptive and self-destructive coping mechanisms. Such issues are also dis-

Table 17–1.   Issues Emphasized in Group Counseling

Acknowledging how hard it is to keep up without group support

Encouraging the use of the "buddy system" with new patients

Encouraging questions and "venting" about psychologic testing

Issues of confidentiality

Discussion of the need to be responsible for own pace

Work ethic

Concerns about returning to work

Fear of pain as punishment

Responsibility regarding medication use

Depression as a part of chronic pain

Reactions to treatment staff and reinforcement for honest and direct feedback

cussed in group counseling sessions. In addition, the training in behavioral stress management and cognitive-behavioral skills aids in this process.

General Education and Support of Other Departments

Because of his or her supportive role throughout the patient's rehabilitation, the psychologist must be able to reiterate and reinforce the treatment techniques and rationale of the other departments. It is imperative that the psychologist be well versed in the "sports medicine" approach, the deconditioning syndrome, scar tissue theory, and other aspects of the program to be able to answer questions and educate the patients. The psychologist also educates the patient on making a commitment, formulating goals, developing realistic expectations about the timetable for recovery, and using new pain control techniques. Explaining the overall progression through the phases of treatment, and preparing the patient for upcoming transitions between phases of treatment, are other important education topics. Because the psychologist works closely with the medical staff to monitor the patient's medication compliance and effectiveness, he or she must also be able to explain the rationale for use of antidepressants, anxiolytics, anti-inflammatories, and the discontinuation of narcotic analgesics and muscle relaxants. While the psychology department members are expected to be able to educate the patient on all aspects of the functional restoration approach, it is important that departmental roles be maintained clearly. Psychology staff members should be supportive of other departments' staff without infringing on their territory, blurring departmental boundaries, becoming competitive with them, or interfering with their treatment plan-timing of interventions.

FAMILY COUNSELING

Besides individual and group counseling, family counseling is also viewed as important and thus provided in the program. Generally, this is done on a weekly group basis for the comprehensive program patients, with their families being invited to participate in the exercises and to tour the facility. They also receive a short presentation on pathophysiology, diagnostics, and surgical procedures, followed by a question and answer session with a program physician.

Table 17–2. Issues Emphasized in Family Counseling

Permission to family members to ignore illness behavior

Suggestions for weekend activities (family exercises, walking in mall, etc.)

Anger of family members that patient "has not pulled his or her share"

Fear of reinjury

Difficulties giving up positive aspects of being disabled (i.e., more time at home with family, etc.)

Discussion of negative impact of chronic pain syndrome on families

Again, the importance of education of patients, as well as family members, is emphasized in the functional restoration approach (Fig. 17–1).

In the psychologic part of the family program, family members receive information about the changes they can expect in their family member, are reassured that the stressors and feelings they have been experiencing are natural, and receive realistic expectations about the increasing function of their injured family member. In general, simply being in the clinic and seeing their family member more active is in itself an extremely important experience.

Topics are generally limited to program-related issues, and how these issues are being helped or hindered by the current marital or family situation. The general issues emphasized in this counseling are presented in Table 17–2.

It should be remembered that many times, because of a patient's chronic disability, family homeostasis becomes significantly disturbed by changes in the patient's personality or behavior. Family members, in turn, begin to change in response to the patient. Indeed, expectations as to how the particular family members should act and feel often change dramatically. Conflicts of expectations arise concerning responsibility, dominance-submission, autonomy, affection, and respect among others. Family counseling focuses on these strains and conflicts created in the family system, and provides support in helping to cope with them more effectively. On occasion, when there is some significant family conflict and pathology, couple therapy and/or family therapy is also offered.

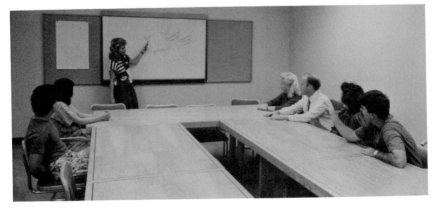

Fig. 17–1. Family counseling session. Involvement of family members in the treatment process is an important component of functional restoration.

BEHAVIORAL STRESS MANAGEMENT TRAINING

In addition to counseling, behavioral stress management training is offered as part of the overall cognitive-behavioral treatment package. This training is designed to increase patients' awareness of stressors, help them recognize the physiologic repercussions of stress reactions, and teach them more effective ways of dealing with these stressors and stress reactions. The rationale for this treatment is explained to the patient using the concept of the pain-stress cycle. Physical and/or mental stress leads to muscle tension, which increases pain, which increases stress. Biofeedback and relaxation training allow the patient to break this cycle, increasing the essence of self-control while decreasing the need for pain medication. Furthermore, these techniques can be used to relieve muscle tension secondary to the physical reconditioning program. Included in this training is initial training in muscle relaxation, followed by exercises in guided imagery in which patients practice relaxing while imagining themselves in various stressful situations. They also achieve daily EMG/temperature biofeedback sessions during which they refine their relaxation skills. Patients are informed that these skills will help them cope more effectively with pain and discomfort.

Indeed, relaxation and biofeedback procedures have been used quite extensively in the treatment of pain (Fig. 17–2). However, when they are used as a *sole* treatment modality, the effectiveness of these procedures has been seriously questioned (Gatchel, Baum, 1983). A major problem with using biofeedback as the sole treatment modality is that one is in effect relying on the erroneous assumption that the etiologic variables and pathophysiology of the pain to be controlled are known and can be voluntarily controlled. It is assumed that biofeedback training will provide subjects with information that will enable them to voluntarily control some aspect of their physiology that purportedly

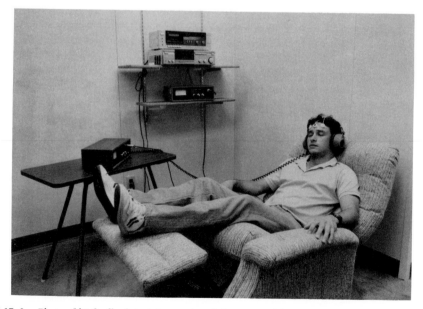

Fig. 17–2. Photo of biofeedback training session. Relaxation and biofeedback procedures are used as adjunctive treatment techniques to help to deal with the anxiety and stress associated with chronic pain.

is causally linked to the pain experience. However, as we have seen, pain is a complex behavior and not merely a pure sensory experience. One cannot expect that dealing solely with some physiologic component of the pain process will totally eliminate the problem behavior. As Gatchel and Baum (1983) have pointed out, it may prove to have as its only active ingredient the ability to reduce anxiety. Since anxiety and pain perception are closely related, relaxation and biofeedback techniques may have an impact on the pain process indirectly through reducing anxiety rather than through any pathophysiology *per se.* At best, then, these procedures should serve merely as adjunctive treatment methods in a more comprehensive therapy regimen. Indeed, this is how they are used in the PRIDE program—as adjunctive treatment modalities.

Table 17–3 lists the various goals of the behavioral stress management training component of the PRIDE treatment program. As can be seen, this component deals with a wide range of stress-related issues.

Cognitive-Behavioral Skills Training

We have also found instruction in a series of educational topics to be extremely helpful in aiding patients to better understand themselves and other factors that can significantly affect their disability. Indeed, as we discussed in Chapter 13, educating the patient as thoroughly as possible about factors involved in his or her disability will greatly aid in improvement. This is in keeping with the philosophy of involving patients in their own treatment and increasing their self-reliance in long-term physical well-being and pain management. In psychology at PRIDE, part of the education process takes place through structured classes that teach some important topics. A series of three classes is administered to all patients: *rational emotive training, assertiveness training* and *selected topics.*

The *rational emotive training* class is patterned after the procedure originally developed by Ellis (1962), who argues that cognitions can produce emotions. He assumes that psychologic problems such as anxiety are caused by faulty or irrational patterns of thinking. Accordingly, he indicates that the focus of treatment should be directed at changing the internal or covert sentences that people say to themselves and that produce negative emotional responses. At PRIDE, the class is designed to teach patients how thoughts affect feelings, and how to change those thoughts when they result in unpleasant or unwanted reactions. Indeed, there has been some experimental support for Ellis' suggestion that irrational beliefs are associated with anxiety (Mears, Gatchel, 1979). By chang-

Table 17–3. Various Goals of the Behavioral Stress Management Component of the PRIDE Treatment Program

Improving the patient's ability to relax physically

Teaching patients to gain better self-control over tense and painful muscles

Improving the patients' ability to relax mentally by gaining control over unwanted thoughts and learning to self-direct thinking

Learning the importance of proper breathing for better relaxation

Addressing individual stress problems and their symptoms

Discussing role of stress and relaxation in symptoms such as sleep difficulties, stiff muscles, bruxism, and emotional distress

ing those irrational thoughts, anxiety can be reduced which, in turn, can have an impact on pain.

The *assertiveness training* class is designed to help improve communication skills and reduce conflict and stress in difficult interpersonal situations. Salter (1949) was the first psychologist to give a great deal of attention to the fact that unassertive behavior often causes anxiety. Many individuals cannot stand up for their rights and greatly regret their inability to do so. This may create a great deal of interpersonal anxiety. Salter developed a method to teach such socially inhibited individuals to express their feelings to others more effectively and assertively. In recent years, numerous investigators have reported the therapeutic effectiveness of assertion training in reducing anxiety and stress in a variety of interpersonal situations (Mears, Gatchel, 1979).

Finally, the *selected topics* class helps patients deal with a number of important issues and situations that they may routinely encounter. These topics include effective time management methods, handling difficult people, recognizing self-defeating behavior, how to have fun in life, and ways of increasing creativity. These topics help patients to better understand and deal with many issues and conflicts they are experiencing or may encounter when they re-enter the workplace.

The information in the above classes is supplemented by one-on-one contact between patient and psychologist during individual and group counseling sessions. The major goal of this educational approach is to impress on the patient that psychologic and emotional factors are invariably involved in the chronic pain syndrome. Figure 17–3 presents a diagram which can be shown to patients to explain this relationship. Physical changes and their effects (such as inability to work, play, financial difficulties, etc.) can lead to emotional changes (such as anger, anxiety, depression, frustration, etc.). These emotional changes, in turn, can lead to increased stress and tension which exacerbates pain. The cycle can also work in the opposite direction, with physical changes and pain leading to increased tension, producing additional stress and irritability, which lead

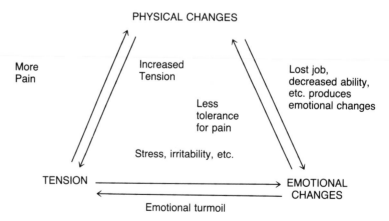

Fig. 17–3. The contribution of physical changes, emotional changes, and tension to the chronic pain process.

to less tolerance for pain. Once the cycle is completed, it can begin at any new point in the cycle and start the whole process again.

Patients are taught that treatment, in order to be effective, must break the cycle at all three sources noted on the diagram. Each source or area is addressed by different aspects of the functional restoration approach: (1) Physical changes and their effects are addressed by medical treatment, medications, physical therapy, and occupational therapy; (2) emotional changes are addressed by psychology and occupational therapy; (3) tension is addressed by the behavioral stress management training.

MAINTAINING THE TREATMENT ENVIRONMENT

Besides involvement in the above four treatment components of MDMP, there is another important role played by the psychologist. Because of the psychologists' training in group processes, and their knowledge of each patient's psychologic characteristics, the majority of the responsibility for maintaining a therapeutic environment also falls to the psychologist. This includes clarifying treatment rationale with the patient, addressing the patient's concerns, correcting misinformation and rumors that frequently circulate within the treatment facility, dealing with disruptive patients, and facilitating communication among the patients.

Part of this therapeutic environment maintenance is accomplished with each patient individually through the counseling and educational interventions already discussed. Additionally, issues impacting the patients as a group are discussed in the daily group support counseling sessions. Patients also attend a similar group one or two times a week during the follow-up phase (Phase III) of the comprehensive program.

It is also essential that frequent and clear communication takes place between each patient's psychologist and all members of the treatment team working with that patient. These meetings may take place informally in groups of two or three, but clear communication about barriers to recovery, disruptive behavior, or non-compliance must also take place in weekly staff meetings so that all staff members can be aware of the issues.

When confrontations are required (particularly regarding disruptive behavior in the treatment facility), responsibility for the confrontation will often fall to the patient's psychologist, since the psychology department is often responsible for dealing with many of the psychosocial and general compliance issues. As in any effective small-group confrontation, the psychologist must clearly express the problem, the reasons for the need to make a change, the expectations, and, when necessary, the consequences of failure to comply.

Functioning as an "Internal Consultant"

The role of "internal consultant" also falls to the psychologists because of their training in consultation and their understanding of transference/counter-transference phenomena. As a "consultant," the psychologist is expected to help other staff members understand each patient's current emotional state, longstanding psychologic issues, preferred coping style, and cognitive functioning. This assists the staff in finding the best way to approach, motivate, and work with each patient. The consultant role is particularly important at times when staff members are having a difficult time working with a patient due to the patient's resistance, or their own countertransference reaction. When staff members better understand the patient and themselves, continued quality of treatment is assured.

Because these patients often exhibit a great deal of anger, they frequently tend to provoke anger in staff members. There is then a strong tendency among treatment staff to revert to viewing these patients as "fakes" and "malingerers" at these times. Helping staff members understand that the patient's current behavior represents a complex interaction of many factors helps to maintain the therapists' respect for the patient. These patients do tend to be somatizers, but only rarely are they truly malingerers.

Psychology staff members also need to make themselves available to other staff for general problem-solving and stress reduction. The rapid pace of program activities, the diverse and difficult patient population, little or no private time for the staff, unpredictability of the daily workload, and the potentially large number of people working in a given area may produce a great deal of opportunity for job-related stress. Besides individual information meetings, psychology staff members occasionally conduct in-service workshops to assist the staff in better understanding and treating the patients, and also in better understanding and dealing with the stressors they face on the job.

THE COMPREHENSIVE PROGRAM

As was done in the previous two chapters, we will now discuss the critical treatment issues that arise during each phase of the overall program.

Phase I: Pre-program

There are a number of education issues that the psychologist is involved in during the pre-program phase. First of all, the basic philosophy of the functional restoration approach is emphasized. Patients are informed that pain may actually increase with increasing activity during the program, but that "pushing through" pain is important and pain does not equal harm. Long-term positive goals such as return to work are also emphasized. The purpose of psychology is presented as helping patients to cope with this temporary discomfort, and to better manage stress and reactions to their disability. Issues concerning proper medication use are also discussed.

During this phase, a counseling consultation is performed in order to initially identify potential barriers to recovery and psychosocial issues including real or imagined losses, fears, anger (at the workplace, insurance company, legal system, medical system, family, and friends), and financial disincentives. The identification of present drug use and/or possible abuse is attempted, as well as the identification of possible medication needs for depression and/or anxiety. Also, if there are signs of significant psychopathology, additional psychologic testing and treatment may be requested.

In terms of general treatment issues, a major goal during this phase is to begin building trust and rapport. In so doing, it is important to defuse possible past negative experiences with the medical treatment system. Potential barriers to recovery are also evaluated, while treatment goals are formulated with the patient. Other important issues dealt with include the following:

    a. Supporting the patient in his or her physical efforts

    b. Maintaining compliance and commitment to the program

   c. Beginning stress management by exploring emotional reactions and build-
      ing new coping skills
   d. Monitoring medication usage and compliance

Table 17–4 presents the advances that the patient is expected to have accomplished by the end of this phase. Failure to accomplish them is considered
cause for concern and needs to be addressed immediately by the treatment
team.

Phase II: Intensive Treatment Phase

During this phase, the comprehensive MDMP reviewed earlier in this chapter
is administered to each patient. The progress of each patient is closely monitored during weekly staff meetings, and appropriate adjustments and recommendations are made whenever patient problems are encountered. As discussed thoroughly in Chapter 13, the comprehensive psychosocial assessment
conducted for each patient helps to guide this treatment process.

Table 17–5 presents the expected patient advances during this phase. Again,
any failure needs to be immediately addressed by the treatment team.

Phase III: Follow-up Phase

Once the patient has completed the comprehensive 3-week program, it is of
great importance to provide continued support in helping the patient move
smoothly from the structured treatment environment to the "real world." Efforts
need to be made to help patients generalize the education and treatment issues
emphasized in the PRIDE setting to the everyday world of work and home. The
patients need to be prepared for return-to-work stressors, with an emphasis on
using the stress management and cognitive-behavioral skills learned during the
comprehensive program.

When patients return for their 6-week evaluation, a brief assessment package
emphasizing self-reported pain and depression is routinely administered to
patients. This helps to monitor changes produced by the treatment program,
and "flags" those patients who are continuing to experience significant negative
emotional reactions to pain.

During this period, as a return-to-work date may approach, a number of
emotional reactions such as fear and anxiety may well increase. They will have
to be dealt with by simple support and by re-emphasizing use of learned coping
skills. It is also important to acknowledge the difficulty of maintaining the
discipline of a home program without the encouragement of the group they
had grown accustomed to at PRIDE. Relatedly, often one must address the
patient's frustration that he or she is not totally pain-free after the 3-week

Table 17–4. Phase I—Pre-program

The patient understands functional restoration philosophy, rationale, and workings of
   PRIDE system

The patient is compliant in attendance

The patient is beginning to trust psychology and look at emotional issues

Medication issues have been addressed—patient tapered off all narcotics and tranquilizers. Antidepressants and anti-inflammatories are stabilized

Table 17–5.   Phase II: Intensive Treatment Program Participation

First Week

Patient understands the day-to-day workings of the program and how to utilize psychology services

Patient is able to separate pain from function

Patient has settled in socially, is comfortable with staff and other patients

Patient is off all narcotics, tranquilizers/muscle relaxants

Medication/sleep problems under control

Patient is focusing on important emotional issues, and family issues—not continual complaints and smoke screens

Patient's physical progression in PT/OT is acceptable

Begin uncovering critical psychosocial issues if not already identified

Second Week

Patient understands return-to-productivity goals and has a plan (Consult with patient's OT therapist regarding this issue)

Patient is dealing with substantive emotional issues, psychologic barriers to recovery

Depression and anxiety decreasing

Patient continues to progress adequately in PT/OT

Patient has received testing feedback, if requested

Third Week

Patient has same return-to-productivity plan as second week and is comfortable with this

Patient's depression or anxiety continues to decrease or is remitted

Patient is preparing for separation from intensive program

Patient continues to deal with substantive emotional issues

Patient is able to begin generalizing what he or she has learned from the program to home/work

Patient's physical progression continues to be acceptable in PT/OT

---

program. Patients must be urged to continue their commitment to the principles of the program, with the emphasis that freedom from pain is a long-term goal.

There are also a number of other issues that are important to continue to monitor during this phase:

a. Continue to support physical conditioning efforts and the learned pain management efforts
b. Reinforce continued commitment and compliance to the principles of the program
c. Continue supporting the patient in obtaining goals
d. Monitor medication usage

Table 17–6 lists those advances expected of all patients at the end of this phase.

Phase IV: Outcome Tracking Phase

This is an important phase for the evaluation of the long-term effectiveness of the program. At PRIDE, we have conducted 1-year and 2-year follow-up

Table 17–6. Phase III—Follow-up

Patient is compliant in attendance, plan, and home program

Patient continues to deal with psychologic issues especially as they affect return to work

Patient is using new skills learned in program in daily life

Patient should be more positive, confident, ready to return to work

Any family issues identified earlier have been addressed

Patient's physical progression in PT/OT continues to be acceptable

Table 17–7. Phase IV—Long-Term Tracking

Patient makes good adjustment to work

Patient continues to use new learning and continue new habits away from PRIDE

Patient is off all psychoactive medication by 6 months

evaluations, in order to document treatment effectivensss and supply much-needed information on long-term outcomes in chronically disabled low back pain patients (Mayer, Gatchel, Mayer, Kishino, Keeley, Mooney, 1987). We have explored outcomes in terms of some realistic outcome criteria such as return to work, surgical treatment, and amount of use of health care professionals. In addition, the self-report psychologic measures are assessed in order to document change in these parameters, and ultimately discover "profiles" of successful or "determinedly disabled" individuals.

In terms of specific treatment issues, efforts need to be continued to be certain that patients are using the appropriate stress management and cognitive-behavioral skills. Checking for relapse is important, with the possibility that a "booster session" or return visit may be necessary for some patients. For some patients, an appropriate referral for ongoing psychotherapy may also be necessary.

Finally, it is also important to check on medication use and compliance on at least a monthly basis up to 6-months during this period. When appropriate, medication levels should be tapered off as lifestyle stressors begin to stabilize. If medication use is still indicated at 6 months, then the patient will need to be referred to a physician for long-term medication maintenance.

Table 17–7 presents those advances that each patient is expected to accomplish by the end of this phase.

CHAPTER REFERENCES

Ellis A: Reason and Emotion in Psychotherapy. New York, Lyle Stuart, 1962.

Fordyce W, Roberts A, Sternbach R: The behavioral management of chronic pain: a response to critics. Pain, *22*:113–125, 1985.

Gatchel RJ, Baum A: An Introduction to Health Psychology, New York, Random House, 1983.

Mayer T, Gatchel RJ, Kishino N, Keeley J, Mayer H, Capra P, Mooney V: A prospective short-term study of chronic low back pain patients utilizing novel objective functional measurement. Pain, *25*:53–68, 1986.

Mayer TG, Gatchel RJ, Mayer H, Kishino N, Keeley J, Mooney V: A prospective two-year study of functional restoration in industrial low back injury. JAMA *258*:1763–1767, 1987.

Mears F, Gatchel RJ: Fundamentals of Abnormal Psychology. Chicago, Rand McNally, 1979.

Salter, A: Conditioned Reflex Therapy. New York, Farrar, Straus, 1949.

Part IV

Long-Term Psychosocioeconomic Implications

Chapter 18

Maintaining Treatment Gains and Productivity

As we have noted throughout this text, chronic low back pain precipitated by work-related causes has traditionally been resistant to both surgical and nonsurgical treatment. These back injuries with resultant disability subsequently become associated with high-cost socioeconomic changes which ultimately impact on consumers, business, and government. While disability itself is generally considered a medical term, its roots are actually embedded in a complex compensation system, creating an array of incentives to management, physicians, attorneys and unions in dealing with it. This often produces some powerful direct financial *disincentives* to the worker to resume competitive employment once again. Together with the superimposed deconditioning syndrome and attendant psychosocioeconomic factors produced by the injury itself, spontaneous return to productivity without high risk of recurrence becomes unlikely. Indeed, the four-times higher incidence of back injury in workers reporting previous back injury testifies to cumulative deficits in physical capacity and work attitudes affecting these individuals.

The functional restoration treatment approach can positively impact on this "disability" system, producing an extremely high return-to-work rate among patients undergoing it (Mayer, Gatchel, Kishino, Keeley, Capra, Mayer, Barnett, Mooney, 1985; Mayer, Gatchel, Mayer, Kishino, Keeley, Mooney, 1987). In reviewing this study by Mayer and colleagues in Chapter 1, we pointed out that, instead of relying solely on measures such as self-reported pain level, medication usage, etc., more realistic outcome measures such as return-to-work should be sought. This is especially important when we are dealing with a problem of major social and economic significance like low back pain. As a consequence, we have focused on outcome measures such as return to work, litigation and additional medical care. This provides information not only on whether the disability has been adequately dealt with, but also the degree to which an individual has become an active, productive member of society once again.

Relatedly, the issue of recurrent injury, which is another important potential outcome measure, has been a traditional fear of industry, prejudicing the injured worker's chances of returning to work for the same employer. As we have previously noted, the improvement in physical functional capacity should also have an effect on recurrence rates. If, as has been suggested, high levels of physical functional capacity correlate with lower risk of reinjury, then many of industry's problems with the returning worker will be resolved, and the prejudices currently noted will slowly disappear. A treatment approach that educates the individual patient to the negative consequences of back disability as a coping mechanism may help the patient deal with more than the physical causes of disability. A recent study by Mayer, Gatchel, Mayer, Kishino, Keeley, and Mooney (1987) has begun to address this reinjury concern, bringing current beliefs into serious question. In this study, it was found that reinjury rates for a non-treatment comparison group was two to three times higher than that of a functional restoration treatment group. Moreover, a 6% reinjury rate found for the functional restoration treatment group over a 2-year evaluation period (or an average of 3% per year) was actually *less* than one would anticipate in the general working population. Since the patients treated in this study were heavily slanted toward a blue-collar, heavy work, previously operated, and chronically disabled population displaying "illness behavior," this result is even more impressive. Clearly, the functional restoration treatment group responded positively to the restoration of increased levels of physical capacity and self-confidence. These positive changes are therefore obviously capable of reversing the anticipated negative statistical consequences of previous back injury. While the replication of these results by other investigators is needed, we may, nevertheless, begin to question the foundation of our prejudice regarding the assumed increased susceptibility to recurrence or reinjury in chronic back pain patients.

Another striking finding of this study was that for those small numbers of treatment group patients who subsequently had surgical procedures at some point in time after completing the functional restoration program, a large percentage of them (75%) were nevertheless working at the 2-year evaluation period. This was in marked contrast to the low 10% rate in the no-treatment comparison group. Thus, these treatment patients appeared to have learned and retained the basic principles of the functional restoration program which continued to be applied even if patients had to undergo surgical treatment. This suggests that such a program can have a significant impact on even that small percentage of patients who eventually succumb to surgery as a treatment alternative.

We thus have an effective treatment program for impacting on low back pain disability, which clearly translates into significant socioeconomic gains. In any evaluation of treatment methods, however, one must look not only at ways of producing immediate positive changes but also at ways of *maintaining* these positive gains. All too often, this latter task is overlooked, so that recidivism rates are quite high when long-term evaluations are conducted. For example, behavioral scientists have developed effective methods for producing short-term reductions in smoking behavior and weight gain assessed during the first 6-months after treatment. However, the statistics on the maintenance of these changes at 2 years post treatment have been far less impressive (Gatchel, Baum, 1983). A major reason for these decreasing gains has been the absence of treatment methods to maintain therapy gains. In order to maintain therapeutic gains, a treatment program must include strategies to ensure compliance or adherence to the basic philosophy and follow-up recommendations. In the remainder of this chapter, we will review the methods that can be used in the functional restoration program to increase the probability of long-term maintenance of treatment gains.

THE ISSUE OF CONTINUED TREATMENT COMPLIANCE/ADHERENCE

Perhaps one of the most thoroughly researched aspects of health behavior is compliance—following a physician's advice or prescribed treatment regimen. *Compliance* is the term generally used to refer to adherence or cooperation—doing as the doctor suggests or following advice to adopt certain attitudes concerning health or health-related behaviors. Taking a prescribed medication when one is supposed to, going on a prescribed diet or exercise program—these are all instances of complying with a physician's advice. *Noncompliance* refers to failure to follow advice—the degree to which a patient does not adhere to what he or she was told.

Despite the great amount of research in this area, progress in improving patient attendance and maintenance of doctor's orders has been slow (Gatchel, Baum, 1983). Apparently, reasons for not following these orders are deeply ingrained and resistant to modification. This is obviously problematic since failure to follow a prescribed regimen may cause a serious breakdown or regression in the treatment process. By not following a prescribed treatment regimen, individuals risk subsequent problems or prolongation of current problems.

For the functional restoration approach, compliance with the physical reconditioning component of the program is an important goal. In order to develop methods of increasing this compliance, we have drawn from the growing research literature on compliance/adherence to physical activity. There has been a rather dramatic resurgence in both the professional and lay community in attention to the therapeutic effects of exercise in preventive and rehabilitative health care. The salience of the "wellness" concept in the health-related industries illustrates this movement. It appears that the current trend of health consciousness in our society emphasizes quality-of-life issues and not just absence of disease.

However, despite the potentially significant health benefits of exercise, together with the statistic that approximately 85% of exercise participants report that they "feel better" while exercising (Morgan, 1981), more than 50% of the individuals embarking on an exercise program will discontinue entirely within the first 6 months (Dishman, 1981). In fact, the rate of dropping out of exercise programs follows a negatively accelerating function across time (Carmody, Senner, Malinow, Matarazzo, 1980). This drop-off pattern is similar to recidivism rates characteristic of smoking, drug and alcohol relapses, and in a variety of medical compliance settings requiring commitment to behavior change (Hunt, Bespelac, 1974). These data indicate that a major question facing health-care professionals no longer is solely isolated to the benefits of exercise, but also to the problem of ensuring that exercise programs are adhered to once they are embarked on.

The Relapse-Prevention Model

Recently, a *relapse-prevention model* has been developed by Marlatt and Gordon (1980, 1981) to address the problem of long-term maintenance of new health behaviors. This model was first developed to aid in the treatment of addictive behaviors such as alcoholism and smoking which, as we noted earlier, are associated with high recidivism rates during long-term follow-up. It focuses on aiding the patient to acquire new coping strategies that will reduce the risk of an initial relapse, as well as preventing any relapse from escalating into a total relapse. The major element of this model, and how it differs from conventional treatment strategies, is that the problem of possible lapses and relapses is neither ignored nor attributed to failures of the treatment program or the patient. Rather, such lapses and relapses are viewed as an important part of the learning required for long-term successful habit change.

The potential usefulness of this relapse-prevention model for improving exercise adherence has generated a great deal of interest. Recently, Bélisle, Roskies, Lévesque (1987) systematically evaluated the efficacy of this model in increasing both short- and long-term adherence to an exercise program. The adherence condition they developed using this model included self-management techniques, high-risk situations, the management of temporary lapses, and relapse-prevention strategies. Results of their research clearly indicated the superiority of adherence in the experimental condition employing the relapse-prevention model relative to a control condition.

At PRIDE, we have incorporated this *relapse-prevention model* as a means of increasing compliance/adherence to the various treatment components after patients have completed the intensive 3-week program. As we have noted throughout the text, it is important for patients to continue the physical conditioning/exercise after leaving the intensive program. One of the reasons for including the extensive patient education component of the program is to engender a better understanding of the chronic pain phenomenon, and factors that can increase or decrease the pain experience, as well as the various effects that the physical reconditioning and exercise can have. Also, the behavioral stress-management techniques patients learn provide them with self-management methods to use especially during crises that may prompt temporary lapses or relapses.

Other Techniques to Increase Compliance

There have also been other techniques that have been shown to contribute to increased compliance and that have been incorporated into the functional restoration program. For example, a number of studies have found increases of up to 60% in general medical compliance as a result of increased contact with medical personnel (e.g., Wilbur, Barrow, 1969). One of the reasons for including a follow-up phase in the functional restoration approach, which we discussed in detail in Part III, is to maintain this contact with patients as a means of increasing compliance. Of course, direct physical contact is the most effective method to use (i.e., having the patient come back to the treatment facility for follow-up evaluations), since such "booster" sessions have been shown to be of critical importance in the maintenance of clinical gains produced by a wide range of treatment programs (Gatchel, Baum, 1983). However, even if the patient cannot physically appear for a follow-up session, there are other methods that can be used to maintain this medical contact. For example, at PRIDE, telephone interviews are conducted on a regular basis as a means of collecting follow-up data on all patients. During these interviews, problems that may have arisen can be discussed, and reminders about learned program skills can be provided. In addition, at PRIDE, a newsletter is sent to all "graduates" of the program on a regular basis. The key factor to remember is that although some forms of contact are more effective than others, *some* regular form of contact is essential to ensure some level of compliance with treatment program prescriptions and achieved goals.

ASSISTANCE AND SUPPORT AFTER THE COMPREHENSIVE PROGRAM

It is therefore obvious that continued contact and support are needed to ensure the maintenance of treatment gains and long-term compliance with the program's philosophy and prescribed lifestyle adjustments. Before discussing in detail the methods employed to maintain physical capacity gains, a review of some additional overall strategies of assistance and support in helping patients re-establish themselves as productive members of their environment will be provided.

One useful support mechanism is the availablilty of a telephone *"hotline service"* in which patients can get in contact with program personnel when a significant problem arises. Issues and concerns can be discussed over the phone, and, if needed, an appointment can be made to have the patient come into the clinic. Also, if a referral is needed, this can also be accomplished over the telephone. The knowledge that this mechanism is available can be reassuring to patients who need to "touch base" with a member of the treatment team after being back "on their own."

Another important assistance mechanism is serving as a *referral source* for patients. After leaving the progam, a patient may encounter a major emotional crisis with which he or she needs help. Referral to an appropriate counseling or therapy facility can be provided. For example, there are many self-help groups in the community such as Alcoholics Anonymous, Weight Watchers, etc., to which individuals can be referred. Likewise, referral to an appropriate health-care professional for related physical problems and concerns can also be made. The important point is that patients come to see the treatment program facility as an important resource if they encounter a significant problem in their lives.

Another area of assistance can be in the realm of vocational rehabilitation. Many times, the employment plans of a patient may suddenly be subject to change. As we noted in Chapter 16, although vocational retraining and/or education is a less desirable goal as it may leave the patient in a dependent "student role," such may be the only alternative available. Part-time employment may be necessary in conjunction with training or school. Additional assistance is usually required in these cases to maintain living standards during the retraining, and the program staff can provide assistance in helping patients get in contact with the appropriate facilities such as the local State Rehabilitation Counseling Agency. We pointed out the important role that Occupational Therapy can play in this process.

We also noted that in some cases, a patient may be too old, unskilled, or severely damaged by multiple operations or cognitive deficits to resume competitive employment. Given sufficient motivation, a wide variety of "home industries" are available, which can supply limited incomes that will decrease the burden to insurers or government for subsidizing this individual. We have constantly been amazed at the ingenuity of many patients in finding self-employed opportunity once conventional employment is recognized to be too difficult to attain or sustain. Support during this transition can be helpful.

MAINTAINING PHYSICAL CAPACITY

Obviously, the maintenance of physical capacity gains is an important goal of functional restoration. In this section, we will discuss how this can be accomplished.

Periodic Testing

The quantitative functional evaluation (QFE), discussed in Part III, is performed post-program on multiple occasions to continue feedback to the patient concerning maintenance of physical capacity. Periodic testing of strength, flexibility, endurance, and task performance capability shows the recovering patient (and athlete) whether physical performance continues to be maintained at a desired level. In Phase IV of the program, increase in patient pain complaints is frequently accompanied by gradual decrease in QFE scores. It is up to the program physician to evaluate whether a setback has been caused by a specific musculoskeletal problem, inattention to exercise protocols, or psychosocial crises. If home exercise protocols are at fault, the feedback afforded by the QFE will permit the physical or occupational therapist to provide advice to the patients for working harder on the specific areas of deficit. If, on the other hand, a major psychosocial stressor has produced the decrement in measured physical capacity and/or effort, appropirate counseling intervention can be arranged to assist with the relevant present crisis intervention. Most organic musculoskeletal problems can be identified specifically, resulting in conventional orthopedic management (injections, non-habituating medications). However, the patient with unusual pain responses maintaining high levels of physical capacity should be thoroughly investigated with appropriate diagnostic tests for previously unsuspected pathologic conditions.

"First Aid" for Recurrent Pain Episodes

Recurrent back pain episodes are endemic among the entire population, and those who have been chronically disabled are certainly no exception. From a pathologic point of view, the scarring or derangement from injury/surgery that originally produced the biochemical dysfunction that led to the chronic low back pain, is still latent to produce additional episodes. However, it is an important function of the "back school" process for the subacute individual, or the full-blown educational process in the comprehensive treatment program, to instruct the patient in dealing with a new acute episode to prevent it from becoming more long-term. If one assumes that the process which led to chronic disability in the first place is a concurrence of maladaptive physical and psychosocial processes for which the patient was not provided with adequate intervention and education, then there is every reason to believe that such future episodes can be prevented as part of the rehabilitation training.

A secondary benefit of the pain increase initially experienced as part of overcoming the deconditioning syndrome is the need to be educated to "work through pain" in overcoming the disability. As such, the groundwork is set for maintaining the highest possible levels of activity with recurrent episodes. Patient self-help measures are taught first, including appropriate stretching exercises, use of anti-inflammatory and over-the-counter analgesics, limited bedrest, and judicious use of heat/cold. Pride in overcoming the episode through self-analysis with calm and patience rather than immediate reliance on health professionals, passive care, or habituating medications is instilled during the follow-up phase of the program. Demonstrated confidence in the patient's ability to handle a new acute episode is one way in which the treatment staff can evaluate the patient's level of understanding of functional restoration.

Home Fitness Programs and Devices

Numerous programs and products are available to help the patient maintain fitness at home. Unfortunately, patients are also bombarded with conflicting advice from the mass media, friends, and a variety of medical and paramedical professionals. At this point, it should be clear to the reader that jogging or riding an exercise bicycle is *not* sufficient to maintain back health if the primary deficit is in true spine mobility or sagittal/rotational strength. Even when all physical capacity deficits noted on initial evaluation have been corrected, those areas of greatest deficiency tend to be those which will recur without attention to home maintenance. It is a truism that people will usually do the things that come easiest to them. The same is true for the injured back patient who will find most distasteful those exercises which are most necessary. For example, many individuals will vigorously pursue aerobic activities in spite of excellent aerobic capacity, but will avoid doing the specific stretching or strengthening exercise most necessary for their functional restoration maintenance.

Most home programs are nonspecific generic fitness programs. It is up to the therapists delivering the instructions at the conclusion of follow-up to provide the patients with specific information on what special areas to emphasize in their own program. The information provided is generally reassessed at the time of each subsequent post-program QFE, with additional recommendations being made if the patient has been unsuccessful in improving the deficient physical characteristic, or if "backsliding" has occurred in a given area. Generally, patients will ultimately reach a "plateau" at which they neither increase nor decrease their physical capacity substantially. At this stage they have reached a balance between their daily activities, exercise, and natural abilities that is usually sufficient to keep their symptoms under control most of the time. Only those individuals motivated to extremely high work or athletic performance will push their physical capabilities beyond this point.

A plethora of home exercise devices is available, with new ones constantly appearing. Exercise bicycles, free weight equipment, roman chairs, dynamic back flexion/extension devices, and a variety of spring- and elastic-controlled tension devices may be obtained to maintain program goals. Such devices in the home have a definite advantage in that their presence tends to act as a constant reminder and motivator about exercise to the program-completing patient. If equipment is available to deal with the specifically deficient dimension and element of performance, it can be useful indeed. Cost, availability, and utility will all be factors in determining purchase of such equipment.

On the other hand, certain individuals may benefit greatly from participation in a health club or fitness center. Such facilities frequently have extensive variable-resistance strength training equipment similar to that on which the patient has trained in functional restoration. Continuation of use of such equipment on a regular basis may continue to build, and then maintain, the patient's high level of function. Such devices are usually far more efficient than those purchased for home use, and in the environment of a health club, the patient's tendency to exert maximally in exercise maintenance is likely to be better than at home. Subtle decreases in capability can be recognized by the patient as a decrease in force/torque generation on a given machine, something that is not usually recognized in a completely unquantified home exercise program. The disadvanatge of such equipment involves persistence with the program. The dropout rate of health clubs and fitness centers is high, due to the inconvenience inherent in the need to drive to the center, change clothes, shower after exercise, etc. The post-program individual must commit significant time to such adventures, and if it is not part of his or her daily routine, adherence to the maintenance program will gradually diminish. Furthermore, as the patient returns to a more normal lifestyle with work, home, and social responsibilities, it becomes more and more difficult to squeeze in the substantial time commitment required for participating in a health club. On the other hand, certain patients will find fitness center participation improves their social lives and will make the necessary commitment. Therefore, a sufficient trial period to evaluate the patient's adherence to such a program should be instituted before recommending a high-cost, long-term membership.

"Reasonable" Ergonomics

One of the disadvantages of current ergonomic training is the teaching of conflicting principles as discussed previously in this text. In attempting to teach "safe" lifting methods, the public has taken advice most properly restricted to the lifting of heavy loads, and translated it as appropriate behavior for all situations. For example, we have previously extensively discussed rationale for the bent back "hanging on its ligaments" as a more efficient way of lifting medium loads than the "straight back, bent knee" position involving substitution of the lower extremity functional unit for the lumbopelvic functional unit. The patient who has paid attention to training principles learned in functional restoration will self-select the style of lifting to provide safety at the highest loads, but also provide efficiency and sufficient training to maintain physical capacity under appropriate circumstances. Most machines cannot be left idle for extended periods of time, nor can they be run at their highest performance levels indefinitely. However, regular running under a variety of speeds and loads is generally felt to provide the highest level of preventive maintenance. In fact, we generally "run in" a new engine by alternating speeds and loads in a prescribed manner for a specified period of time. It is likely that the "human machine" is no different, and that each patient who has completed functional restoration needs to continue a prescribed "run-in period" for a similar period of time. Athletes talk of getting their bodies "in the groove" for specific activities. Restoring function of the human spine in coordination with other parts of the body and in relation to its multiple physiologic determinants would appear to be equally important parts of the maintenance process.

We have now concluded our discussion of the treatment program and the outcome criteria for program discharge. However, the important issues of the pace of reconditioning and the limitations of our measurement devices remain. These issues can be dealt with only through a home program.

Pace of Reconditioning

No one is certain how quickly either deconditioning or reconditioing can be expected to occur in the lumbar spine under a variety of conditions. In previous extremity work, it has been estimated that immobilization results in a 3%/day loss of muscle bulk; however, given the motivational factors in strength assessment, the correlation of atrophy with loss of strength may be imperfect, and complicated by attendant loss of joint motion. It has similarly been empirically observed that the pace of muscle strengthening is relatively slow when building a normal muscle to supernormal levels, as in body building or weight lifting training. Again, there are limitations to our ability to obtain knowledge in these areas, since muscle bulk measurements may vary with minor measurement errors, state of hydration, etc., while weight lifting is a complex, whole-body task involving both strength and technique. The technique, involving body position and agility, may substantially alter an individual's total weight-lifting ability, even though the subject's strength (as measured by isometric or isokinetic lifting devices) is identical to that of someone capable of lifting only a fraction of the weight moved by the trained lifter.

It has also been noted empirically in a treatment program that remarkably rapid increases in strength can be accomplished in short periods of time, particularly in motivated individuals showing low levels of strength or effort on initial testing. It now appears evident that spinal muscular atrophy will occur only to a limited extent, providing the individual with even prolonged disability a "bottom line" of about 50% of predicted strength. Patients initially performing below this level generally do so on the basis of limited effort, due either to pain, neuromuscular inhibition, or fear of injury. Given sufficient motivation, education and training, these individuals will make rapid increases of physical capacity into the middle ranges of their capability. However, progression beyond this level is a much slower process, dealing as it does with true neuromuscular incompetence or atrophy. Individuals whose great inactivity, surgical injury or disuse have led to profound degrees of neuromuscular dysfunction in the spine, can expect that they will still not have achieved optimum functional capacity even after a standard follow-up period. They must thus expect to continue with a home program which continues to build on their gains to achieve higher levels of functional capacity without the supervision and group encouragement that motivated them in the functional restoration environment.

Another maintenance problem revolves around pre-injury attitudes toward physical activity. Most individuals who have become chronically disabled back patients have not had premorbid exercise as part of their lifestyles. Many of the patients were high school or college athletes, but had subsequently become much less fit, while others have absolutely no athletic background whatsoever. Thus, expecting these individuals to continue to maintain their physical capacity rather than see it drift back to pre-program levels may be unrealistic. Even patients who have noted substantial gains in pain perception and functional abilities may find it difficult to keep regular exercise as part of their lives once they have returned to a full day's work and customary interaction in family life. In the case of the "blue collar" worker during strenuous daily physical activities, considerable exercise may be maintained simply by performing the tasks on the job. However, for more sedentary individuals or especially those doing *intermittent* heavy manual tasks (truck drivers unloading their trucks, etc.), a return to the pre-morbid lifestyle may result in decreasing physical capacity, increasing pain perception, and, potentially, a predisposition to recurrent injury.

LIMITATIONS OF PRESENT MEASUREMENT TECHNIQUES

As we have discussed in Part II, we have come a long way in the recognition of our visual limitations to observation of spine function. Similarly, technology has provided important new tools for quantification of physical function through indirect means, allowing comparison of one individual's performance to that of another. However, there remain significant areas of performance which cannot be measured by our current techniques. Moreover, there are areas of deficiency which will require additional research and experience to clarify.

One area of limitation is the small number of subjects currently available in the normative database. Ultimately, large groups of normal subjects must be tested and job-, age-, gender-, and weight-specific normalizations must be tested. Weight normalization has depended on empirical observation that muscle bulk is related to weight, and strength is related to muscle bulk. However, in the over- or underweight individual, this form of normalization may be distorted, making delineation of test profiles of pain-free but overweight individuals a necessity. It is already noted empirically in a small number of patients that individuals who are only mildly overweight will demonstrate increased trunk strength in proportion to their weight, even though this increased weight does not come from increased muscle bulk. It is as though they are constantly "carrying a load" on their backs in daily life, which may provide regular training to the spine musculature. On the other hand, it appears that significiant decrements in weight-normalized physical capacity are noted in the extremely obese subject.

A second area requiring clarification utilizing current technology is definition of the "effort factor" more objectively. Certainly, the principle that consistency of performance on multiple repetitions documents good effort appears to have face validity. However, it has also been shown that a trained individual, given optimum circumstances of fixed anatomic position, visual feedback, and sufficient practice, may "fool the system." Thus, there is a need for objectively defining the performance variability produced by suboptimal effort with specific protocols that remove opportunities for inadvertent deception. While the software for such testing appears to be available in at least two of the presently available devices, numerical limits of curve variability in large normal populations have yet to be defined.

A third technologic necessity which may be just emerging is the protocol for measurement of endurance/recovery potential. Isolated strength tests themselves do not speak to the issue of worker performance through the course of an 8 to 12 hour day. Measures of aerobic capacity through ergometric testing can give a partial answer to the endurance problem, insofar as it is affected by circulatory deficits. However, until specific endurance/recovery time protocols are established for spine/abdominal musculature and lifting performance, knowledge of personal capability in this area remains incomplete. It is hoped that, once endurance profiles are known for incumbent workers in specific job categories, knowledge of the appropriate end-point for training the injured worker will be sufficient to gauge his or her actual work capabilities from a short addition to present test protocols. Presumably, however, it will take considerably longer to develop muscular endurance, including time actually "training" on the job, before this dimension of human performance is acquired once again.

Finally, the most complex dimension of human performance remains elusive to all researchers in sports medicine. This is the dimension of coordination or agility, which every training athlete knows comes only after a specific training period in the "sport" itself. No technique for measuring such complex tasks has yet emerged, other than the level of performance produced by the athlete himself. Thus, a baseball pitcher must ultimately leave the gym where he has been working on mobility and weights, and move on to practice throwing motions at gradually increasing speed and number of repetitions. The only known measure of his performance will be the return of his speed, accuracy, repetition capability, and "stuff" in actual pitching against batters. Similarly, a non-athlete returning from a back injury will be measured on his performance in life activities: job productivity, lost time, home contributions, and recreational pursuits. At the present time, patient outcome reports appear to be the best way of judging this performance dimension.

CHAPTER REFERENCES

Bélisle M, Roskies, E, Lévesque JM: Improving adherence to physical activity. Health Psychology, 6:159–172, 1987.

Carmody TP, Senner JW, Malinow MR, Matarazzo JD: Physical exercise rehabilitation: long-term dropout rate in cardiac patients. J Behavioral Med, 3:163–168, 1980.

Dishman RK: Prediction of Adherence to Habitual Physical Activity. In FJ Naggle, HJ Montoye (Eds.). Exercise in Health and Disease Springfield, Charles C Thomas, 1981, pp. 259–275.

Gatchel RJ, Baum A: Introduction to Health Psychology. New York, Random House, 1983.

Hunt WA, Bespelac DA: An evaluation of current methods of modifying smoking behavior. J Clin Psychol, 30:431–438, 1974.

Morgan WP: Psychological Benefits of Physical Activity. In FJ Naggle, HJ Montoye (Eds.). Exercise in Health and Disease. Springfield, Charles C Thomas, 1981.

Marlatt GA, Gordon JR: Determinants of Relapse: Implications for the Maintenance of Behavior Change. In PO Davidson, SM Davidson (Eds.). Behavioral Medicine: Changing Health Lifestyles. New York, Bruner/Mazel, 1980.

Marlatt GA, Gordon JR: Relapse Prevention. New York, Guilford, 1981.

Mayer TG, Gatchel RJ, Kishino N, Keeley J, Capra P, Mayer H, Barnett J, Mooney V: Objective assessment of spine function following industrial injury: a prospective study with comparison group and one-year follow-up. Spine, 10:482–493, 1985.

Mayer TG, Gatchel RJ, Mayer H, Kishino N, Keeley J, Mooney V: A prospective two-year study of functional restoration in industrial low back injury. JAMA 258:1763–1767, 1987.

Wilbur JA, Barrow JG: Reducing elevated blood pressure. Minnesota Med, 52:1303, 1969.

Chapter 19

Socioeconomic Implications: Re-employment and Impairment Evaluation

There is no doubt that the functional restoration approach, if competently and systematically administered, will have a significant positive effect on low back pain disability. We have documented how it can have a significant impact on realistic outcome variables such as return to work. It should be clearly noted, though, that the laudable outcomes of return to work and case settlement involve many processes outside the direct control of the medical treatment facility. Other participants in the "Disability System" (including attorneys, insurance companies, employers, unions, and state/Federal workman's compensation adjudicators), play an active role in setting the incentives or disincentives for the quality of the outcome. Indeed, re-employment issues are dramatically influenced by attitudes of the participants in the "Disability System." The widely held perception that a previous back injury inevitably predisposes to a far higher incidence of subsequent back injury often leads employers and their insurance carriers to dissuade the injured worker from returning to his previous employer. This perceived "prejudice" has led, over time, to liberalization of the disability evaluation process with increased benefits to guard against the negative impact on re-employment. These changes may then result in further disincentives to a return to productivity. In this final chapter, we will review some of these important issues. Such issues are extremely important for treatment facilities to be aware of.

RE-EMPLOYMENT ISSUES

Vocational Rehabilitation

Ideally, a patient, even one with prolonged disability, will continue to retain a position in a company by virtue of employer enlightenment or union rights. A suitable "light duty" transition period will be succeeded by the patient's return to full employment with the same employer in the same position. Under other circumstances, patients may be forced to seek employment elsewhere, but will succeed in accomplishing this in a favorable economic environment. Patients with multiple skills, permitting them to select work of lower job demand, may choose alternative employment. These individuals may even be compensated for accepting such work at lower wage-earning capacity. However, patients with low skills, qualifying them only for high job demand positions, may occasionally be unqualified for return to such positions by virtue of age

294

or severity of underlying structural pathologic condition, and may thus be a candidate for vocational rehabilitation.

A variety of services are customarily available through a multitude of private, state and Federal resources. Trained counselors provide vocational evaluation services, identifying employment opportunities within the worker's physical and mental capabilities. Counseling services may assist the patient in developing suitable job behaviors, techniques for finding jobs, and "job clubs" in which similarly injured workers share experiences in seeking re-employment. The work ethic is strongly reinforced, and the many positive aspects of work as a social activity and producer of self-esteem are encouraged.

A network of employers willing to provide on-the-job training may be available through such agencies. They may support such employers with tax incentives or funding to encourage new careers for injured workers. Finally, more long-term retraining in alternative occupations may be available. Such efforts must be instituted with extreme caution, however, as the long-term recidivism and failure to complete such programs is high. Problems of wavering interest in retraining may be ameliorated by insistence that the program be accompanied by part-time gainful employment in a position of which the patient is physically capable. This activity has the dual benefits of maintaining high levels of physical activity and reintroducing the patient to work responsibilities.

Job Design

An innovative concept just beginning to emerge, but not yet practical for "real world" industry, is the amalgamation of worker re-entry and job redesign. Ergonomic engineering has made inroads over the last decade in promoting modification of the work site to improve worker safety, though some other areas of ergonomic training have been shown to have limited value (i.e., training workers in "proper" lifting techniques). Workplace redesign to decrease erratic or asymmetric loading appears to make good sense. Centralizing loads by raising them off the floor onto pallets and off high shelves to shoulder level, repackaging materials into lighter bundles of appropriate dimension, redesigning work sites to avoid asymmetric loading, and "tuning" truck suspensions to alter vibration frequencies are just some of the engineering modifications being evaluated in an effort to prevent back injuries in high risk jobs. Hopefully, in the future, enlightened employers will consider implementing such modifications in conjunction with accepting the injured worker back to his or her employment.

Re-employment Discrimination

Prior to 1973, the Equal Employment Opportunities Commission (EEOC) was empowered under Title VII of the Civil Rights Act of 1964 as amended by the Equal Employment Act of 1972 to require that there be significant evidence that a battery of tests is predictive of future injury risk and/or job performance. EEOC guidelines stated that the predictive value should be statistically significant at the $p<0.05$ level, and that appropriate validation be performed. Chronic low back pain patients with permanent partial impairments are considered handicapped persons. Prior to 1973, such individuals had no recourse against discrimination experienced in re-employment. The Congressional passage of the Rehabilitation Act of 1973 led to a change in this situation. However, discriminatory practice has continued to be widespread, and the effectiveness of protective legislation remains difficult to assess (Rehab Act, 1973; Vietnam Act, 1974).

Regulations specifically provide for an employer to offer equal employment opportunities to all workers. In addition, the employer must pay for "reasonable accommodation" in order to provide those opportunities that are necessary to permit the "handicapped" worker (i.e., one with a permanent partial impairment) to perform the essential functions of work. Such accommodation may be limited by the "undue hardship" provision in which employers can be excused from accommodation obligations they would otherwise be required to submit to.

However, the law provides for a specific defense: The Bona Fide Occupational Qualification (BFOQ) test. If an employer can demonstrate that a particular class of individuals cannot perform specific tasks required of them, they may be excluded from employment. If business necessity perceived by employers prompts them to exert such a defense against the class of back-injured workers, regulations constrict their ability to devise pre-employment tests. In particular, pre-employment inquiries on application forms or at interviews regarding presence, nature, and severity of handicap are prohibited. An important caveat, however, is that such inquiries are prohibited only prior to an offer of employment, not prior to the date commencing employment. Requiring a medical evaluation in which specific historical information is obtained from the patient after an offer of employment may evade the intent of the regulations. Finally, specific regulations provide for standards for both hiring and promotion. These specifically refer to any selection criteria or screening tests which tend to discriminate against handicapped persons. The only acceptable tests must fulfill the following qualifications: (1) The test or selection criteria must be shown to be *job-related* for the position in question; or (2) if there are alternative job-related tests or criteria that do not select out the handicapped person, the more discriminatory test is prohibited.

Prevention Programs

Industry, as the ultimate resource "where the buck stops" in paying for low back disability, is understandably highly motivated to grasp at anything (real or imagined) to prevent an unnecessary financial drain. In some cases, such efforts might be perceived as beneficial to the worker, as when education programs are instituted or medical benefits are paid. However, worker selection methodology is considerably more controversial, and is often perceived to be highly discriminatory (Rockey, Fantel, Omenn, 1979). As in most other things, while it may make greater intuitive sense to prevent a problem before it arises, "treatment" systems are usually set up to solve the problems once they arise. Such systems become self-sustaining, and generally show little interest in avoiding problems which might obviate the need for a solution. In the low back pain disability system, the medical industry, the legal industry, and the insurance industry all benefit directly or indirectly from dealing with problems once they arise. Thus, unfortunately, strong economic motivations for prevention can be expected to come only from the victims of the low back system: the employer and the injured worker. Thus far, prevention has had relatively little impact on the planning or actitivies of either of these groups. As is common to most systems, the motivation of the "host" for active defense (because of ignorance, misinformation, misplaced priorities, or misperception of harm) is usually far less than that of the "parasites" for aggressive offense.

One of the problems inherent in more widespread prevention interest revolves around the many issues discussed in Part I of this book. Contributions to the enigma include: (1) absence of a specific pain source; (2) problems in definition of low back disease; (3) inability to select out criteria separating the high cost chronic back injury from self-limited, extremely common acute back pain; and (4) impaired ability to identify functional capacity deficits. While it may be an accepted medicolegal decision to define low back pain in the work place as "an injury," deciding from an epidemiologic point of view whether it is an injury, a disease, or a psychosocial phenomenon is difficult, and by its nature hinders our ability to identify risk of disease. Thus, it becomes extremely difficult to develop tests or selection criteria with any predictive value.

A second problem arises in defining cost-benefit ratios for prevention. Education and training programs, inexpensively provided to a mass audience of workers, have been the mainstay of back care for a decade. Unfortunately, they have proved to be neither effective in reducing injury rates after a 6-month period, in preventing injury, nor cost-efficient (Bigos, Spengler, Martin, Zeh, Fisher, Nachemson, Wang, 1986; Spengler, Bigos, Martin, Zeh, Fisher, Nachemson, 1986). When individual tests are given to prospective asymptomatic employees, considerably higher expense is incurred, with no statistical evidence to show that such tests can discriminate either the incidence of acute injury, or of high cost chronic cases (Bigos, Spengler, Martin, Zeh, Fisher, Nachemson, Wang, 1986; Spengler, Bigos, Martin, Zeh, Fisher, Nachemson, 1986).

As we have already seen, disability management attempts to identify and overcome a series of educational and psychosocioeconomic "barriers to functional recovery" which greatly affect the low back healing process. Relatively little work has been done to isolate these variables in a prevention, as opposed to a therapeutic, domain. There is some evidence to show that the Minnesota Multiphasic Personality Inventory (MMPI) may help to discriminate patients who will become chronic patients from symptomatic acute patients (as well as surgical failures), but attempts to apply this in a systematic fashion have not proved feasible under clinical conditions. Clearly, however, we must distinguish which disease we are talking about: *(a)* asymptomatic workers displaying age-related degenerative changes as documented radiographically; *(b)* acute back pain (with 80% population prevalence over a lifetime); *(c)* recurrent, episodic back pain; or *(d)* chronic unremitting, disabling back pain. If we are speaking of the latter, with its high human and financial cost, no effective predictors have yet emerged. Episodic recurrent pain occurs in 40 to 50% of all acute pain sufferers with a similar absence of predictor variables.

Another problem in prevention is the multifactorial nature of chronic low back pain and its relatively low prevalence in any specific population. Because it is a dynamic phenomenon involving structural defects, physical capacity deficits, and multiple psychosocioeconomic variables, no single predictive test can be expected to have a high degree of both sensitivity and specificity in identifying the problem. For example, of the multiple variables tested over years in the Boeing study, only a poor work performance report by a supervisor was found to have statistically significant correlation with injury rates. The worst reports occurred in the high-cost injuries. However, use of such a test would probably involve both low predictive value and discriminatory aspects. Despite these difficulties, tests and inquiries are being utilized in industry, and workers facing re-employment will have to face those aspects which impact on their re-employment opportunities. Pre-employment inquiries were discussed above. Medical examinations and worker selection techniques will be discussed in the next section.

Worker Selection Tests

Andersson and Lehmann identify four characteristics of appropriate screening procedures: safety, predictive value, practicality and legality (Andersson, Lehmann, 1984). These tests are used by them to evaluate all screening procedures. With respect to predictive value, they recognize three other characteristics of a test: the accuracy of the measure, its sensitivity, and its specificity (Table 19–1) (Andersson, Lehmann, 1984).

One unfortunate statistical quirk, however, clouds the horizon of such worker screening. The predictive value is highly dependent, not only on accuracy, sensitivity, and specificity of a test, but also on the prevalence of the condition under study. Epidemiologists recognize that prevalence rates under 50% are associated with progressive decrements of prediction even on highly sensitive/specific tests. A superb test may have a predictive value of only 67% when there is a prevalence rate of the disease of only 10%, or a predictive value of 16% with prevalence of only 1%. As an example, the low prevalence rates for situations in which a high predictive value is desirable are as follows: *(a)* asymptomatic workers have lost-time injuries annually of 3 to 4%; *(b)* asymptomatic workers becoming chronic, high-cost cases annually have a rate of 0.2 to 0.3%; and *(c)* acutely injured workers who will become chronic have a rate of 5 to 10%. The statistical uncertainty introduced by such low prevalence rates places many worker selection programs, particularly those dealing with

Table 19–1. Test Characteristics

Category	Definition	Formula
Accuracy	Ability of a test to provide a valid and relevant measure of a specific quantity	
Sensitivity	Ability of a test to identify patients with a particular disease	$\dfrac{\text{True positives} \times 100}{\text{True pos.} + \text{False neg.}}$
Specificity	Ability of a test to identify non-disease so that negative results occur in patients free of disease	$\dfrac{\text{True negatives} \times 100}{\text{True neg.} + \text{False pos.}}$
Predictive value	Ability of a test to predict both presence and absence of disease, affected by both sensitivity and specificity; and prevalence of the disease.	$\dfrac{\text{True positives} \times 100}{\text{True neg.} + \text{False pos.}}$

low-risk jobs, on shaky footing indeed. This statistical fact is often overlooked by the informed. Obviously, it has great implications for evaluating the effectiveness of any screening devices.

In terms of specific screening tests, they are usually performed as part of a medical evaluation and involve three phases of various degree of emphasis depending on industry criteria, physician and employer: *(a)* medical history/physical; *(b)* radiographic examination; and *(c)* strength testing.

Medical History/Examination

The history primarily focuses on delineating previous back and neck difficulties. Certainly, the high incidence of recurrence has been documented for both low back pain and sciatica (Rowe, 1963; Rowe, 1965; Pedersen, 1981; Troup, Martin, Lloyd, 1981; Bierring-Sorensen, 1983; Magora, Taustein, 1969). Many of these authors suggested that recurrence (implicitly noted with a positive response on screening history) would predict a higher number of lost work days and additional episodes of back pain, thus making these candidates less desirable as employees. This assertion remains controversial, however, as one group suggested that acute episodes caused by true "accidents" (as opposed to back pain simply arising on the job) failed to predict recurrence.

Efforts are also usually made in the history to identify episodes in which litigation or compensation may have played a role. Work history information, as well as that of intercurrent diseases, may be included. The length and severity of previous episodes, including surgical procedures, will also be closely scrutinized. Inquiries made during the examination, once a job has been offered, are *not* prevented as discriminators by Federal law.

The occupational physical examination, following the same pattern, will search for evidence of prior surgical procedure or lumbar dysfunction. Height, weight, age, and gender are carefully observed as predictors of performance in manual tasks, while attitude and demeanor are subtly assessed. Spine dysfunction is evaluated through muscular development, posture, general fitness mobility, and neurologic tests (Cady, Bischoff, O'Connell, Thomas, Allan, 1979). As we have discussed many times previously, the predictive value of many physical examination findings has been shown to be nil (obesity, age), while others are suggested but not proven (evidence of regular smoking, use of alcohol or drugs).

Radiographic Assessment

Safety and practicality questions are not usually major issues in radiographic assessment (though they probably should be), but the predictive value of these tests certainly is. We have previously discussed much of the difficulty with these tests. Asymptomatic patients over age 40 demonstrate a 35% incidence of "herniated nucleus pulposus" on CT scans (Wiesel, Tsourmas, Feffer, Citrin, Patronas, 1984; Bell, Rothman, Booth, Cuckler, Garfin, Herkowitz, Simeone, Dolinskas, Han, 1984). It has been estimated that up to 70% of x rays were read as "abnormal," and up to 26% of workers were rejected or restricted in multiple studies based on radiographic assessment (Foote, 1982). In a prospective study, there was no significant correlation identified between subsequent incidents of back pain and two groups of workers selected by x ray (Gibson, Martin, Terry, 1980). The trend over the past decade, based on such evidence (or lack of it), has therefore been to reject pre-employment x rays as a relevant or accurate tool for predicting low back injury (Montgomery, 1976; LaRocca, MacNab, 1969; Rockey, Fantel, Omenn, 1979). Furthermore, since radiographs are static documents of *past* events, perfectly asymptomatic findings of no clinical significance may be used to disqualify workers, thus bringing up both legal and ethical objections to routine radiographic assessment.

Physical Capacity Tests

Historically, "strength" tests used to select workers have been whole-body lifting rather than isolated lumbar strength tests (Ayoub, Mital, Bakken, Asfour, Bethea, 1980; Snook, Campanelli, Hart, 1978; Keyserling, Herrin, Chaffin, 1980; Kroemer, 1970; Chaffin, Park, 1973; Chaffin, Herrin, Keyserling, 1978). The techniques usually involved either isometric, isoinertial, or psychophysical lifting associated with ergonomic analysis of the job. The worker seeking re-employment is increasingly likely to be exposed to such tests during the screening process. However, their predictive value for employment remains controversial. We have previously discussed many of the issues regarding isolated lifting tests as sole quantifiers of physical functional capacity during the rehabilitation process. The same problems remain when evaluating sensitivity and specificity in worker selection.

Moreover, those methods involve other difficulties. The ergonomic analysis tends to set "minimum standards" for a job in terms of lifting and cardiovascular function. Because of the limits of practicality, the tests are generally relatively simple and nonspecific. They generally eschew normalizing factors, so they tend to select the largest, healthiest male specimens as successful test completers. This built-in tendency may be considered discriminatory. Conversely, the tests generally fail to identify the individual workers's capabilities relative to his or her anticipated ability, thus frequently disqualifying smaller but fit individuals while passing larger applicants, possibly post-injury, functioning at much less than their full capabilities.

While such issues continue to cloud the scientific validity of screening procedures, the demand for "something" to limit the cost of low back pain will continue to stimulate introduction of these techniques into the workplace. It is anticipated that the implications for worker re-employment will be a gradually more arduous pre-employment evaluation. With a sluggish economy and relatively high unemployment, growing industries can afford to put some emphasis on worker selection as a means of injury prevention. As has occurred before, it will do so even without a scintilla of scientific backing.

IMPAIRMENT/DISABILITY EVALUATION

Compensation is the issue of primary importance to the legal establishment, and is a vital part of the psychosocioeconomic pattern of chronic low back pain. Compensation for actual damage to "the body as a whole" is a part of the fabric of all state and Federal workmen's compensation statutes. It also plays a role when perceived negligence prompts personal injury or product liability litigation. Such compensation may be a potent incentive for a variety of behaviors and, as such, it is not surprising that compensation is involved in the majority of disabling chronic back pain cases. In the minds of many observers, compensation itself is the overwhelming cause of such disability, but the large number of patients who continue to be disabled even after all compensation issues have been resolved argues against this hypothesis. Rather, compensation incentives/disincentives may merely accompany other factors which generate the disability; subsequently, the disability becomes self-propagating. By their nature, the workmen's compensation statutes are most closely tied to issues of work absence and compensation.

Workmen's Compensation

The workmen's compensation laws represent a compromise between rights of the employer and employee, in which the latter obtains prompt, fair and reliable treatment in exchange for limiting the liability of the employer. Though the laws have frequently been challenged since their importation from Europe nearly a century ago, the trend has been for a gradual liberalization of benefits and interpretation in favor of the injured worker. The state for this progressive social legislation was set during the heady days of rapid industrial expansion in Europe. The first laws were passed in Germany in 1884, coming to the United States after the turn of the century. The injured worker, faced with a task of suing his or her employer for negligence, was often unable to mount the financial resources to do battle. Medical care was frequently not obtainable, the old job was lost, and the worker "blacklisted." If the case was lost, the worker frequently became a financial burden to his or her family or to society's charity.

While provision of medical benefits that are "necessary and reasonable" to workers is a major benefit of the system, we are here most interested in understanding the dynamics of direct financial compensation to the injured worker. These benefits are considered "temporary or permanent" and "partial or total." Supplementary benefits may be available in terms of both short-term and long-term disability (LTD). These benefit issues will be considered below.

Temporary Total Disability (TTD)

All states, as well as the Federal Government, provide this benefit, usually beginning after a statutorily determined "waiting period," with benefits retroactive to the first day of disability. There is a great deal of variation in the amount of benefit paid, though there has been a tendency, over the last decade, to bring up the benefits in states that historically maintained the lowest weekly supplement. Most benefits are gauged to two-thirds of the individual's previous income up to a fixed maximum, and the benefits are generally tax-free. They continue until the patient is no longer disabled, is only partially disabled, or the condition becomes permanent.

Permanent Total Disability (PTD)

Such a rating, though generally intended for the most catastrophic cases, is not rare in low back disability, particularly the multiply operated patient. Workers may be so identified, depending on state regulations, if either: *(a)* they cannot return to any employment whatsoever; *(b)* they cannot return to employment for which they are qualified; *(c)* they are judged unable to "obtain or retain" employment in the future; or *(d)* vocational rehabilitation is unable to make them capable of developing an employable skill. These workers may receive a lump sum or periodic payment equal to a fixed percentage of their preinjury wage, often associated with a specific time limit. In many cases, long-term disability (LTD) benefits, relief from a variety of long-term personal ob-ligations (home and auto loans, etc.), and Social Security Disability Income (SSDI) are linked to "achieving" such a status. Because of the financial risk associated with giving up their "claimant" status, individuals already declared medically "P and T" patients are extremely difficult to rehabilitate, even if they previously possessed a strong work ethic.

Permanent Partial Disability (PPD)

When the patient has reached a "medically stable" plateau, he or she may be eligible for benefits related to a persistent partial disability. This benefit, in particular, shows extremely wide variation in payment for identical disabilities (Larson, 1982). This situation arises from the controversial necessity for a phy-sician to rate the impairment. A disability rating is derived from the impairment rating and applied to benefit schedules provided for in the law. Besides these scheduled benefits related to physical function, nonscheduled benefits com-pensate the worker for lost wages as determined by decreased earning capacity related to disability. Such payments may also be periodic or lump-sum. Attor-neys are frequently called on to negotiate for such benefits on behalf of a patient/claimant, generally on a "contingency fee" basis. Their fee is usually deter-mined by statute as a percentage of the ultimate recovery. In some states, it may also include a percentage of the temporary total benefits.

Impairment Rating

Programs such as Social Security Disability Income (SSDI) and long-term disability (LTD), as well as many supplemental insurance policies for mortgage and car payments, require documentation of ongoing disability. Workmen's compensation and Social Security generally recognize permanent partial dis-ability, while a variety of suits involving negligence necessitate actual rating of the disability to determine payment. Some PPD determination is performed according to fixed schedules set by statute. Certain industries involving seamen and railroad workers (Jones Act and FELA) may combine features of both compensation systems.

There is currently no general agreement on the "right" system for rating impairment or disability. Impairment is considered solely a medical judgment and implies the rating of anatomic or functional loss. On the other hand, dis-ability is a loss of the capacity to engage in gainful employment. Disability is caused by impairment, and takes into consideration such factors as previous work skills, age, education, previous job demands, motivation, and psycho-social barriers. Disability is considered to be an administrative rather than a medical issue. The distinction between disability and impairment is based on the legal perception that medicine, as a science, can quantify the degree of loss of bodily function objectively, thus guiding the more subjectively determined rating of disability. The "whole man" concept artificially divides the body into a series of anatomic units, each of which is expressed as a percentage of the putative whole man. Thus, even complete loss of a major part of the anatomy cannot represent more than a fraction of the "whole man." In some venues, a general injury may allow total disability to be declared even with only a partial injury if the attendant function is considered indispensable to "whole man" activities.

The physician is the central figure in the determination of impairment. As such, he or she has a major responsibility for assisting the patient engaged in functional restoration in resolving ongoing compensation issues at the conclusion of rehabilitation treatment. There are four central issues in this process, as noted in Table 19–2, and discussed below.

Healing Period

The legal concept of a "healing period" does not resemble the healing period associated with tissue reconstitution. Tissue healing generally occurs in a matter of days or weeks. Even fractures heal in a matter of a few months. However, healing period in terms of disability evaluation refers to the time during which spontaneous improvement in the patient's condition (generally implying subjective symptoms) can still be expected to occur. At the conclusion of that period, the patient becomes "medically stable," or is determined to have reached "maximum medical recovery." This point is generally considered the time for determining medical impairment and setting permanent partial disability benefits. Under ideal circumstances, applying current knowledge of tissue healing, this point should be reached in most cases of unoperated low back pain in 4 to 6 months. In operated cases, an approximately identical period should transpire for healing after the surgery. Unfortunately, many such cases continue in the "Disability System" as neglected cases for many years.

Cause of Impairment

In some cases of litigation based upon a precipitating event, a causal relationship must be established by the physician between the "injury" and subsequent low back symptoms. In fact, such a relationship is often difficult to determine scientifically. However, in practice, such relationships are only infrequently challenged. In most cases, these challenges are not appealed in the courts, and over the decades a progressively more liberal interpretation of this causal relationship has evolved. Since the patient's initial history and physical findings are usually the standard by which this relationship is judged, to deny the statement of relationship would be tantamount to doubting the word of the patient who gave the history. While such doubts may be justified in some cases, they are rarely sustained by the actions of a jury. Physicians who casually ignore or doubt their patient's verbal statements usually note a drop in patient visits and referrals.

Determine Functional Limitations or Capacity for Work

Traditionally, this has been done by a physician working alone with little idea of what the patient's actual job requirements or actual physical capability

Table 19–2. Physician Actions in Determining Impairment

1. Determine conclusion of "healing period"
2. Determine causal relationship between injury and impairment
3. Determine the residual functional capacity or functional limitations
4. Determine extent of any permanent impairment

are. All too often, the relatively low state of the art in impairment evaluation allows patients' subjective report of their job description and estimate of their own physical capabilities to be used directly, or with slight interpretation by the physician. The result is frequently extremely low limitations, well below the patient's actual occupational tolerances and/or job demand. This mismatch between job requirements and limitations set by the physician may have a damaging effect on the patient's prospects for return to his or her previous job. The patient may have perceived advantages to encouraging such a mismatch, as compensation may sometimes be enhanced if patient limitations are set at such a low level that return to work in the same or similar position is not feasible. The worker may weigh such benefits against loss of employment or opportunity for advancement. In any case, it is clear that such secondary gain issues may influence this report of symptoms and cloud the evaluating physician's judgment. It is in this area that quantification of physical capacity technology can be most useful. The actual documentation of capacity to perform lifting and other activities of daily living, as well as documenting the renewed capacity of the "biomechanical chain" in low back mobility and strength, may improve the patient's work capacity. In addition, it also documents the patient's motivation and eagerness to get well, in spite of a permanent partial impairment. On the other hand, depending on state statutes, the patient may recognize that determination of even partial work tolerance may disqualify him or her from compensation with permanent total benefits. However, this is not usually a great sacrifice, as such benefits are only infrequently distributed.

Determination of Permanent Partial Impairment

Though there is no uniform rating system for impairment, there are guidelines (American Medical Association and American Academy of Orthopedic Surgeons) to techniques for determining impairment in most parts of the human anatomy. Unfortunately, the low back rating uses the most incomplete and arbitrary methods, which is noteworthy and paradoxical in view of the frequency with which such impairment ratings are required. Even though this impairment rating is supposed to document the damage to structural body parts in an objective way, problems alluded to in Part I of this book often lead to a subjective determination of impairment in this area. The patient's subjective reporting may enter strongly into the impairment evaluation process, as may the results of radiographic tests which document pre-existing and not "injury-related" factors. In some cases, it may even be necessary to distinguish pre-existing from "injury-related" factors as part of the rating process. However, rather than providing a useful, accurate tool to the legal profession, such opinions become purely subjective on the part of the physician and show extreme variations depending on the philosophic bent of the "expert witness."

Actual clinical practice of impairment rating is interesting to examine. In one survey, it was found that a group of orthopedic surgeons showed a range of low back impairment ratings from 0 to 50%, but that the "average rating" was 13% (Brand, Lehmann, 1983). By contrast, another survey showed an "average award" by a compensation board to be closely matched (14%) (White, 1969). These "traditional" ratings have come to be widely accepted by compensation administrators with relatively small variation from state to state. However, under most litigation procedures, a contesting side can request an independent medical examination from "their doctor," whose testimony presumably "neutralizes" the inflated or deflated rating of the treating physician. To halt the practice of marching an army of testifying "expert witnesses" through the courts, most administrators and third party carriers will generally accept the treating physician's impairment rating if it is "in the ball park." Attorneys and claims personnel may subsequently attempt to educate the errant physician.

There are flaws in all methods of determining impairment. Certainly, the error of relying on simple angular measures of the spine, as proposed in American Medical Association guidelines as "objective data," should be apparent to readers of this chapter, and this technique should be altered. California has already taken steps to incorporate new technology into its disability evaluation procedures by specifying accepted techniques and giving greater credence to evaluation done with more reliable instruments and techniques.

Similarly, the confusion of pre-existing or aggravating conditions with the low back pain episode (as in higher ratings for spondylolysis or spondylolisthesis) should be carefully scrutinized, as these radiographic findings may not be predictive of future difficulty or in any way related to the compensable event. Certainly, however, ablative surgical procedures, leading to additional scar and biomechanical disruption, is traditionally accepted as causing greater impairment. This fact is generally recognized by most adjudicators, who typically grant considerably higher payments when surgery has been performed. This widely known policy may act as a monetary disincentive to nonoperative treatment with rehabilitation, promoting "surgery as the last resort" even after multiple consultants have previously ruled it out as a rational alternative. Thus, in at least one state, a policy of assigning statutory impairments nearly identical for operative and nonoperative treatment of low back pain has recently been put into practice. It remains to be seen whether this will provide a solution to problems of low back disability, or arbitrarily punish those who have undergone major surgical intervention.

One must be certain, if using physical capacity tests as part of the impairment evaluation process, that an accurate, valid, relevant test is utilized in which an effort factor is concurrently evaluated. Given the nearly simultaneous motivations of seeking employment and determining disability for compensation, patients have been seen to perform dramatically differently in each of these scenarios. Such findings may be anticipated in any dynamic process measured at a single point in time. Therefore, it is doubly important that the clinician be certain that the point of "maximum medical recovery" has been reached prior to evaluating disability. All reasonable passive and active interventions should have taken place prior to this assessment.

As new evaluative techniques become available, legislators must be careful to avoid the trap of rewarding the individual displaying the lowest physical capacity, as this is also the individual with the lowest effort in functional restoration. This disabled claimant places himself or herself at lowest risk for reinjury by refusal to return to competitive employment. Rather, creating positive reinforcements through greater rewards for those working harder to achieve higher levels of physical capacity, in spite of underlying permanent structural defects, is in the best interest of the society. The evaluating physician can best assist this process by evaluating higher disability based primarily on recognized structural damage to the body. This could be modified upward based on effort shown by the patient in his or her own rehabilitation.

CHAPTER REFERENCES

Andersson G, Lehmann T: Worker Selection. *In* Occupational Low Back Pain. Ed. Pope M, Frymoyer J, Andersson G. New York, Praeger Publishers, 1984, pp. 218–232.

Ayoub M, Mital A, Bakken G, Asfour S, Bethea N: Development of strength and capacity norms for manual materials handling activities. The state-of-the-art. Human Factors *22*:271–283, 1980.

Bell G, Rothman R, Booth R, Cuckler J, Garfin S, Herkowitz H, Simeone F, Dolinskas C, Han S: 1984 Volvo Award in Clinical Sciences: a study of computer assisted tomography II. Comparison of metrizamide myelography and computed tomography in the diagnosis of herniated lumbar disk and spinal stenosis. Spine *9*:552–556, 1984.

Bierring-Sorensen F: The Prognostic Value of the Low Back History and Physical Measurements. Unpublished Doctoral Dissertation. University of Copenhagen, Copenhagen, 1983.

Bigos S, Spengler D, Martin N, Zeh J, Fisher L, Nachemson A, Wang M: Back injuries in industry: a retrospective study II. Injury factors. Spine *11*:246–251, 1986.

Bigos S, Spengler D, Martin N, Zeh J, Fisher L, Nachemson A, Wang M: Back injuries in industry: a retrospective study III. Employee-related factors. Spine *11*:252–256, 1986.

Brand R, Lehmann T: Low back impairment rating practices of orthopaedic surgeons. Spine *8*:75–78, 1983.

Cady L, Bischoff D, O'Connell E, Thomas P, Allan J: Strength and fitness and subsequent back injuries in fire-fighters. J Occup Med *21*:269–272, 1979.

Chaffin D, Park K: A longitudinal study of low-back pain as associated with occupational weight lifting factors Am Indus Hyg Assoc J *34*:513–525, 1973.

Chaffin D, Herrin G, Keyserling W: Pre-employment strength testing. An updated position. J Occup Med *20*:403–408, 1978.

Foote G: Pre-employment radiography of the lumbosacral spine. Radiology in health screening. Australas Radiol *26*:25– 29, 1982.

Gibson E, Martin R, Terry C: Incidence of low back pain and pre-employment x-ray screening. J Occup Med *22*:515–519, 1980.

Keyserling W, Herrin G, Chaffin D: Isometric strength testing as a means of controlling medical incidents on strenuous jobs. J Occup Med *22*:332–336, 1980.

Kroemer K: Human strength. Terminology, measurement and interpretation of data. Human Factors *12*:297–313, 1970.

LaRocca H, Macnab I: Value of pre-employment radiographic assessment of the lumbar spine. Can Med Assoc J *101*:383–388, 1969.

Larson A: The Law of Workmen's Compensation. New York, Matthew Bender, 1982.

Magora A, Taustein I: An investigation of the problem of sick-leave in the patient suffering from low back pain. Industr Med Surg *38*:398–408, 1969.

Montgomery C: Pre-employment back x-rays. J Occup Med *18*:495–498, 1976.

Pedersen P: Prognostic indicators in low back pain. J Royal Coll Gen Pract *31*:209–216, 1981.

Rehabilitation Act of 1973, statutes at large, v. 87, Public Law 93–112, 355–394, 1973.

Rockey P, Fantel J, Omenn G: Discriminatory aspects of pre-employment screening: low back x-ray examinations in the railroad industry. Amer J Law and Med *5*:197–214, 1979.

Rowe M: Preliminary statistical study of low back pain. J Occup Med *5*:336–341, 1963.

Rowe M: Disc surgery and chronic low back pain. J Occup Med *7*:196–202, 1965.

Snook S, Campanelli R, Hart J: A study of three preventive approaches to low back injury. J Occup Med *20*:478–481, 1978.

Spengler D, Bigos S, Martin N, Zeh J. Fisher L, Nachemson A: Back injury in industries: a retrospective study I. Overview and cost analysis. Spine *11*:241–245, 1986.

Troup J, Martin J, Lloyd D: Back pain in industry. A prospective survey. Spine *6*:61–69, 1981.

Vietnam Era Veterans Readjustment Assistance Act of 1974, statute at large, v. 88, Public Law 93–508, 1578–1602, 1974.

White A: Low back pain in men receiving workmen's compensation: a follow-up study. Canad Med Assoc J *101*:61–67, 1969.

Wiesel S, Tsourmas N, Feffer H, Citrin C, Patronas N: 1984 Volvo Award in Clinical Sciences: a study of computer assisted tomography I. The incidence of positive CAT scans in an asymptomatic group of patients. Spine *9*:549–551, 1984.

ADDITIONAL REFERENCES

American Medical Association Guides to the Evaluation of Permanent Impairment. Chicago, AMA, 1983.

Pope M, Frymoyer J, Andersson G: *Occupational Low Back Pain.* New York, Praeger Publishers, 1984.

APPENDIX

Equipment and Manufacturers

Name of Device	Manufacturer	What Measured?
Med Design Inclinometer	Med Design, Ltd. Liverpool, England	Spine range-of-motion
MIE Inclinometer	MIE, Ltd. Leeds, England (Importer: Chatteck, Inc. Chattanooga, TN)	Spine range-of-motion
EDI-320	Cybex/Lumex, Inc. Ronkonkoma, NY	Computerized spine range-of-motion
OrthoRanger	MI Technologies, Daytona Beach, FL	Spine range-of-motion
Metrocam	FARO Med. Tech. Inc., Montreal, CN	Range-of-motion, limb length
Cybex TEF (Trunk Extension/Flexion)	Cybex/Lumex, Inc. Ronkonkoma, NY	Sagittal trunk isokinetic strength/endurance
Cybex Torso Rotation	Cybex/Lumex, Inc. Ronkonkoma, NY	Axial plane trunk isokinetic strength/endurance
Kin-Com System	Chatteck Corp. Chattanooga, TN	Sitting sagittal isokinetic trunk strength
B-100, B-200	Isotechnologies, Inc. Hillsboro, NC	"Isodynamic" multiplanar trunk strength
Lido System	Loredan, Inc. Davis, CA	Standing/sitting sagittal isokinetic trunk strength/endurance
Biodex Back Attachment	Biodex, Inc., Shirley, NY	Sitting, semi-reclining isokinetic sagittal trunk strength/endurance
ISTU (Isometric Strength Testing Unit)	Dynadex Corp., Ann Arbor, MI	Isometric lift capacity
Cybex Liftask	Cybex/Lumex, Inc. Ronkonkoma, NY	Isokinetic/isometric lifting
Electronic Resistance Systems (ERS)	Digital Kinetics Danville, CA	Isokinetic/isotonic lifting
WEST 2	Work Evaluation Systems Technology Huntington Beach, CA	Isoinertial lifting

Equipment and Manufacturers *Continued*

Name of Device	Manufacturer	What Measured?
Biodex Lift Simulation Attachment	Biodex, Inc. Shirley, NY	Isokinetic lifting
Fitron	Cybex/Lumex, Inc. Ronkonkoma, NY	Aerobic capacity/lower extremity endurance
UBE	Cybex/Lumex, Inc. Ronkonkoma, NY	Aerobic capacity/upper body endurance
Versa-Climber	Heart Rate, Inc. Costa Mesa, CA	Aerobic capacity, climbing strength/endurance
BTE	Baltimore Therapeutic Equipment, Inc. Baltimore, MD	Upper extremity strength/fatigue work simulation
WEST 4	Work Evaluation Systems Technology Huntington Beach, CA	Upper extremity strength/fatigue
Cad Tex	Physio-Tek, Inc. Martinez, CA	Isokinetic/isotonic work simulation

INDEX

Page numbers in *italics* indicate illustrations; numbers followed by *t* indicate tables